GLOBAL DIMENSIONS OF CHILDHOOD OBESITY

GLOBAL DIMENSIONS OF CHILDHOOD OBESITY

RICHARD K. FLAMENBAUM
EDITOR

Nova Science Publishers, Inc.
New York

For permission to use material from this book please contact us:
Telephone 631-231-7269; Fax 631-231-8175
Web Site: http://www.novapublishers.com

Library of Congress Cataloging-in-Publication Data

ISBN 1-60021-037-6

Published by Nova Science Publishers, Inc. ✢New York

CONTENTS

Preface		**vii**
Chapter 1	Childhood Obesity in Transitional Countries: A South African Perspective *J. Mukuddem-Petersen and M.A. Petersen*	**1**
Chapter 2	Child Overweight and Obesity in Global Perspective: Emergent Risks Related to Household Wealth, Social Status and Urbanism in Developing Countries *Alexandra Brewis and Mary C. Meyer*	**51**
Chapter 3	Childhood Obesity in the Eastern Mediterranean Region *Roya Kelishadi*	**69**
Chapter 4	Adolescent Obesity: An Increasing Problem. Turkey and Other Countries' Status *Naci Öner*	**89**
Chapter 5	Magnitude and Possible Contributors of Childhood Obesity in Iran: Implication for Action *Behnoush Mohammadpour-Ahranjani, Arash Rashidi, Majid Karandish, Mohammad-Reza Vafa*	**99**
Chapter 6	The Endogeneous Obesity we Still Don't Recognize *Geni Balaban and Gisélia Alves Pontes da Silva*	**127**
Chapter 7	Childhood Obesity: The View from the Family *Anders Lindelof*	**139**
Chapter 8	Development of Child Food Preferences: The Role of Age, Experience and Exposure *Meredith S. Dolan, Michael Henderson and Myles S. Faith*	**123**
Chapter 9	Obesity: Current Research and Dilemmas *Roger J Harris, Sophie Aubrey, Rebecca Gibbs and Ambreen Clement*	**169**

Chapter 10 Childhood Obesity: Caregivers' Perceptions, Attitudes and Behaviors Related to Physical Activity and Inactivity **199**
Mozhdeh B. Bruss, Timothy J. Michae, Joseph R. Morris, Linda L. Dannison, Jackie A. Quitugua and Rosa T. Palacios

Index **255**

PREFACE

Children become overweight for a variety of reasons. The most common causes are genetic factors, lack of physical activity, unhealthy eating patterns, or a combination of these factors. In rare cases, a medical problem, such as an endocrine disorder, may cause a child to become overweight. This book presents ongoing and new research on a public health problem in virtually all developed countries.

In modern times, overnutrition in humans is a very complex and common eating disorder that normally results in obesity. In some regions in the world, this multifactoral condition has reached pandemic proportions in both adult and child populations. In particular, the fact that obesity is on the increase during the earlier stages of human life is of grave concern. In this regard, the prevalence of childhood adiposity is largely attributable to the obesogenic culture that has become entrenched in contemporary society. Although this is mainly true for developed countries, recently, countries in developing regions such as South America (studies conducted in Brazil and Mexico), the Middle East, Asia (investigations done in China, India, Indonesia, Nepal and Mongolia) and Central and Southern Africa (for instance, Kenya and South Africa, respectively) have experienced similiar trends. Chapter 1 mainly involves the latter mentioned Southern African country where obesity is confounded by rapid demographic, nutritional and epidemiological transition. In South Africa, one in three men (30 %) and more than one in two adult women (57 %) can be considered to be overweight. Specifically, in this geographic region, childhood obesity is creating a burden that co-exists with malnutrition and nutritional deficiencies. We complement our discussions about aspects of the obesity pandemic in South Africa by reviewing related studies on this phenomenon conducted in the developing countries mentioned above and developed countries. In either case, it is clear that obesity and its co-morbidities offer a serious long-term challenge to governments and health care organizations alike. In addition to the issues raised above, we take our lead from the 2000 World Health Organization (WHO) Report on preventing and managing obesity, that identified the relationship between adiposity in children and retarded linear growth (stunting) as a research priority. As a result we provide an in-depth discussion on the association between stunting and obesity in South Africa. In the formulation of a strategic response, towards the end of the current chapter, we propose that the prevention of obesity in childhood via appropriate interventionary programmes is the best strategy to control its prevalence in adulthood.

Very little is known currently about the pattern of risk for early childhood overweight and obesity in the least developed countries, where child under-nutrition remains very common and a pressing concern. We use standardized anthropometric and interview data pertaining to seventeen nationally-representative samples of 37,714 children aged between 30 and 60 months to model that risk. We particularly consider in Chapter 2, the possible roles of changing social and economic status of households and urban residence, and take into account such factors as variations in family size, in maternal nutritional status, and children's histories of under-nutrition (observed as growth stunting). The relationships among these variables are quite different across world regions except for mothers' overweight status, which was a strong predictor in all. In sub-Saharan Africa, overweight children are extremely rare and the only strong predictor is having a mother who is overweight. In Northern Africa urban residence is a risk factor. In the Americas, increasing wealth and social status of households raises risk substantially. Stunting places children in Africa, but not the Americas, at significantly increased risk of being overweight, and in northern Africa this effect is particularly pronounced in cities. We find every indication in these trends that child obesity and overweight might very quickly emerge as the modal nutritional status of children worldwide. The model suggests that childhood overweight in many ways embodies relative poverty as national wealth rises, just as child stunting reflects the conditions of absolute poverty. As economic growth accelerates in the poorer countries, the least advantaged sectors of their populations can remain absolutely poor while their relative poverty also increases. This means that risk for childhood obesity will grow, and probably rapidly, and it will increasingly co-exist with and so be intensified by under-nutrition.

The potential increase in non-communicable disease (NCD) is escalating much more rapidly in developing than industrialized countries. In this regard, a potential emerging public health concerning developing countries may be the increasing incidence of childhood obesity and as a result , an enormous socioeconomic and public health burden for poorer nations in the near future. However, little is known about its prevalence because of limited number of national studies, various definitions used and different age groups studied that make the comparisons difficult.

In the last decades, the countries located in the Eastern Mediterranean region (EMR) have experienced a transition from a traditional to a Westernized lifestyle and has undergone a rapidly occurring epidemiologic transition. The Middle- East located in this region has the highest dietary energy surplus of the developing countries. As a result, a rapid rise in NCD risk factors is according in different age groups, but very limited data exists about children living in this part of the world.

Through a systematic review, Chapter 3 compares surveys on the prevalence of overweight and obesity among children and adolescents living in the EMR, not only to review the differences, but also to assess the quality of methodologies, to explore the most important environmental influences, and to scrutinize the variations among sub-groups of the population.

The prevalence of overweight (based on WHO definition) among preschool children varies from near 3% in United Arab Emirates (UAE), Iran and Pakistan to 8.6% in Egypt. Among older children and adolescents (6-18y), the prevalence of overweight among girls ranges between 6.3% in Bahrain to 31.8% in Kuwait; among boys, it ranges between 4.9% in Saudi Arabia to 30% in Kuwait. The prevalence of obesity in girls is reported from near 3% in UAE and Iran to 35.1% in Bahrain; among boys, it ranges from 2.1% in Iran to 21% in Bahrain and 14.7% in Kuwait.

Overall, the prevalence of childhood overweight and obesity in Iran is reported much lower than in Arab countries of the EMR that is suggested to be because of underlying genetic and lifestyle differences. However, the recent national survey in Iran found a higher prevalence of obesity among the younger than older children, and is alarming for the rapid increase in childhood obesity.

Few studies performed in the EMR have assessed the environmental influences on childhood obesity, but the few studies addressing this matter emphasized that sedentary lifestyle, especially in girls and in urban residents, along with low nutrient but energy dense foods consumed, as well as the public belief considering fatness as a sign for health and beauty are the major factors in the high prevalence of obesity in this region.

It should be acknowledged that many of reviewed studies do not reflect national data, and include various age groups with different cutoffs used for overweight, making the comparison difficult.

Nevertheless, in spite of these limitations, the findings of the present study provide alarming evidence-based data for health professionals and policy makers about the considerable prevalence of childhood obesity in the EMR countries, many of them still grappling with the public health effects of malnutrition and micronutrient deficiencies.

Introduction: Obesity is currently regarded as a chronic and recurring disorder and it is closely associated with various chronic disorders such as cardiovascular diseases, metabolic syndrome, anxiety and mood abnormalities. Adolescence appears to be high risk period for the development of obesity and obesity in this period is more likely to track into adulthood. The prevalence of childhood and adolescence obesity in Europe and the USA has doubled during the last 10 to 15 years. There are only a few conducted studies related to adolescent obesity in Turkey, therefore, we tried to evaluate the features that represents our region. We also aimed to evaluate the last obesity and overweight prevalence status of the adolescents throughout Europe and the world.

Methods: This was a cross-sectional study, including a representative sample of 928 adolescent girls and 1004 adolescent boys in rural and urban area of Edirne, Turkey. For this study, the body weight and height of adolescents were measured using standard procedures. BMI (kg/m^2) was calculated as the ratio of the body weight to square body height. Prevalence of obesity and overweight was defined as age and gender specific BMI in excess of the 95th and 85th percentiles, respectively.

Results: The prevalence of overweight and obesity among adolescent girls of in our region was found to be 9.6 % and 3.8 %, respectively, while it was 7.8 % and 0.7 % among adolescent boys. Adolescent obesity prevalence was found to be higher in girls than in boys ($p<0.05$), although there was no gender difference in overweight prevalences between adolescent girls and boys. In the urban area, the prevalence of overweight and obesity among adolescent girls was 9.3 % and 0.9 %, while it was 8.6 % and 0.6% among boys, respectively. In the rural area; among adolescent girls, overweight and obesity prevalence was 9.9 % and 3.4 %, while it was 6.0 % and 0.6 % among boys, respectively.

Conclusions: Chapter 4 has showed that obesity prevalence of our adolescent population was lower than European adolescents and this difference is even higher when it was compared to the adolescents in the USA. The reason for the lower rate of obesity among our adolescents are largely unknown. However, one of them may be Mediterranean type of diet which contains more vegetables and less meat and carbohydrate.

Chapter 5 is intended to propose potential strategies and programmes based on the magnitude of overweight and obesity problem among Iranian children as well as an analysis of its possible contributing factors. The chapter includes four sections. In section one, we present international and (sub) national evidence on the prevalence of overweight and obesity in children and adolescents. This will allow us 1) to show the magnitude and trend of the problem; 2) to conduct a comparative study between current figures and the corresponding results reported from other countries (both developing and developed); 3) to make comparison between Iranian children and the reference population; and 4) to draw a geographical map of childhood overweight in Iran. In section two a brief discussion on possible contributing factors of overweight and obesity found by different studies is presented. In the third section, based on the facts and findings presented in the section two as well as available studies and statistics on biological and socio-economic variables and characteristics in Iran, an analysis towards determination of the most relevant contributing factors for overweight and obesity among Iranian children is discussed. Finally in the last section, we briefly suggest potential strategies and programmes aiming at prevention of childhood and adolescence obesity.

Introduction: Obesity etiology is multifactorial, including genetic and environmental factors. Traditionally, obesity is classified as endogenous (due to genetic syndromes and endocrine diseases) and exogenous (due to excessive intake in relation to energy expenditure). It has been related that endogenous obesity is responsible only for a small percentage of the total of obesity cases. We defend the idea that this approach is too much simplistic and reflects a gap between clinical and research settings. We believe that this small endogenous obesity percentage is actually due to our still limited knowledge about the energy balance regulation and the several obesity causes. Objective: Chapter 6 reviews the literature concerning energy balance regulation, genetic and neuroendocrine factors involved in obesity etiology and future perspectives for obesity treatment. Sources of data: articles published in indexed scientific journals, books, dissertations and thesis. Most articles were obtained from Medline and Scielo databases using the keywords “obesity”, “energy balance”, “genetic”, “hormone”, “treatment”, for the period between 1985 and 2005. Results: here we discuss the following topics: energy balance regulation, obesity genetics and gene – environment interactions, metabolic imprinting and future perspectives for obesity treatment. Conclusion: The recent advances in our understanding of neuroendocrine energy balance regulation, obesity genetics and gene – environment interactions demand a paradigm shift in obesity classification and therapeutic approach. In the future, patients previously classified in the same group, as having exogenous obesity, may have their obesity cause identified and individualized at the endogenous level. An individualized approach of the different obesity causes may lead us to safer and more effective treatments.

Chapter 7 is based on a qualitative study exploring overweight and obese children and their families’ perceptions and understandings of the child’s obesity. The study involved 60 obese children and 40 parents. Three analytical areas of interests are elaborated. 1) Which factors do the child and his or her family believe initially to have caused the child’s obesity? 2) How does the child’s obesity influence the daily life of the obese child and its parents? 3) How does the family try to help and support the child towards weight loss?

The results showed that many families either partly or not at all believed that factors related to diet and exercise had caused the child’s obesity. However, these families were aware of the medical explanation of obesity but believed that their child was an exception from this. As these families did not associate the obesity with diet or exercise they believed that external and non-adjustable factors had caused the obesity. Compared with families associating the child’s obesity with diet and exercise these families were less affected by the child's obesity and were thus less willing to achieve weight loss by changing their way of living.

I relate the empirical findings to the currents Danish ways of treating childhood obesity. I show that these weight reducing strategies are characterized by a goal of changing the child's eating and exercising habits regardless of the perception of the family. I propose that this imbalance between the families' perception of the obesity and the strategies focus on diet and exercise might explain the depressing results weight reducing strategies are generating.

This leads to my final supposition that future intervention programs aiming at reducing the child's weight must deal with the perceptions of the family simultaneously or even prior to traditional focus on diet and exercise.

The main objective of Chapter 8 is to summarize the literature on early determinants and development of child food preferences. The chapter begins with a literature review of the earliest flavor preferences for sweet, salty, and bitter tastes during infancy and the effect of early exposure to infant formulas on the later taste preferences. The effects of exposure frequency, food experience, role modeling, parenting styles, and mass media are followed by behavioral techniques to modify children's food preferences. The final section of the chapter covers commonly used assessments of infant and child food preferences.

As outlined in Chapter 9, there is a worldwide epidemic of obesity, with prevalence rates reaching alarming proportions in some western countries, but also in many parts of the developing world.

Hunger and weight gain are controlled by a complex group of interactions between the gut and brain. Recent advances have highlighted some of the main appetite control hormones, but these only help our understanding of the physiological processes controlling weight gain. Although there are a few extremely rare medical conditions causing childhood obesity, the main cause is a change in diet, with a high intake of energy dense, fatty and sugary food and drink, coupled with a dramatic decline in the amount of exercise being taken.

The long-term effect of this increase in obesity is likely to be an increase in cardiovascular mortality, as well as a massive rise in children with Type 2 diabetes, already being seen in many overweight teenagers from some racial groups.

A number of treatment strategies have been designed. Most are a combination of dieting, life style changes and family behaviour therapy. Medical and surgical interventions are reserved for those children who are morbidly obese, and likely to suffer life threatening events, such as sleep apnoea.

Unfortunately, intervention only has limited success, and the end result may well be a decline in the current increasing longevity, especially in the developed world.

The purpose of Chapter 10 was to investigate primary caregivers' perceptions, attitudes and behaviors related to physical activity and inactivity among 6-10 year old children in order to better understand factors related to childhood obesity. This exploratory study used qualitative methods to identify sociocultural and familial factors related to physical activity and inactivity among different Asian/Pacific Island groups resident in the Commonwealth of the Northern Mariana Islands. Results suggest that among caregivers there are distinct sociocultural beliefs, attitudes, and behaviors related to physical activity and inactivity. Gender differences were observed with relation to caregivers' perceptions of physical activity. Benefits and disadvantages of physical inactivity were highlighted by the caregivers. An important finding was the view held by caregivers that children need other children to stay physically active. Additionally, different ethnic groups gave different meaning to weight normalcy, physical activity and inactivity. Familial differences were also observed among ethnic groups, with regards to preventive strategies related to childhood obesity and factors that influence their understanding of weight status. With regards to community support for the prevention of childhood obesity, caregivers perceived environmental changes as a necessary condition for increasing physical activity among families. In addition, caregivers identified the need for nutrition education programs that offer awareness and skill-building workshops in bringing about food-related behavior modification among families.

In: Global Dimensions of Childhood Obesity
Editor: Richard K. Flamenbaum, pp. 1-50
ISBN 1-60021-037-6

Chapter 1

CHILDHOOD OBESITY IN TRANSITIONAL COUNTRIES: A SOUTH AFRICAN PERSPECTIVE

J. Mukuddem-Petersen[1]**and *M.A. Petersen*[2†]
[1]Northwest University, Potchefstroom X 6001, SA,
[2]Northwest University, USA

Abstract

In modern times, overnutrition in humans is a very complex and common eating disorder that normally results in obesity. In some regions in the world, this multifactoral condition has reached pandemic proportions in both adult and child populations. In particular, the fact that obesity is on the increase during the earlier stages of human life is of grave concern. In this regard, the prevalence of childhood adiposity is largely attributable to the obesogenic culture that has become entrenched in contemporary society. Although this is mainly true for developed countries, recently, countries in developing regions such as South America (studies conducted in Brazil and Mexico), the Middle East, Asia (investigations done in China, India, Indonesia, Nepal and Mongolia) and Central and Southern Africa (for instance, Kenya and South Africa, respectively) have experienced similiar trends. This contribution mainly involves the latter mentioned Southern African country where obesity is confounded by rapid demographic, nutritional and epidemiological transition. In South Africa, one in three men (30 %) and more than one in two adult women (57 %) can be considered to be overweight. Specifically, in this geographic region, childhood obesity is creating a burden that co-exists with malnutrition and nutritional deficiencies. We complement our discussions about aspects of the obesity pandemic in South Africa by reviewing related studies on this phenomenon conducted in the developing countries mentioned above and developed countries. In either case, it is clear that obesity and its co-morbidities offer a serious long-term challenge to governments and health care organizations alike. In addition to the issues raised above, we take our lead from the 2000 World Health Organization (WHO) Report on preventing and managing obesity, that identified the relationship between adiposity in children and retarded linear growth (stunting) as a research priority. As a result we provide an in-depth discussion on the association between stunting and obesity in South Africa. In the formulation of a strategic response,

*E-mail address: wskjmp@puk.ac.za; Telephone +27-18-299 2553; Fax: +27-18-299 2570 (Corresponding Author)
†E-mail address: wskmap@puk.ac.za

towards the end of the current chapter, we propose that the prevention of obesity in childhood via appropriate interventionary programmes is the best strategy to control its prevalence in adulthood.

Key Words: Childhood Obesity, Nutrition Transition, Double Burden, South Africa.

1 Introduction

Excess bodyweight is one of the most important risk factors contributing to the overall burden of lifestyle disease globally. Statistically speaking, 1.1 billion adults and 10 % of children are now classified as either being overweight or obese. In particular, childhood obesity among school-going children has reached epidemic proportions globally with 155 million of such children suffering with this condition. More specifically, the rate of overweight children in South Africa is 12 %, with the USA at 14 %. Childhood obesity is linked primarily to unhealthy eating habits, but is also related to the fact that children today are a lot less active than in the past. In this regard, in developing countries where both these habits have taken root, 7 to 10 % of children aged between 3 and 9 are obese. More generally, evidence based on epidemiological research has suggested that this surge in the prevalence of childhood obesity in such countries can be attributed to the following factors. In this regard, vulnerable periods of life (for example, maternal nutrition and metabolic factors, inadequate early nutrition), physical inactivity (for example, reduced physical activity among urban populations), genetic and environmental factors (for example, a nutrition transition to lipid-rich diets), socioeconomic factors and ethnic and gender differences are some of the most studied and relevant factors to be considered. In our discussion, we specifically highlight and expand upon these issues impacting the obesity problem.

Based on recent advances in the literature involving developing countries, it seems appropriate to have as the centerpiece of this chapter a critical discussion on childhood obesity and its array of co-morbidities in South Africa. In this context, the complex pathological processes involved reflect environmental and genetic interactions with individuals from disadvantaged communities seeming to be at greater risk than the more affluent. Often called the "Rainbow Nation", South Africa is a country in transition that is known for its diversity with an array of creeds and cultures found within its borders. Since its 1994 political transformation, South Africa (estimated 2005 population of 42 million) has undergone simultaneous social, epidemiological and economic transitions. In particular, variation in dietary patterns, access to health care, weather patterns, food availability and levels of economic growth are evident. Unfortunately, in recent times, lifestyle diseases like obesity have escalated in different age and gender groups, various ethnic groups and urban and rural dwellers (see [168]). Data published in the 2002 South African Youth Risk Assessment Survey by the South African Medical Research Council, show the prevalence of overweight (including obesity) among young people aged 13 to 19 years to be 17 % overall affecting more girls (25 %) than boys (7 %). Moreover, the 1999 National Food Consumption Survey (NFCS) in South Africa found that 7.6 % of children in the 1 to 9 year age group is overweight in the urban areas with a higher prevalence among children of well-educated mothers (12.5 %). Nationally, 6 % of children in the 1 to 9 year age group was found to be overweight. The South Africa Demographic and Health Survey (SADHS) of 1998 found that 5.3 % of adolescent males and 17.6 % of adolescent females are overweight while 2 % of adolescent males and 5.9 % of adolescent females are obese. In addition, this chapter will explore the relationship between stunting and obesity which has been postulated in countries undergoing the nutrition transition. Prevalence was highest (over 20 % for boys and girls combined) in white and Indian children. Another key factor revealed in the NFCS in South Africa was that approximately 20 % of children under the age of 9 had suffered from stunting, related to chronic undernutrition early in life, and ironically, the problem was worst among small children raised on commercial farms (see [173]). These children may be particularly vulnerable to developing abdominal obesity with energy-dense Western diets. Also, we will provide a comparison of studies conducted on children in South Africa with other studies on children in transitional countries such as Brazil, China, Russia, the Philippines and Mexico. Finally, trends for this pandemic in children are also provided as a backdrop to better understand the South African situation in the global context.

The contribution in this chapter is organized as follows. The current section is introductory in nature, while Section 2 offers an overview of the nutrition transition and double burden experienced by developing countries like South Africa. Section 3 contains the main discussion and highlights certain key aspects of obesity. The fourth section considers how roleplayers in the health and medical community can respond to the obesity crisis in developed and developing countries. Within the South African context, conclusions are drawn and directions for future research suggested in Section 5. Finally, we provide a two-part appendix that contains abbreviations for terms related to childhood obesity, overweight and stunting and furnish a summary of information from studies about childhood obesity in South Africa.

2 Nutrition Transition & Double Burden

This section provides a discussion of two of the most characteristic obesity-related issues in a developing country such as South Africa. Firstly, we look at aspects of the change in nutritional status being experienced in the aforementioned country. Furthermore, we identify the double burden that involves the co-existence of nutritional states related to under- and overnutrition.

2.1 Nutrition Transition

The term "nutrition transition" refers to the sequence of changes in dietary patterns and nutrient intake associated with social, cultural and economic shifts accompanying an amendment of the demographics of a country or region. In essence, two processes of change occur concurrent with or prior to the nutrition transition. The first is the demographic transition which is the shift from a pattern of high fertility and mortality to one of low fertility and mortality. This shift is characteristic of a modern industrialized country. The other process of change is the epidemiological transition which was described, for instance by Omran in [125], as the change from a pattern of high prevalence of infectious disease associated with malnutrition, periodic famine and poor environmental sanitation to one of high prevalence of chronic and degenerative disease associated with urban-industrial lifestyles (see, also [124]).

Researchers found that most countries in Latin America, Asia, the Middle East, Northern Africa and the urban areas of sub-Saharan Africa have all experienced a change in the overall structure of its dietary pattern with related disease patterns over the last few decades (see, for instance, [84], [110], [132], [133] and [197]). Regarding sub-Saharan Africa, by virtue of its economic growth, South Africa is considered to be one of the countries that is undergoing rapid demographic and nutritional transition (see [20]). In this regard, the dietary patterns in the said country seem to be characterized by high intakes of saturated fats, sugar and refined foods but low consumption of fiber-containing foods. These patterns coincide with the so-called "Western diet" and usually accompany lifestyles characterized by lower levels of activity (see, for instance, [20], [142], [171], [172] and [199]).

2.2 Double Burden

In the ensuing analysis, the double burden is seen from a global and South African perspective. Also, we discuss the occurrence of dual burden households in the context of developing countries.

2.2.1 Global Perspective

The double burden of nutritional diseases refers to the co-existence of malnutrition and micronutrient deficiencies on the one hand and chronic, noncommunicable diseases on the other. At the turn of the century, malnutrition was the cause of almost 4 million deaths and contributed to many more on the continent of Africa and such regions as South East Asia. Chronic diseases, especially heart disease, stroke, cancer and chronic respiratory diseases, make up approximately 60 % of global mortality and 50 % of the global burden of disease (see, for instance, [136]). Unfortunately, the global response to these major public health problems has been inadequate.

Generally, the public health focus of a country with a relatively low gross national product (GNP) will be on underweight and undernutrition. However, in countries with a higher GNP, policy makers are more likely to be concerned with the rising prevalence of obesity and chronic disease. A recent overview by Popkin (see [136]; also [133]) confirms that when a country with a low GNP experiences economic growth, the population's diet structure shifts, and combined with reduced physical activity, a rapid rise in obesity and subsequent chronic disease levels occur (see [48]). The double burden emerges where underweight and overweight coexists due to this transition. Furthermore, these changes impact nutritional outcomes, such as shifts in average stature (e.g. stunting), body composition (e.g. overweight, obesity) and morbidity (increase in chronic diseases leads to increased death rate).

2.2.2 South African Perspective

The co-existence of stunting and overweight in school children reflect an aspect of the South African nutritional transition (a transition from a traditional African diet to a more Western-type diet), where the already stunted and underweight become both stunted and overweight, a double burden. In South Africa, this burden may exist in the same household (dual burden household) and has emerged as a new concern (see [48]). The aforementioned factors independently or collectively may contribute to the dual burden phenomenon in South Africa.

A study conducted by Bourne and co-workers in the Cape Peninsula in South Africa, serves as a good example of a population displaying the dual burden phenomenon. The aim of the said study was to investigate the nutritional status of 3-6 year-old African children. The method involved obtaining dietary information and taking anthropometric measurements and blood values. Their findings confirmed that growth retardation and wasting in the said population coexisted with emergent obesity. The blood analysis revealed that the undernourished and obese children consumed a diet low in micronutrients. More specifically, most subjects were deficient in calcium (80 %), iron (77 %), vitamin A (64 %), riboflavin (52 %), niacin (53 %), vitamin B6 (58 %) and vitamin C (76 %). The dietary analysis showed that many children received adequate portions of meat and foods from the cereal group and more than 120 % of the RDA for folic acid (68 %) and for vitamin B12 (63 %). Macronutrient energy distribution fell within prudent dietary guidelines: 28.1 % of energy from total fat, 63.7 % from carbohydrates, and 13.2 % from protein. Furthermore, Bourne and co-investigators show that 44.8 % percent of children had only 2 meals with more than 600 kJ, 9.2 % had only 1 meal. The anthropometric measurements suggested that 27.6 % were stunted, 7.7 % were underweight, 7.9 % were wasted and 20.1 % were obese. However, the diet was deficient in milk (median intake, 0.5 portion vs. 2-3 portions as recommended by the department of national health and population development guidelines), fat (2.5 portions vs. 4 portions), vegetables and fruit. These findings are indicative of a population undergoing the nutrition transition, where acute and chronic undernourishment coexists with obesity (see [21]).

2.2.3 Dual Burden Households

Research completed in 2005 by Doak and co-workers (see [48]) suggested that a considerable proportion of households in developing countries, such as South Africa, have undergone the nutrition transition in which over- and underweight coexist. Previously, these households were called "under/over" (see [50]), but are now known as "dual burden" households. This term refers to a household in which one person is overweight while another is underweight. In one household, infectious disease may explain why one person is underweight and another overweight in spite of sufficient food. On the other hand, a different dual burden household might occur as the result of an eating disorder, such as anorexia nervosa or bulimia. As a result, the dual burden of overweight and undernutrition clusters within a single household. Empirically, stunting among children was found to coexist with overweight and obese mothers in several developing countries (see [66]). Prior studies have shown the dual burden household to be associated with socio-demographic factors such as income and urban residence (see [47] and [49]) in countries experiencing rapid changes in diet and physical activity. In this regard, the percentages of dual burden households in Brazil, China and Russia were 44 %, 23 % and 57 %, respectively. An investigation to determine the corresponding percentage of such households for South Africa was initiated in 2005. Furthermore, research by Doak and colleagues challenges the notion that underweight and overweight are opposing public health concerns and illustrates the need for public health programmes that are able to simultaneously address underweight and overweight (see [50]).

3 Perspective of Childhood Obesity, Overweight and Stunting

Childhood obesity is an emerging public health problem throughout the world (see [199] and [200]). It is associated with several risk factors for later heart disease and other chronic diseases including hyperlipidaemia, hyperinsulinaemia, hypertension (see [162]), and early atherosclerosis (see [14], [15] and [101]). These risk factors may operate through the association between child and adult obesity, but they may also act independently (see [117]). In this section, we define and give an overview of childhood obesity. In addition, we discuss the root causes of this phenomenon and the trends that are evident. Furthermore, we consider the most important factors that influence the prevalence of obesity. Finally, the association between stunting and obesity among children is discussed.

3.1 Definition and Overview

In studies conducted under South African conditions, the following definitions for obesity and overweight are generally used. Obesity is characterized by excessive or abnormal fat accumulation in adipose tissue with the related undesirable positive energy balance, weight gain and possibility of impaired health status (see [67]). This condition is present when total body weight is more than 25 percent fat in boys and more than 32 percent fat in girls (see [98]). On the other hand, overweight may be defined as a weight-for-height $>$ 2 standard deviations (SD) from the National Centre for Health Statistics/World Health Organization international reference median (see [200]). In addition, Cole and collaborators (see [30]) defined internationally acceptable cut-off points for body mass index (BMI) for overweight and obesity in children. Here the appropriate cut-off point was defined in BMI units in young adulthood and extrapolated to childhood, conserving the corresponding centile in each dataset. This definition was less arbitrary than others and encourages direct comparison of trends in child obesity worldwide.

3.2 Etiology of Childhood Obesity

In the developing world, the etiology of the obesity pandemic involves rapid shifts in diets and a decline in physical activity in leisure, transportation and work associated with modern-day living. Regarding the latter, increased levels of sedentary behavior associated with the worldwide use of mass media compound these effects (see [140]). In addition, results from twin studies (see [10] and [22]) suggest that the tendency to obesity is inherited, at least in part, and that responsiveness to dietary intervention is genetically determined (see [129]). While childhood obesity does not necessarily indicate adult obesity, epidemiological studies have found that about a third of obese preschool children and a half of obese school-age children become obese adults (see [166]). This means that children with overweight or obese parents have a greater risk of being obese themselves (see [92] and [195]). Therefore, during the early years of life, focus should remain on sustaining proper growth and development. Ultimately, the regulation of the energy balance is highly complex and forms an integral part of societal, behavioural, genetic, hormonal, and neural influences (see [100]). Several studies have verified that the aforementioned causes of obesity are also evident in the South African situation (see, for instance, [88], [90], [91] and [102]).

3.3 Childhood Obesity Trends

In the ensuing analysis, trends in obesity are viewed from a global, developing countries and South African perspective.

3.3.1 Global Perspective

Globally, the rapidity of obesity is unprecedented in the history of mankind. This escalating rate of obesity in youths and adults is a frequent outcome of modernisation or acculturation (see [68], [86], [109], [136], [137], [152], [192] and [200]). There is enormous heterogeneity in the patterns, trends and timing of obesity among developing countries. In particular, an increasing prevalence of obesity in many countries, including those that have traditionally had high rates of undernutrition (see [139] and [200]) are being reported. Countries in economic transition from underdeveloped to developed, such as South Africa, China and Brazil, are particularly affected and, in fact, have an increasing prevalence of obesity across all economic levels and age groups (see [133] and [138]). Essentially, this worldwide phenomenon can be considered to be a result of social, economic and cultural problems being encountered by developing and newly industrialised countries, as well as ethnic minorities and the disadvantaged in developed countries (see [53], [89], [140], [164] and [165]). Furthermore, the current levels of overweight in countries as diverse as Mexico, Egypt, and South Africa are shown to be equal or greater than those in the United States (see [192]). The impact of abdominal visceral fat accumulation on metabolic derangement is now under extensive study in adults. Abdominal visceral fat has recently been measured in children (see [4], [6], [59] and [115]). These studies have suggested that deleterious effects of visceral adipose tissue on blood lipid risk factors seen in adults are already present in children.

3.3.2 Developing Countries Perspective

The rapid changes in dietary patterns and lifestyles occuring in many developing countries warrant close monitoring of overweight prevalence in children so that preventative measures can be taken in a timely manner (see [41]). A recent study investigating adolescent obesity dynamics was undertaken across four longitudinal studies (see [192]). Nationally representative data from Brazil (1975 and 1997), Russia (1992 and 1998), the United States (National Health and Nutrition Examination Survey (NHANES) I (1971-1974) and NHANES III (1988-1994)), and nationwide survey data from China (1991 and 1997) were used. The results of this study suggested that trends and current prevalence of overweight varied substantially across the four countries. Once again it was evident that the burden of nutritional problems was shifting from energy imbalance deficiency to excess among older children and adolescents in Brazil and China. These changes and differences may relate to changes and differences in key environmental factors across countries. Similar to adults, the changes in youth obesity in these four countries varied across levels of household income.

3.3.3 South African Perspective

A recent national study by Puoane and co-workers, on childhood obesity in South Africa, showed that 56.6 % of girls aged 15 years and older were overweight or obese (see [149]). There is evidence to suggest that in many cases this disposition subsequently manifests itself in adulthood. According to the secondary anthropometric data analysis of the NFCS in South Africa, Steyn and fellow researchers showed that 6.7 % of 1 to 9 year-old children nationally were classified as being overweight (1 to 2 SD WAZ) and 3.7 % as obese (> 2 SD WAZ), where WAZ is the abbreviation for Weight-for-Age z-score. As a result, the conclusion is that 10.4 % of South African children are overweight and/or obese (see [173]).

3.4 Factors Influencing Childhood Obesity

Genetic predisposition, vulnerable periods of life, socioeconomic background and emotional factors, as well as ethnic and gender differences are some of the factors that influence overweight/obesity. Diet is determined by cultural and socioeconomic background and as such plays a role in the development of obesity.

3.4.1 Vulnerable Periods of Life

Critical or susceptible periods of development have been identified for many behavioral and developmental processes. In particular, numerous studies have shown the importance of nutrition during certain periods of life when an individual may be more vulnerable to the development of future obesity. Obesity occurs during the following critical periods: prenatal period (intra-uterine life), infancy, adiposity rebound (4 to 7 years), adolescence, early adulthood, pregnancy and menopause (see [37]). The onset of obesity during these periods appears to increase the risk of persistent obesity and its complications. The literature suggests that a series of biological factors, such as the timing of adiposity rebound and parental obesity, which might relate to both behavioural and biological causal mechanisms, affect carryover of fatness from childhood into adulthood (see [71], [143] and [195]). In this regard, there is evidence to suggest that adiposity in childhood and adolescence influences adult mortality and morbidity (see [117]).

In South Africa, Steyn and collaborators conducted a national study aimed at determining the nutritional status of children. These authors found the highest prevalence of overweight in 1 to 3 year-old children living in urban areas (see [173]). Various hypotheses proposed that nutritional insults during pregnancy or infancy may have long-term effects on a wide range of metabolic and other physiological relationships (see [9]). In particular, Barker and his colleagues have shown that adults with low weight at age 1 year or low birth weights have a greater tendency to store fat abdominally (see [9]). In addition, it was found that males who experienced famine during the first half of gestation were more likely to become obese as young adults. Detection of individuals at high risk during childhood may help to establish healthy lifestyles and prevent the development of obesity before 2 critical periods: the adiposity rebound and adolescence (see [37]).

Rapid growth during infancy in children who have not been suffering from intrauterine insult and are not small for gestational age (SGA) has been the focus of more recent research (see [25], [93], [126] and [127]). Several authors identified rapid growth in infancy, which they term catch-up growth, to be associated with an increase in childhood risk factors for overweight and obesity. Such children had significantly greater weights, heights, and fatness later in childhood and a more centralized fat distribution (see [126]). Cameron concluded (see [25]), in an analysis of South African urban children, that the majority of such children were overweight by 2 years of age and more likely to be classified as obese by 9 years of age. Although SGA children who demonstrate rapid weight gain in infancy are known to enter puberty earlier (see [32], [108] and [167]), no information is yet available on children who had birthweights that were appropriate for gestational age (AGA) nor on skeletal maturity. Obesity and overweight are associated with advanced sexual and skeletal maturity in normal children (see [186] and [187]). Such advancement in AGA children with rapid weight gain in infancy would account for their greater size during childhood and thus not necessarily pose a threat of greater risk during adolescence and early adulthood. The outcome of the South African study by Cameron revealed that rapid weight gain was experienced by 21.8 % and normal weight gain by 78.2 % of children. The proportions of boys and girls within the groups were not significantly different. In common with previous analyses (see, for instance, [126]), children with rapid weight gain were significantly lighter at birth (2982 grams vs. 3206 grams) and significantly taller and heavier from age 1 to 9 years and fatter (greater subcutaneous skinfolds) from 5 years of age. At 9 years, they were 3.8 cm taller and 3.8 kg heavier with 3.7 % greater body fat. Also, the rapid weight gain group had significantly greater subcutaneous fat, total body fat, and lean tissue for equivalent BMIs. Chronological age at 9 years were not significantly different. They were also not significantly different between the sexes in either rapid weight gain or normal weight gain groups. Because these children have a greater risk of overweight and obesity (see [25], [93], [126] and [127]) but are not advanced in skeletal maturity, later adolescent adjustments toward relatively lower weight and fatness values are unlikely. The identification and monitoring of such children is, therefore, of importance in reducing their risk of morbidity.

As was mentioned before, several studies suggest that childhood is a key period to identify those at risk of becoming obese adults. Most studies that examined the persistence of obesity from childhood and adolescence to adulthood found that fatter children were more likely to be overweight later in life (see [143]). As a result, the development of overweight in childhood is also related to subsequent overweight or obesity in adulthood (see [71]). Prevention may be more effective and should occur when adult overweight starts to develop in childhood (see [72]). Obesity not only persists from infancy into adulthood, but has been associated with an unfavourable cardiovascular risk profile in the first 20 years of life (see [3], [45] and [131]).

The development of obesity may start during the adolescent growth spurt period, which is one of the critical periods for the development of obesity identified by Dietz (see [37]). In girls, menarche indicates that the adolescent growth spurt has been completed and can be used to indicate a new stage of development (see [104]). Maturation can be assessed through a variety of approaches including skeletal age, appearance of secondary sexual characteristics and menarche. However, many studies of adolescents only report menarche (see [104]). The high obesity prevalence in adolescents is shown to be persistent into adulthood with high incidence in the transition to adulthood. We see from studies conducted in the US that the increase in obesity from adolescence to adulthood is marked. Other countries, like South Africa, following this trajectory are likely to see substantial adult obesity and its associated co-morbidities if this trend is not reversed (see [140]).

3.4.2 Physical Activity

Physical activity is important for achieving proper energy balance, which is needed to prevent or reverse obesity. Such activity on a regular basis can improve body composition and have a positive effect on resting metabolic rate and the maintenance of weight loss. Moreover, physical activity may affect the distribution of body fat independently of its effect on body weight (see [180]). Properly designed activity programmes may preserve or even increase lean muscle mass during weight loss. Several large, cross-sectional studies in the United States, Canada, and Europe (see [180] and [163]) have reported an inverse relationship between levels of physical activity and indirect measures of body fat distribution (for example, waist-to-hip ratio). South African children are even more inactive than their counterparts abroad because many schools lack sporting facilities or offer insufficient physical activity.

Changes in physical activity appear to be changing swiftly worldwide especially in the developing countries. In this regard, there are several linked changes in such activity occurring jointly. One is a shift away from the high-energy expenditure activities such as farming, mining, and forestry towards the service sector (see [134]). Reduced energy expenditures in the same occupation are a second change. Other major changes relate to the modes of transportation and activity patterns during leisure hours. The concept of engaging in physical activity during leisure time is not recognised in many cultures and communities in which energy conservation has historically been a prime concern during times of food shortage. The improvement in food availability has done little to change such attitudes. In contrast, the Nordic countries and some other cultures prize fitness and vitality and thus have a positive attitude to physical activity; they devote considerable amounts of leisure time to vigorous activity at the expense of more sedentary pursuits (see [199]). In addition, in Hispanic and Asian cultures, strenous physical activity may not be considered feminine, or there may be a greater emphasis on academics (see [196]).

It is difficult to know whether obese individuals are less active because of their obesity or whether a low level of activity caused the obesity (see [78]). Results from some studies, however, suggest that low and decreasing levels of activity and a rise in sedentary behaviour are primarily responsible for obesity. For instance, this condition is absent among elite athletes while those athletes who abandon their sport frequently experience an increase in body weight and fatness. This conclusion is further supported by prospective data by Dietz and Gortmaker in [40]. As far as the developing countries are concerned, in a study carried out on shantytown children from Sao Paulo, Brazil, the authors found that low energy expenditure may be a risk factor for weight gain in susceptible populations. In particular, low energy expenditure may help to explain the increased risk of excess weight gain leading to obesity among shantytown girls compared with shantytown boys (see [78]). A study conducted in China provides an interesting example of the change in physical activity seen in many other countries in transition. In this context, the proportion of urban adults (male and female) working in occupations where they participate in vigorous activity patterns has decreased. In rural areas, however, there has been a shift towards increased physical activity linked to holding multiple jobs and more intensive effort. For rural women, there is a shift towards a larger proportion engaged in more energy-intensive work, but there are also sections where light effort is increasing. In contrast, for rural men there is a small decrease in the proportion engaged in light work effort. In China, 14 % of households acquired a motorized vehicle between 1989 and 1997. Also, these authors showed that the odds of being obese were 80 % higher ($P < 0.05$) in households for men and women who owned a motorized vehicle compared to those who did not own a vehicle (see [12]).

Activity may also decrease in response to social or biological cues. As girls age they may become more interested in appearance and pursue more sedentary social interests, or they may adopt sedentary, adult-modelled behaviour patterns (see [169]). Therefore, parental modelling influences the adoption of physical activity by offspring in childhood and adolescence and beyond (see [155]). Consequently, the decline in physical activity levels of parents has a direct negative effect on the activity levels of the children.

The trends mentioned above also play themselves out in the South African context. For example, a study in the North-West Province of South Africa by Kruger and co-workers (see [88]) reported that a large percentage of stunted girls were in the mostly inactive category (72.5 %) and deposited relatively more subcutaneous fat compared with non-stunted girls (66.1 %). Published data from the "Birth-to-Twenty" study conducted by the University of Witwatersrand in Johannesburg, South Africa, showed that less than one-third of black South African children are offered physical education at school. More than 40 % of South African youth in the age group 9 to 11 years old, do not get enough exercise (see the website http://www.wits.ac.za/birthto20/news301.php).

3.4.3 Genetic and Environmental Factors

Garn and colleagues (see [63], [64] and [65]) demonstrated that as a result of the interaction between genetic and environmental factors, children whose family members are obese are four times more likely to be obese themselves than children whose family members are lean. By comparison, Locard and colleagues in [97], reported a threefold increase in childhood obesity when a parent is overweight. Moreover, Whitaker and colleagues (see [195]) reported that parental obesity increased the risk of childhood obesity by twofold to threefold at all ages. Ultimately, a treatment plan for the parents as well as the child may need to be considered if many family members are obese.

The role of epidemiological, genetic and molecular factors (see [200]) in weight gain is currently the focus of much research. A series of studies over the past decade strongly support the view that many genes are involved in causing a susceptibility to obesity. Based on the evidence accumulated > 600 genes, markers, and chromosomal regions have been associated or linked with human obesity phenotypes (see, for instance, [130]) Also, the discovery of leptin has led to a renewed interest in genetic and metabolic influences in the development of obesity. While it is possible that single or multiple gene effects may cause overweight and obesity directly, and indeed this is so in some individuals, this does not appear to be the case in the majority of people. Instead, it is currently considered that the genes involved in weight gain increase susceptibility or risk of an individual to the development of obesity when exposed to an adverse environment (see [199]). Many more years of research will be needed before the important genes and the critical mutations are finally defined for both excess body fat content and upper body and abdominal fat accumulation.

3.4.4 Socio-Economic Factors

The rapid increases in obesity rates over recent years have occurred in too short a time for there to have been any significant changes within populations. This suggests that the primary cause of the rapid global rise in obesity lies in environmental and societal changes that are now affecting a large proportion of the world's population (see [200]). The process of modernization and economic transition has seen most countries of the world move towards industrialization and an economy based on trade within a global market. This has brought about a number of improvements to the standard of living and services available to people throughout the world. However, it has also had a number of negative consequences that have directly and indirectly led to deleterious nutritional and physical activity patterns that contribute to the development of obesity. Changing societal structures resulting from this transition have given rise to new problems associated with unemployment, urban crowding, and family community breakdown (see, for instance, [200]). A review of the literature revealed that socioeconomic status (SES: composite index combining income, education, occupation and in some developing countries, place of residence (urban/rural)) and obesity, in women, were consistently inversely related. By contrast, SES and obesity tended to be directly proportional to each other in populations of developing countries. However, a 1998 WHO study on men in developing countries reported an inverse association, whereas a substantial minority (30 %) reported a direct association (see, for instance, [199]).

In traditional societies from developing countries, as per capita income increases, the nature of the diet tends to change in a pervasive and well-documented manner. In particular, intakes of animal fat and protein and sugar increases, while the consumption of vegetable fat and protein and complex carbohydrates decreases. An increase in income may be associated with increased away-from-home consumption of high-fat food items (as in the Phillipines) or with increased consumption of meat (as in China). However, the overall effect points to a greater intake of total fat and an associated increase in the prevalence of obesity (see [200]). In particular, Popkin and colleagues showed a strong positive correlation between income and a high weight-for-height in Brazil and also a significant inverse relationship between undernutrition and income (see [142]). In Thailand, although in transition from an agronomy-based to an industrial-based economy, the obesity-socioeconomic relation is like that of developing countries (see [111]).

In the immediate sequel, we highlight the outcomes of three studies conducted on child populations in South Africa that explores the relationship between socioeconomic status and obesity. Monyeki and fellow researchers conducted a study in the rural community of Ellisras in the Limpopo Province of South Africa which explored the occurrence of obesity in 3 to 4 and 5 to 10 year-old children during their preschool years and first years of formal schooling, respecitively (see [112]). Very few children (0-2.5 % of males and 0-4.3 % of females) had BMI values above the NHANES III 85th percentiles, indicating a very low prevalence of overweight children in the area. These researchers concluded that few Ellisras rural children had above normal values for BMI, indicating a low prevalence of obesity in this community. Also, Mukuddem-Petersen and colleague showed that children from urban areas tended to have higher mean BMI and triceps and subscapular skinfold thicknesses (TSF and SSF, respectively) than children (10 to 15 years) from rural areas and informal settlements in the North-West Province of South Africa (see [113]). Clearly the place of residence and, in turn, socioeconomic status directly influences the nutritional status of populations. Based on the secondary anthropometric data analysis of the NFCS in South Africa, Steyn and investigators showed that the highest prevalence of overweight and obese children resided in informal urban areas (see [173]). Overweight and obesity together (> 1 SD WAZ) was 10.4 %, with the highest prevalence in children living in such areas. Furthermore, 1 in 13 children aged 1 to 9 years living in formal South African urban areas are obese. Different outcomes from other studies conducted in other regions of South Africa and places of residence (urban/rural) reflect the complexity and diversity of the nutrition transition within one country. Evidently, the individual components of SES may have independent and even antagonistic effects on dietary intake and physical activity patterns so it is often very difficult to make generalizations about the relationship between SES and obesity (see [199]).

3.4.5 Ethnic Differences

Some ethnic groups in industrialized countries appear to be more susceptible to the development of obesity and its complications than others. This problem seems to arise from a combination of genetic predisposition, a change from the traditional to a more affluent sedentary lifestyle and its accompanying diet (see [199]). In the discussion below, we consider the differences between ethnic groups on a global level and compare this with the results of studies conducted in South Africa.

From data collected by the Pediatric Nutrition Surveillance System (PedNSS) it is evident that nutritional status varies among different race and ethnic groups worldwide. Black children have the highest rates of low birth weight and anemia, Hispanic and native American children have the highest rates of overweight; and the Asian children have the highest rate of shortness. There also exists ethnic variation, with girls of Asian or Mexican origin having relatively more subcutaneous fat on the trunk than girls of European or African origin (see [13]). In these populations, fat-rich energy-dense diets are likely to be cheapest, and reduced levels of activity stem from unemployment. Other factors associated with poverty may also be involved. In general, the prevalence of obesity is higher among Americans of African heritage than among Americans of European heritage (see [54] and [181]). Cardiovascular disease mortality is significantly higher in black than in white women. The black mortality rate is between two and four times that of white women, a difference that translates to an excess of 80 000 annual cardiovascular disease deaths for black women under 65 years of age in the USA. Because differences in body fat and BMI between black and white girls appear to occur sometime between childhood and young adulthood, the age of 9 to 10 years was chosen as the entry age range for the National Heart, Lung and Blood Institute Growth and Health Study Research Group (NHLBIGHSRG). This pre-pubertal stage of development is also the age at which little differences between blacks and whites in prevalence of obesity is expected. Differing rates of maturation may explain some of the observed black-white differences in BMI, although other factors may also contribute (see [118]). In this regard, the mid-upper arm circumference measurements of black children should be interpreted cautiously as excess subcutaneous fat may obscure the detection of muscle wasting (see [1]). In cross-sectional analysis, black girls are further in the maturation process than white girls at both ages 9 and 10. This earlier onset of maturation may have a primary role in the development of obesity differences between the races (see [118]). The etiology of the difference in obesity between races remain unknown (see [118]).

Some time ago, Walker and Walker (see [191]) conducted a study aimed at determining the weight, height and triceps skinfolds of black, Indian and white 18 year-old high school pupils in South Africa. This study revealed that the said anthropometric values were significantly lower for black boys when compared with white boys. Yet, obesity was far more prevalent among the black girls compared with their white counterparts. Values on Indian boys were similar to those of black boys, although the former were far more favourably placed socioeconomically. Indian girls, compared with black girls, had highly significantly lower values for weight and skinfold thickness, but not for height. However, mean weight for height values for black and Indian boys were similar to values for white boys. Weight-for-height values for Indian girls were similar to data for white girls, although values on these two ethnic groups were significantly lower than those for black girls (see [191]). Black women are fatter than white women from their twenties onward both in terms of skinfolds and BMI, whereas white girls in elementary and junior high school tend to be similar to or fatter than their black counterparts. Similarly, this difference in black and white girls from the North-West Province of South Africa was evident in the study by Mukuddem-Petersen and colleague. In particular, 10 to 15 year-old white girls (14.2 %) were more overweight than their black (7.1 %) counterparts (see [113]). Also, Indian children (6.4 %) and children of mixed ancestry (2.9 %) had the lowest prevalence of overweight in this population (10-15 years). Contrary to other studies, [60] and [118] showed that overweight and obesity, as well as earlier onset of maturation, were more prevalent in white subjects than black ones. It is possible that other confounding factors, such as the low income of most black families, could have played a role in this outcome (see [148]).

3.4.6 Gender Differences

A number of studies have indicated that females are more prone to obesity than males. In this regard, there are a number of physiological processes that are believed to contribute to an increased storage of fat in females. For instance, females have a tendency to channel extra energy into fat while males utilize more of this energy for protein synthesis. This pattern of energy usage or nutrient partitioning in females contributes to further positive energy balance and fat deposition for two reasons. First, the storage of fat is far more energy-efficient than that of protein, and second, it will lead to a lowering of the lean-to-fat ratio with the result that the resting metabolic rate (RMR) does not increase at the same rate as body mass. Such fat deposits are believed to be essential in ensuring female reproductive capacity. Studies in humans and animals indicate that girls exhibit a stronger preference for carbohydrate prior to puberty while boys prefer protein. However, after puberty, both males and females display a marked increase in appetite for fat in response to changes in the gonadal steroid levels. This rise in fat appetite occurs much earlier in females (see [95]).

The analysis in the previous paragraph is related to a study conducted by Monyeki and fellow researchers among preschool children and childen who were in their first years of formal schooling in Ellisras in the Limpopo Province of South Africa (see [112]). They found that 7 and 8 years old childrens mean BMI was statistically significantly higher in males compared to females ($P < 0.05$). The log transformed supraspinale skinfold thickness was larger in females compared to males at ages 4 to 7 years; the log transformed SSF was larger in girls compared to boys aged 7 to 10 years. About 15 % of the males showed overfatness at ages 3 to 4 years, while low prevalence was found at older ages. Mukuddem-Petersen and a fellow investigator conducted a study in the North-West Province of South Africa which demonstrated that the mean TSF is smaller at a later age in boys than in girls (10 to 15 years). This related to girls entering puberty sooner than boys. Furthermore, waist circumference (WC) in boys is slightly smaller at 14 years; however the girls WC suddenly increased at 14 and 15 years of age (see [113]). This could be explained by the increased muscularity of boys and increased adiposity of girls at the onset of puberty (see [37]). Similarly, in other studies, it was found that girls had almost 50 % greater skinfold thickness than boys at all ages (see [123] and [174]) and the percentage body fat was lower in obese boys than in obese girls (see, for instance, [6]). Cameron and Getz (see [27]) described a gain in fat among South African adolescent girls occurring after peak height velocity. Among boys there was a gradual increase in skinfold thickness from age 7 to 18 years and virtually none of the boys could be classified as overweight. The skinfold thicknesses of girls increased more per year, with a clear acceleration in subcutaneous fat deposition from age 14, the mean menarcheal age of the study group. As elluded to previously, this period is associated with hormonal changes that may increase the susceptibility of the female child to fat deposition (see [27]).

3.4.7 Assessing Obesity

In the discussion below, we consider the methods of measurement of obesity that are commonly used in South Africa. There are many procedures available to determine body fat levels or adiposity. The most reliable method of body fat determination is by studying cadavers that involves the dissection of components of the human body (see [30]). Assessment of adiposity may be estimated through in vivo body composition methods such as underwater weighing, deuterium oxide dilution and radioactive potassium counting (see [192]). However, these methods are expensive and/or invasive and not well suited to large epidemiological studies. In addition, the assumptions underlying these methods are population- and age-specific and may not be equally valid for different age and ethnic groups (see [42] and [192]).

By contrast to the previous paragraph, indirect anthropometric estimates of body composition have proven useful for clinical practice, large population-based field studies and epidemiological surveys. Simple anthropometry is appealing due to its simplicity, practical nature; non-invasiveness and cost-effectiveness. For large-scale screening of obesity, measures based on anthropometry are essential. The main contenders are the BMI (measured in kg/m^2) and selected skinfolds. Specifically, among all anthropometric measurements, the BMI represents the most frequently used index for evaluating nutritional status. Despite the fact that the value of the BMI is generally interpreted as a measure of body fatness, it can also reflect differences in fat-free mass. BMI is more reproducible than skinfolds, but its correlation with body fat is weaker. In addition to assessing body fat distribution accurately, two or more skinfolds or possibly body circumferences may be required (see [143]). For instance, both arm muscle circumference and area (see [74]) are regarded as an indicator of body muscle mass. Skinfold thickness is a more direct indicator of adiposity than BMI. In this regard, TSF thickness has been found to be the single best indicator of the percentage of body fat in women and children (see [153] and [34]). Despite this, previous studies on children and adults demonstrated strong correlations between TSF and BMI. The correlation of TSF and BMI is weaker in males since BMI is altered more by muscularity than it is in females (see [116]). In terms of acceptability though, BMI still has the edge over all types of skinfolds, including TSF. Weight-for-age is one of the most widely used nutritional parameters (see [174]).

Although, WHO and the Centers for Disease Control and Prevention both recommend BMI as a fatness indicator across populations (see [29], [30], [116], [165] and [198]), recent findings have challenged the assumption that BMI has the same meaning in all ethnic groups (see [150]). In a situation that is particularly relevant for South Africa, [39] warned that, until more studies include ethnic groups other than whites, BMI should be used cautiously in assessing fatness across populations (see [39]). Estimates of the prevalence of overweight and obesity in population groups are typically based on BMI, and BMI centile curves have been developed for use in paediatric population for clinical and possibly epidemiological purposes (see [31]). The latter mentioned study of Cole and co-workers included all ethnic groups with the BMI cut-points for adults of 25 kg/m^2 and 30 kg/m^2 for overweight and obesity being established worldwide. However, there was no commonly accepted standard of determining overweight and obesity in children until Cole and co-workers (see [30]) published reference curves for children aged 2-18 years based on pooled data from several countries. This included cut-points for BMI at 6 monthly increments in age which correspond to the percentiles of children with a BMI of 25 kg/m^2 (overweight) or 30 kg/m^2 (obese) at 18 years of age. A recent meta-analysis of the relationship between BMI and percentage body fat (BF) among Chinese, Ethiopians, Indonesians, Polynesians, Thais, American blacks and American whites revealed that people of different ethnic groups had significantly different BMIs at the same levels of BF, age, and gender (see [44]). Differences in the relationship between BMI and percentage BF have also been shown when comparing populations from Singapore (see [43]), Japan (see [43]), Hong Kong ([62]) and American whites. Within the USA, the NHLBIGHSRG found that the BMI for lean 9-year-old black children was 3 % higher than that for lean white children of the same age (see [85]). Possible reasons for ethnic differences in the relationship between BMI and percentage BF include differences in fat-free body density, the distribution of subcutaneous fat and limb length relative to trunk size ([192] and [85]). These findings suggest that estimates of BF from anthropometric indicators may produce systematic errors across different ethnic groups (see [116]).

It has been suggested, however, that BMI may be a less sensitive indicator of fatness amongst children (see [151]) and BMI gives no information about fat distribution. In a study that included a consideration of South African variations, Eckhardt and collaborators attempted to address this gap by exploring the ability of a variety of anthropometric indicators to predict body fatness in youths from four different countries: South Africa, the Philippines, China, and Russia. Two different indicators of body fatness were explored as standards against which the anthropometric measures were compared (see [51]). This study highighted the complex nature of body composition research. Furthermore, these authors concluded that the changes in BMI represent changes in fat free mass (FFM) in addition to changes in fat mass (FM). In children undergoing dramatic changes in body composition, BMI is a poor proxy for adiposity. BMI is a better indicator of adiposity in adults, in whom dramatic changes in FFM are not common (in the absence of major disease), and weight changes mainly reflect shifts in FM. Also, they suggested that future studies that relate anthropometric indicators to more direct measures of BF need to explore further the influence of maturation levels. In particular, it is important to consider that sexual maturation and age at menarche affect total fatness and regional fat distribution. The timing of growth spurts influence changes in subcutaneous fat accretion (see [13]). In particular, sexual maturation has also been reported as an important factor producing variations of BMI so that caution is essential when using BMI in adolescence. It was observed that the percentage body fat/BMI relationship was influenced by stage of pubertal development to a greater extent than it was by age (see [17]). In addition, when interpreting BMI data collected from populations with stunted children, we need to be cautious especially in countries like South Africa undergoing nutrition transition since as the relationship of BMI to adiposity may be altered.

Despite all of the objections raised in the above discussion, in South Africa, BMI is most commonly used because of the relative ease and accuracy of the basic measurement (see [75]). Consequently, it is widely recommended for epidemiological and clinical evaluation of obesity in children and adolescents. Age-dependent reference data for BMI are necessary for children, as changes in body composition occur during growth (see [17]). Thus tailored estimating equations that take such differences into account should be used when studying body composition in youths from the different ethnic groups present in South Africa (see [51]).

3.4.8 Consequences of Childhood Obesity

Overweight and obesity in childhood and adolescence are associated with significant physical and psychosocial health problems (see, for instance, [38] and [58]). Its consequences are greater than those associated with many other chronic physical health conditions. Adolescent overweight is associated, for instance, with increased adult morbidity in men for gout, and in women for arthritis. Among women, childhood overweight may be associated with menstrual problems in early adulthood (see [92]). Men who were overweight in adolescence were three times more likely to develop gout when compared with their lean counterparts (see [117]). Research shows that overweight/obesity in children, particularly during adolescence, persists into adulthood and is associated with an increased risk of many diseases including atherosclerosis, cardiovascular disease (see, for instance, [131]), hypertension (see, for instance, [162]), cancers, diabetes, respiratory disorders, gall bladder disease, infertility and several non-fatal but debilitating conditions (see [200], [30], [200], [106], [188] and [70]). More specifically, hyperlipidaemia, characterized by an increase in the serum triglyceride (TG) level, hyperinsulinaemia and an elevation of serum transaminase level due to fatty liver, are considered to be the three major abnormalities in clinical laboratory data associated with childhood obesity (see [5]).

A number of studies have shown that glucose tolerance falls with decreasing birth weight and that people with low birth weight and high BMI as adults are those at greatest risk of developing Type II (non-insulin-dependent) diabetes mellitus. Crowther and investigators (see [35]) conducted a study in a group of 7-year-old black South Africans for whom longitudinal anthropometric data were available. Oral glucose tolerance tests (OGTTs) were carried out and inverse correlations were found between birth weight and the total amount of insulin secreted during the first 30 min ($r = -0.19$, $p = 0.04$) and last 90 min ($r = -0.19$, $p = 0.04$) of the OGTT. This correlation was also evident between birth weight and the 30 min glucose concentrations ($r = -0.20$, $p = 0.02$). Children born with low birth weights but who had high weights at 7 years had higher insulin concentrations and indices of obesity compared with those with low birth weights and low weights at 7 years. There were also positive correlations between weight velocity and BMI ($r = 0.24$, $p = 0.02$) and weight velocity and insulin resistance ($r = 0.18$, $p = 0.04$) as measured using homeostasis model assessment (HOMA). Crowther and co-workers concluded that low birth weight in conjunction with rapid childhood gains in weight in the form of subcutaneous fat, produces poor glucose tolerance in 7-year-old children and can make them susceptible to the development of Type II diabetes later in life (see [35]).

3.5 Stunting and Overweight

In this subsection, we consider the relationship between stunting and overweight. In South Africa, several studies have already been conducted on this issue (see, for instance, [88], [113] and [142]). Our discussions on the link between stunting and obesity centre around a definition and overview, etiology and mechanism, trends and the factors influencing their association.

3.5.1 Definition and Overview

Short stature, also known as low length-for-age, growth retardation, or stunting, can be defined as a height less than the 5th percentile of the age- and sex-specific length or height reference population defined by the National Centre for Health Statistics (NCHS) of the US Department of Health and Human Services Centre for Disease Control and Prevention (CDC) (see [36]). Stunting may be an indication of the long-term health and nutritional history of a population and may reflect the normal variation of growth within a population, taking into account that 5 % of children that are expected to fall below the established cut-off defines this phenomenon (see [198]). In essence, on a population level, an increased prevalence of shortness (above the expected 5 % level) suggests that the growth of some children in the population is retarded. Besides percentiles, z-scores are also used to classify or quantify degrees of stunting. In this context, it was estimated that 2.5 % of children in developed countries are shorter than -2 z scores and are, thus, classified as being stunted. In this regard, z-score is a SD score and is defined by WHO (see [198]) as the "deviation of the value for an individual from the median value of the reference population, divided by the SD from the reference population". Particularly, in South Africa, almost 20 % of children in urban areas are stunted by 2 years of age (see [26]). The WHO (see [199]) regards a population as being moderately affected if 25-50 % of children under the age of 5 years are stunted, and severely affected if more than 50 % are stunted.

In the past, there was a clear association between stunting and access to food; the more food that was available the less the incidence of stunting. In recent times, this association may not be as apparent (see [142]). The condition of being overweight coexists with under-nutrition in many developing countries. Previously, most stunted children in South Africa grew up under conditions of food shortage and had little opportunity to become obese. However, the nutrition transition has caused shifts in dietary composition and activity patterns that have lead to the development of overweight (see [141]). In response to this type of transition, the 1998 WHO Report (see [199]) identified the relationship between BMI and adiposity in children with retarded linear growth (stunting) as being a research imperative. Consequently, numerous researchers have started to investigate this association with many issues still to be elucidated (see [113], [142], [160] and [161]). The age at which stunting relates to the development of obesity is unclear but may be during the four critical periods identified by Dietz (see [37]).

3.5.2 Etiology and Mechanism of Stunting Leading to Overweight/Obesity

Low height-for-age is indicative of stunting, which is a result of chronic, long-term dietary inadequacy, reflecting socio-economic deprivation. In particular, stunting in children is a consequence of many adverse factors, including poor nutritional status of pregnant mothers and children, low birth weight due to inadequate food intake (see [11]), parents' short stature (see [2]), low income, exposure to infection and other diseases, emotional stress (see [189]), lack of physical activity and perhaps the stressful physiologic effects of high altitude (see [103] and [61]). Within child development, stunting and overweight/obesity were manifested by dietary patterns that had shifted from the traditional diets composed of high-fiber, low-fat foods to Western diets of low-fiber, high-fat, high-energy, low-cost foods. It was subsequently hypothesized that the combination of nutritional stunting and exposure to cheap high-fat foods was a major contributing factor to concurrent stunting and overweight/obesity. Specifically, data from Brazil appear to indicate that mild stunting might be associated with a greater susceptibility to the effects of high-fat diets (see [161]). In this regard, excess weight gain among lower-income groups is believed to be the result of a change from a traditional "healthy" diet to a high-fat diet in addition to decreased levels of physical activity (see [46] and [82]).

There are several possible mechanisms for the relationship between stunting and overweight in children. Essentially, a number of highly speculative explanations for the said relationship stem from the work of Barker in [9] and none seem to be mutually exclusive. Barker proposes that hormonal changes and their physiologic responses, such as abdominal obesity stem from fetal or infant undernutrition facilitating long-term changes based on metabolic adaptations (see [9]). In particular, Barker suggests that an infant's major adaptation to undernutrition is reduced growth rate and related changes in fetal hormone production that yield long-term effects including changes in insulin and growth hormone. In addition, in a series of studies on small samples of English adults, Barker showed that low birth weight was related to subsequent abdominal obesity and a wide range of hormonal changes associated with the metabolic syndrome (see [131] and [114]). Furthermore, he has shown that growth retardation is associated with later obesity and a range of hormonal changes. Although the mechanism by which stunting may predispose to overweight or obesity remains largely undefined. It has been postulated that nutritional stunting is associated with impaired fat oxidation (see [77]) which could predispose stunted children to excessive weight and fat gains at excessive energy and fat intakes. This was evident in another study where nutritionally stunted children had measurably impaired fat oxidation compared with non-stunted control children living in the same environment. Specifically, stunted children had significantly higher respiratory quotients (RQ) and lower fat oxidation in the fasting state and 30 minutes after a meal (subsequent postprandial meals remained higher but not significantly so). These findings may help to explain previous observations of increased prevalence of overweight among stunted adolescents and adults in developing countries, because fat that is not oxidized must be stored (see [160]). Another study suggested that the diet early in life has a significant effect on later metabolism and health (see [77]). A further postulate is that nutritionally stunted children may have an impaired regulation of energy intake, which increases the risk for obesity (see [76]). It has been proposed that stunted children have lower energy requirements and should have lower total energy intakes than non-stunted children (see [77]).

There appears to be a coexistence of stunting and overweight in low-income populations undergoing the nutritional transition. Although no association between stunting and energy expenditure was found among children ages 8 to 11 y in Brazil, (see [78]) fasting fat oxidation was significantly lower in the stunted group than in the non-stunted group (see [77]). This finding may help to explain the increased prevalence of obesity among stunted adolescents in developing countries. As in South Africa, stunted children and, in particular, those recovering from protein-energy malnutrition, are programmed to accumulate greater body fat at central sites during adolescence (see [113]).

3.5.3 Trends of Stunting and Overweight/Obesity

The United Nations International Children's Education Fund (UNICEF) has estimated that approximately one out of three children younger than five years of age are chronically malnourished. This malnourishment makes them susceptible to poor linear growth early in life (see [11]). A decade ago the United Nations sub-committee on Nutrition estimated that one-third to two-thirds of children in developing countries may be considered to be of short stature (see [159]). A high weight-for-height is emerging as a growing nutrition concern among children in communities undergoing nutritional transition (see [133] and [161]). Body composition, especially fat mass, could also be an important component and determinant of long-term outcome of stunting. A distinct association exists between stunting and overweight/obesity and with few exceptions, the types of determinants for these two nutritional disorders appear to be the same but directionally opposite in affording risk for a given nutritional disorder. Stunted children have nearly twice the risk of being overweight (BMI = 25 kg/m^2). Doak and collaborators concluded that if under- and overweight can occur in the same household, common underlying causes of both conditions may be identified (see [46]).

In 1996, the percentage of 3 to 6 and 7 to 9 year-old children that were stunted among black and mixed-ancestory South African children was close to 30.6 % (see [142]). The NFCS of 1999 showed that at least 21,6 % of children between the ages of 1 and 9 years old are stunted, indicating chronic past undernutrition (see, for instance, [90] and [91]). At the national level in South Africa, stunting was prevalent in 19.3 % of 1 to 9 year-old children, with the highest prevalence in those of age 1 to 3 (24.4 %), in rural areas (23.8 %) and on commercial farms (25.6 %) (see [173] and [91]). Younger children (1 to 3 years of age) were found to be most severely affected as well as those living on commercial farms and in tribal and rural areas (30,6 %). Also, a 2003 study conducted by Zere and colleague claimed that stunting was the most prevalent form of malnutrition in South Africa (a reflection of long-term undernutrition = -2 SD HAZ). Here the rate of stunting (for children under-five years) was found to be the highest in the South African provinces (Eastern Cape and Limpopo Province) with the highest prevalence of poverty (see [202]). Research in the last decade, notably by Popkin and collaborators (see [142]), provided evidence for concurrent stunting and overweight or obesity in some developing countries. These countries (South Africa, Russia, China, and Brazil) were linked by their classification as transitional countries in that they were transiting through both economic and social changes. Similarly, Sawaya and colleagues showed a relationship between stunting and obesity in countries undergoing the nutritional transition (see [161]). This has been found at the community level in South Africa (see [170] and [21]) and Brazil (see [55]). Recently, Jinabhai and collaborators conducted a study in the KwaZulu-Natal province of South Africa on rural primary school children aged 4 to 5 and 8 to 11 years (see [81]). The outcome of the study showed that there was moderate stunting in 10-25 %, wasting in 1-6 %, 5-24 % were overweight and 1-10 % obese. An increasing prevalence of overweight and obesity was seen in both the 4 to 5 and 8 to 11 year age-groups. The finding that moderate stunting co-exists with overweight and obesity suggests that patterns of under- and over-nutrition in South African children are changing and might indicate the early stages of a complex nutritional transition. The cross-sectional study conducted by Mukuddem-Petersen and Kruger in the North-West Province of South Africa showed no significant association between stunting and overweight in 10 to 15 year-old children. However, there was a tendency for the stunted girls older than 14 years to start to gain subcutaneous fat even though at these ages they were still underweight (see [113]).

3.5.4 Factors Influencing Stunting and Overweight/Obesity

In the following discussion, we consider vulnerable periods of life for stunting and obesity. Babies of abnormally short length at birth are also at risk for short stature later in life. This indicates that intrauterine growth is important for a child's subsequent growth (see [198]). There are several reasons for stunting being prevalent in the first 2 to 3 years of life and not later. During early childhood, nutritional needs are greater in relation to weight than at any subsequent stage in life since the rate of growth is the highest that it will ever be. Thus, the opportunity for growth retardation is great in early childhood, partly because more growth is taking place (see [104]). Also, the interactive effects of poor energy and nutrient intakes, infection (see [189]) and the child's dependence on others for nutrition early on in life cannot be ignored. Specifically, African populations, especially preschool-aged children, are exposed to malnutrition, and this may have a major effect on growth and development. Height retardation may be regarded as an index of past and chronic malnutrition over a long period (see [13]) which leads to a reduction in final stature. In this regard, in the NFCS, stunting decreased with an increase in age. It was lowest in the

7 to 9 year-old group which does reflect catch-up growth with time (see [90] and [91]). The ability of children to demonstrate catch-up growth has been recognized for almost four decades (see [145]) and is characterized by an increased growth velocity in height and/or weight after the removal of some constraint on normal growth. This increased velocity brings the child's height-for-age or weight-for-age status back toward the normal centiles, and in the best-case scenario, actually returns the child's growth pattern to its preinsult status (see [176]). Evidently, children who are stunted in childhood are likely to have short stature in adulthood (see [156]) although evidence suggests that some catch-up growth may occur (see [99], [104] and [194]). In addition to catch-up growth occurring after the removal of an insult in childhood and adolescence, such growth also occurs during infancy. In this case, the rationale is that the growth of the fetus had been constrained, and when freed from this constraint, the affected infant demonstrates rapid growth to reach its genetically determined growth canal (see [177]). The focus of previous research on catch-up growth in infancy has generally been on children who were SGA (see [145]) at birth and who were thus thought to have suffered from intrauterine growth retardation as a result of factors other than maternal size. The period from childhood to adolescence and then from adolescence to adulthood is also considered a particularly nutritionally vulnerable time. Not only does significant physical change take place during these times, but food habits and lifestyles also evolve that form the basis for long-term health (see [37]). The growth spurt associated with adolescence is a universal phenomenon. However, this spurt differs in intensity and duration from child to child. It usually occurs in boys between 12.5 and 15.5 years while in girls it generally occurs about two years earlier. Before the growth spurt boys and girls only differ by about 2 % in height, whereas this difference increases to about 8 % after the spurt. This increase in height is mainly due to an increase in the growth of the trunk rather than leg growth (see [175]).

A greater central fat distribution has also been found in children stunted early in childhood (see [49] and [158]). In particular, studies on three continents showed that nutritional stunting, which is usually caused by chronic undernutrition (see [194]), is positively associated with adult fatness (see [160] and [161]). In addition, an association between excess weight gain and dietary fat content in stunted Brazilian children was observed. This trend was not detected in non-stunted control children (see [161]). Clearly, children ages 1 to 3 years are most vulnerable to undernutrition and overnutrition. If stunting takes place at this age, it is postulated that these children may be at greater risk for being overweight (see [142] and [135]). A diet low in nutrient density may lead to this outcome. It is apparent that interventionary steps should take place early in life for those at risk of being overweight and stunted (see [96]).

The factors affecting stunting in South Africa include age of menarche in girls, low birthweight, undernutrition during critical periods of development and lack of physical activity. Specific studies conducted in South Africa discussing these factors are outlined below. In a recent study conducted by Mukuddem-Petersen and colleague in the North-West Province of South Africa, it was confirmed that stunting at 14 and 15 years of age in girls could be related to the late onset of menarche (see [113]). Stunted girls had a significantly higher age at menarche (13.37 years, 95 % CI 12.80, 13.95) than nonstunted girls (12.73 years, 95 % CI 12.58, 12.89). Here CI is the abbreviation for confidence interval. This can be explained by the fact that menstruation usually begins a little more than 1 year after peak linear growth is attained (see [17]), and stunted girls apparently reached peak velocity in linear growth later than nonstunted girls. As was stated previously, stunting in this population could be due to low birthweight and/or short length, growth retardation at 2-3 years of age, growth retardation at puberty or combinations of the above mentioned phenomena (see [113]. Research has suggested that undernutrition in early life may play a role in promoting adult obesity. Recently, Mamabolo and collaborators conducted a study (see [102]) to determine the prevalence of stunting, wasting and overweight and their determinants in 3-year-old children in the Central Region of the Limpopo Province in South Africa. Height-for-age z-scores were low, with a high incidence of stunting (48 %). The children also exhibited a high prevalence of overweight (22 %) and obesity (24 %) with 19 % being both stunted and overweight. Gaining more weight within the first year of life increased the risk of being overweight at 3 years by 2.39 times (95 % CI 1.96, 4.18) while having a greater length at 1 year was protective against stunting (odds ratio (OR) 0.41; 95 % CI 0.17, 0.97). Furthermore, it is important to realise the importance of normal length and weight being attained at 1 year of age, since these in turn predict nutritional status at 3 years of age (see [102]).

Furthermore, Cameron and fellow researchers investigated stunting at 2 years in relation to body composition at 9 years in a mixed-longitudinal study of prepubertal African children from Soweto-Johannesburg, South Africa. These investigators found that the children who were stunted at 2 years were significantly shorter and lighter than non-stunted children at 7 to 9 years, but there were no differences in their BMI or centralization of body fat. Previously, stunted status significantly predicted reduced weight and height at 7 to 9 years but did not predict BMI, body composition, or fat patterning after controlling for potential confounding factors. Cameron and co-workers concluded that greater BMI in stunted infants does not demonstrate a tendency toward overweight or obesity but is a reflection of the greater reduction in height rather than weight in stunted children. Stunted children may be programmed to accumulate greater body fat at central sites during adolescence, but these authors were unable to show that these changes are evident before the initiation of pubertal development (see [28]).

Mukuddem-Petersen and colleague (see [113]) showed that stunted girls (10 to 15 years) from the North-West province in South Africa had a tendency to have more subcutaneous fat and to gain fat at the umbilical level compared to the nonstunted girls (10 to 15 years). Popkin and co-investigators (see [142]) and Benefice and co-researchers (see [13]) found that girls stunted at infancy catch up in body weight and subcutaneous fat during puberty but do not catch up with respect to stature. Stunted girls tended to accumulate more subcutaneous fat on the trunk and arms than did non-stunted girls (see [13]). The same seems to be true for the study by Mukuddem-Petersen and colleague (see [113]). However, because the birth weights were unknown in this population, it was not possible to assess whether stunting was the effect of recent malnutrition, intrauterine growth retardation, or a combination. In developing countries such as South Africa, many children become stunted during infancy due to inappropriate weaning practices, poor diet, and repeated infections (see [91]). The diets of these children may have been limited in essential nutrients required for an increase in height and muscle mass but not in energy for an increase in body fat. Early nutritional programming may result in hormonal effects that limit linear growth but not fat deposition (see [142] and [13]). Critical periods of development have been well recognized for many behavioural and developmental processes.

Next, we consider physical activity and the affect it has on stunting. In the study by Torun and Viteri (1994) it was found that mild-to-moderate exercise combined with a good diet enhances linear growth (see [179]). This may be mediated by endocrine growth factors, of which synthesis is prompted by exercise. A study in a group of malnourished children showed that the group with greater physical activity grew more in height and lean body mass than did the less active control group. The investigators suggested that inactivity often accompanies severe malnutrition and may contribute to stunting (see [179]).

In a recent cross-sectional study conducted in the North-West Province in South Africa researchers showed that stunted subjects were less active than the non-stunted ones (see [88]). Furthermore, it has been proposed that chronically malnourished children have less lean body mass, resulting in decreased metabolic rate and physical activity (see [8]). Hoffman and co-workers (see [78]) found significantly lower resting energy expenditure (REE) in stunted children than in non-stunted children, but no significant differences between REE adjusted for body weight or FFM of the stunted and non-stunted groups. Low energy expenditure in physical activity predicted excess weight gain in children (see [69]). In the North-West Province of South Africa a study conducted by Kruger and investigators showed the mean energy intake per kilogram of body weight in the stunted girls (10 to 15 years) to be significantly higher than that of the non-stunted girls (see [88]). In this context, the stunted girls had a relatively greater energy intake and deposited relatively more subcutaneous fat than did the non-stunted girls. A higher percentage of the stunted girls were in the mostly inactive category (72.5 %) compared with non-stunted girls (66.1 %), which could have contributed to the tendency to deposit adipose tissue. Older inactive stunted girls in the North-West Province of South Africa were relatively fatter than younger inactive stunted girls. Also, older inactive stunted and non-stunted girls had a greater mean sum of skinfold thicknesses than did their younger counterparts, but the difference between the two means was greater for stunted than for non-stunted girls (see [88]). In particular, the stunted 15 year-old girls had the same mean sum of TSF and SSF and a similar mean waist circumference as non-stunted girls of the same age group; however, after adjustment for dietary factors, activity and body weight, the adjusted sum of SSF and TSF was higher in stunted than in non-stunted girls. The higher adjusted sum of skinfold thicknesses in stunted girls may indicate a tendency for stunted girls to store body fat in favor of oxidation of fat for energy. This corresponds with the results of Hoffman and co-investigators (see [77]). Linear growth in these girls seem to be limited, but the potential for body fat deposition, especially abdominal fat, is not. Because stunted children may have impaired fat oxidation, (see [77]) it is even more important for them to be physically active in order to improve energy use and to prevent excessive fat deposition.

Genetic and environmental factors play a major role in stunting. While genetic factors are obviously the major determinant of linear growth potential, reaching this potential is dependent on a number of environmental factors of which nutrition is of great importance (see [11], [99], [159] and [194]). In this regard, the macronutrient components of foods like protein, carbohydrate and fat, which are the sole contributors to energy intake, are the principal determinants of growth rate. Therefore, anthropometric determination of nutritional status is indicative mainly of the availability of protein and energy foods. Recent studies suggests that micronutrients may also be involved in determining growth rate. In particular, zinc, iron and calcium seem to play a very prominent role. A study done on urban Chinese children to ascertain the effects of zinc and micronutrient repletion on growth, confirmed the essentiality of zinc for the growth of children (see, for instance, [128]). Zinc supplemented infants demonstrated improved linear growth velocity. Marginal and moderate growth impairment in children as a consequence of inadequate zinc intake has been reported from many developed and developing countries. The clinical manifestation of zinc deficiency include growth retardation. In addition, zinc is required for DNA synthesis, cell division and protein synthesis. Several hundred zinc containing nucleoproteins are probably involved in gene expression of various proteins (see, for instance, [146]). Furthermore, zinc supplementation is effective for inducing growth in short children with a zinc deficiency (see [119]). Harris and co-workers (see [73]) found the proportion of children with stunted growth was greater in rural areas than in urban areas in Tibet. There is some evidence to suggest that physiological mechanisms promote the accretion of body fat rather than protein after nutritional deprivation (see [7], [52] and [157]).

In a study done on Kenyan primary school children, it was found that the provision of iron supplements resulted in improved growth (see [94]). Also a randomized, double-blind, placebo-controlled trial carefully studied the intake of calcium-enriched foods and bone mass growth in pre-pubertal girls. The results suggest a possible positive effect of calcium supplementation on skeletal growth in pre-pubertal girls (see [18]). Similarly, in the study by Mukuddem-Petersen and collaborator which was conducted in the North-West Province of South Africa, they found that stunted growth was most prevalent in the rural areas (boys: 26.7 %, girls: 23.7 %) and the least prevalent in urban areas (boys: 17.1 %, girls 11.6 %) (see [113]). About half (51 %) of the stunted girls and 43 % of the stunted boys came from the rural areas. Other research set within the urban environments of developing countries has suggested that stunting in infancy may increase the future risk of greater fatness and overweight in later childhood (see, for instance, [13]). It is within the urban environment that transition is most evident. These environments are characterized by a rapidly increasing population density and concomitant changes from traditional low-fat to Western high-fat diets. This may interact in poorer families, in which stunting is endemic, to increase the susceptibility to excess body fat gain in children who are stunted (see [160], [161]). Sawaya and co-workers (see, for instance, [160]) described a prevalence of 30 % undernutrition (low height-for-age, low weight-for-age) among children in a shanty town in Sao Paulo, Brazil compared with concurrent prevalences of 21 % and 8.6 % for adolescent female and male overweight, respectively. Studies by Mukuddem-Petersen (see [113]) and Kruger (see [88]) conducted in 10 to 15 year-old children in the North-West Province showed no significant association between stunting and overweight in this population. However, there was a tendency for urban stunted girls to gain more subcutaneous fat at the onset of menarche than stunted girls from informal townships. Therefore, this outcome could predict possible problems of overweight as they get older. Futhermore, in this population the differences in measures of weight status between stunted and nonstunted children were more pronounced in the rural areas, (see [113]). It should be noted that this province is in a stage of rapid economic transition; people in rural areas live in traditional African villages with a tribal chief, whereas urbanized people live under Westernized conditions (see [185]).

Socio-economic factors have a major part to play in stunting. The prevalence of stunting is high in less-developed countries with low socioeconomic standards. This situation reflects the high frequency of undernutrition observed in such countries. However, the occurrence of stunting can be significantly reduced, but by no means eliminated (see [203]), with improvements in socioeconomic conditions such as better and more accessible health care facilities. In addition, studies have shown that among children from low socioeconomic levels, a short period of breastfeeding is associated with a higher risk of complications and or early primary undernutrition with both factors determining growth retardation (see [178] and [184]). Gross national product was related negatively to stunting and positively to overweight. In countries where maternal and child malnutrition exist alongside rapid economic development, abdominal obesity and associated chronic diseases seem likely to increase (see [79]).

Recent research done in the Central Region of the Limpopo Province of South Africa revealed that having a mother as a student increased the risk for stunting at 3 years by 18.21 times (95 % CI 9.46, 34.74) while having a working mother increased the risk for overweight by 17.87 times (95 % CI 8.24, 38.78) (see [102]). All these factors also appeared as risks or as being protective in children who were both overweight and stunted, as did living in a household having nine or more persons (OR 5.72; 95 % CI 2.7, 12.10). The emergence of the nutrition transition with its rapid shifts in the composition of diet and activity patterns and subsequent shifts in body composition may lead to considerable obesity over the next several decades. This may affect individuals living in environments in which current infant feeding and morbidity patterns during infancy are associated with extensive stunting (see [133]).

Ethnic differences are related to the prevalence of stunting. In the USA, the high prevalence of short stature among black infants aged less than 12 months (14.8 %) probably reflects the relatively high rate of low birthweight among this group (see [29]). Also, there are several other research studies involving different ethnic communities that exhibit a correlation between stunting and obesity. In particular, investigators have noted that Mexican-American children, when compared to non-Hispanic whites, are shorter but heavier for their heights. This is a paradoxical situation, as was pointed out by Trowbridge in [182], in that short stature is generally associated with poverty and chronic undernutrition whereas overweight is associated with overnutrition. Since many Mexican-Americans are poor, one would expect them to be short and thin, not short and plump. In addition, poor children in rural areas of Mexico and Central America are considerably shorter than Mexican-Americans. Also, maturational differences between black and white girls have been reported in the past (see [60]). It was clear from cross-sectional studies that black girls are further in the maturation process than white girls at both ages 9 and 10 years. This earlier onset of maturation may have a primary role to play in the development of obesity differences between the races (see [118]).

Contrary to the result from some studies (see [60] and [118]), in [113], Mukuddem-Petersen showed that overweight and obesity, as well as earlier onset of maturation, were mostly found in white subjects in the North-West Province of South Africa rather than black subjects. It is possible that other confounding factors could have played a role in this outcome. For example, low income of most black families in the aforementioned geographical region (see [148]). Also, the mean age at menarche of white girls was earlier (12.53 years-old, 95 % CI 12.24, 12.82) than in black girls (12.95 years-old, 95 % CI 12.77, 13.15). As in South Africa, impaired fat oxidation was shown previously to be a risk factor for excess weight gain in several populations known to be susceptible to obesity (refer to the case of the Pima Indians explained in [196]).

Gender differences have a vital part to play in stunting. Jinabhai and collaborators conducted a study in KwaZulu-Natal, South Africa, on rural primary school children aged 8 to 11 years (see [81]). The investigation suggested that 4 to 11 year-old girls in the National Schools Study and in the primary datasets had a significantly higher prevalence of overweight than boys; girls (1.4 %) were also more obese than boys (0.9 %) and boys significantly more stunted than the girls. Evidently, results from the cross-sectional study conducted in the North-West Province of South Africa by Mukuddem-Petersen and a co-worker showed that distinct gender differences exist. In particular, mean TSF is smaller at a later age in boys than in girls (10 to 15 years). Furthermore, WC in boys is slightly smaller at 14 years old with the girls' WC suddenly increasing at 14 and 15 years of age (see [113]). An explanation for this is that boys exhibit greater muscularity whereas girls show increased adiposity at the onset of puberty (see [37]). Linear growth slowed down a bit for 10 year-old boys, and at 15 years of age in girls. The increase in the TSF and SSF in the girls coincides with the onset of menarche. The stunting at 14 and 15 years of age in girls could be related to a late onset of menarche. Stunted girls had a significantly higher age at menarche (13.37 years, 95 % CI 12.80, 13.95) than nonstunted girls (12.73 years old, 95 % CI 12.58, 12.89). This can be explained by the fact that menstruation usually begins a little more than 1 year after peak linear growth is attained (see [17]) and stunted girls apparently reached peak velocity in linear growth later than nonstunted girls (see [113]). In girls, menarcheal status furnishes reference data that are less detailed but easier to collect. In order to evaluate puberty-related BMI. O'Dea and Abrahams (see [123]) reported significantly lower BMI of age-matched premenarche vs postmenarche girls. However, multivariate tests demonstrate that menarcheal status did not influence BMI when corrected by pubertal stage and age (see also [17]). They demonstrated that degree of pubertal maturation has a greater influence on BMI than age in both genders, but that this is more evident in girls (see also [17]).

Next, we consider a few consequences of stunting and obesity. Evidence from both human and animal studies support the hypothesis that chronic undernutrition, severe enough to cause permanent growth retardation, is associated with later risk for chronic metabolic diseases (see [77], [142], [158], [161] and [190]). In addition, substantial evidence supports the significant role of growth retardation in impaired cognitive functions (see [16] and [107]), physical capacity for labor (see [121], [122] and [154]) and impaired immune function (see [83] and [183]). Taken together, it is clear that preventing or treating growth retardation in countries with precarious economic conditions may play a major role in promoting future productivity and overall social and economic development (see [57]). The extensive investigations by Fogel on the ways in which height, independent of weight and BMI, relates to morbidity and mortality patterns and trends give more relevance to a biological hypothesis (see [56]). For example, stunting during the developmental stages has far reaching effects into adulthood by increasing the risk of chronic diseases. In particular, stunting during early childhood has been associated with excess weight gain in later life (see [166]) and with the development of certain chronic diseases including type 2 diabetes and hypertension (see [162] and [201]). It is claimed that stunting among children and adults from developing countries induces functional impairment on a wide spectrum of biological, behavioural and social dimensions (see [193]). In particular, being shorter than average may not seem to be an important clinical problem or public health issue, but the factors that cause stunting have adverse consequences. These include impaired development, lower intelligence, poorer academic performance and a reduced capacity for work in adults. These factors, in turn, have a negative effect on economic productivity. Shorter women are at greater risk for obstetrical complications and there is an intergenerational effect of stunted growth (see [61] and [103]). Stunting at school age and in adolescents may be less reversible than in younger children (see [104]).

Childhood stunting has been suggested as a factor contributing to high rates of adult obesity in developing countries (see [142] and [160]). Scientific research on stunting and obesity and their relationship has developed in several directions in recent times. The results from previous studies suggest that the type of obesity changes with age in obese children. The older obese children tended to gain more fat at the umbilical level than the younger ones, and this was considered as the general worsening of body build during growth in obese children (see [4]). Similarly, Mukuddem-Petersen and colleague confirmed this deterioration in body build in 10 to 15 year-old children of the North-West Province of South Africa. Specifically, the stunted girls' mean WC gradually increased up to the age of 13 years and then there was a sudden increase at age 14 and 15 years. This coincided with a rapid increase in BMI and TSF+SSF at ages 14 and 15 years of age in the stunted girls (see [113]).

4 Strategic Response

In this section, we highlight some of the strategic responses to the problem of childhood obesity and its ramifications in South Africa. In this regard, a clear understanding of the nutrition transition and the double burden phenomenon is of primary importance when trying to find a solution to a problem of such magnitude. Also, we consider the strategies being implemented to combat overweight and obesity. Finally, we discuss the interventionary programmes being developed to address the problem of stunting and obesity.

4.1 Double/Dual Burden

The cumulative effect of the double burden of apparently related nutritional disorders in South Africa needs to be evaluated to develop satisfactory interventions for their prevention and management. In this regard, detailed quantitative and qualitative information is being compiled in several ongoing studies. These investigations are an imperative if a better understanding of the underlying causes of the dual burden condition in a particular household is to be developed. Preliminary indications are that individuals in a household may have very different energy density needs related to physiological changes throughout the life cycle. Furthermore, an underweight child may be independently predisposed to becoming overweight or obese later in life. Environmental factors, such as activity patterns and food availability, could contribute to differences in energy intake and expenditure. Individuals with shared genetic and household environmental risk factors may have sufficiently different lifestyle patterns related to external social, cultural and physiological factors. A programme of education at every level of society is important to increase awareness of the health risks related to the double burden. In this regard, prevention programmes should consider, not only the nutrition concerns of a single individual, but of the whole household. More specifically, nutrition interventions targeting "at-risk" individuals should be cautioned against making recommendations that would alter household diets and jeopardize vulnerable persons within the same household. Instead, prevention programmes should transmit health messages that contribute to the optimal weight and good health of all persons in the household.

One of the objectives of the WHO programmes to combat obesity is to advance public health worldwide. This goal can only be met through decisive and coherent action which in many developing countries requires complex interventions in both mal- and overnourished communities. For instance, investigation of both under- and overnutrition have important clinical and public health implications for planning Primary Health Care (PHC) services and health promotion strategies to prevent chronic diseases in adulthood. Such investigations in developing countries require a shift in the focus from under-nutrition and food security, to the assessment of trends in overweight and obesity (see [200]). The nutritional transition facing developing and middle-income countries also has important implications for preventative strategies to control chronic degenerative diseases (see [200]), [133] and [112]). Dual burden households are most prevalent in countries that are experiencing the chronic disease phase of this transition.

Like many other countries, in South Africa, there is an urgent need to address non-optimal diets and physical inactivity via multi-sectoral and multidisciplinary approaches. Further avenues that are worth exploring are life course approaches, addressing poverty, gender and culture sensitivities and making stakeholders accountable. Also, the South African government should adopt a prominent role in altering the environment to support the entire nation as well as individuals in their attempt to improve their nutritional and physical activity patterns. In this context, national legislation and appropriate infrastructure are critical for introducing effective policies. Ultimately the main policy recommendations of the strategy for South Africa should be to develop national dietary and physical activity guidelines. Furthermore, health organizations should provide accurate and balanced information to consumers, in particular with regard to nutrition labelling, nutrition and health claims and address issues related to marketing of foods for children. In addition, assessment and evaluation of South Africa's food and agriculture policies should be consistent with a healthy and adequate diet. Also, it is of paramount importance to build on the existing structures and national mechanisms rather than create new ones. Thus, an effective response requires sustained political commitment, and broader, multi-level involvement with all relevant stakeholders in South Africa.

4.2 Childhood Obesity

Prevention of obesity is a public health priority, where much of the attention should focus on childhood and adolescence (see [75]). These public health interventions are required because expensive and technologically advanced treatment for obesity would exhaust public health resources. The problem of obesity in ethnic minorities demonstrates the need for targeted prevention and intervention strategies (see [13]). Dramatic increases in obesity have been followed by epidemics of non-communicable diseases, such as cardiovascular disease. This has relevance for policymakers, health planners and communities to implement appropriate actions to prevent and control the emergence of these epidemics at an early stage. Sensitivity to weight gain may be amplified by certain factors such as the development of a disease, or by therapy with drugs which promote weight gain as a side-effect (see [199]). Furthermore, genetic, biological and other personal factors such as, gender and age interact to determine an individual's susceptibility to weight gain (see [200]).

Obesity cannot be prevented or managed solely at the individual level. Communities, governments, the media and the food industry need to work together to modify the environment so that it is less conducive to weight gain. Such partnerships are required to ensure that effective and sustainable changes in the diet and everyday levels of physical activity can be achieved throughout the community. According to WHO, three settings for implementing obesity management interventions aimed at children can be identified as family-based, school-based and primary-care based programmes (see [199]). As regards health promotion programmes, many studies recommend that regular, enjoyable physical activity, a healthy diet and acceptance of the normal range of body shapes should be encouraged. Children should be encouraged to increase physical activity by helping to set their own activity goal, monitor activity performance and provide incentives for reaching the activity goal. Family activity patterns should be reviewed and improved (see [23] and [147]). In addition to this, regular monitoring of the anthropometric status of children and adolescents should be conducted (see, for instance, [19]). This approach will allow obesity prevention and management strategies to be harmonized with existing public health policies and programmes for control of all non-communicable diseases (NCDs) (see [199]).

The impact of the rapid process of socio-economic development during the 1990s on the nutritional status of South African children is poorly understood (see [105] and [24]). Clearly, in South Africa, obesity in childhood is one of the most complex and least understood clinical syndromes in pediatric medicine practice. The scale of the problem suggests that only a concerted sustained effort by health professionals in collaboration with many other disciplines and organizations will reverse this trend for future generations. In South Africa where overweight/obesity co-exist with undernutrition, there is an urgent need to prevent or reverse unhealthy trends in diet and physical activity patterns (see [199]). Regular clinical and epidemiological monitoring of nutritional status needs to be undertaken to examine possible future trends of overweight/obesity and their relationship with stunting. This may also be compared with global trends. The South African Heart Foundations Community Childrens Programme (SAHFCCP) was initiated in 1997, and by 2005, had already affected the lives of 2 million children countrywide. The initial focus was on children aged between 3 and 6 years with this being extended to primary school children from previously disadvantaged areas. The main objective of the programme is to educate the children as well as the teachers, parents and child caregivers. Study units include a consideration of nutrition, exercise, the effect of smoking, basic hygiene and HIV awareness. With South Africa being a multilingual country (11 official languages), the material is presented in four languages: English, Afrikaans, Xhosa and Zulu.

4.3 Stunting and Overweight/Obesity

It is clear that a paradigm shift is needed for future strategic responses. When examining the type of determinants of stunting and overweight, in the context of poverty and rapid nutritional transition, it becomes apparent that neither nutritional disorder be treated in isolation but should, by necessity, be afforded equal priority in terms of health resources. The analysis of the relationship between stunting and overweight among children has important implications for policy-makers in developing and planning public health interventions, and for monitoring the nutritional transition. Intervention early in life by targeting children are likely to have lasting effects on health behavior and may reduce risk of disease in these populations. Nutritional interventions in stunted children should focus not only on nutrient supplementation but also on measures to increase physical activity and prevent overweight.

Despite the stumbling blocks identified previously, some encouraging programmes have already been implemented in South Africa by various roleplayers. For instance, in 1995, the South African Medical Research Council (MRC) recognized the lack of health facilities within a rural village in the KwaZulu-Natal Province of South Africa. This prompted the establishment of a growth-monitoring programme for preschool children. This community-based project is run by nutrition monitors (local people specifically trained for the project) through home-based centres (called Isizinda) within the community. As part of their contribution towards the initiative, families make their homes available on a voluntary basis to serve as growth monitoring points. The various aspects of the programme are managed and coordinated by the headmaster of the local primary school. Activities at the Isizinda include monthly growth monitoring, nutrition education, and recording of morbidity and mortality data. Children who are in need of medical treatment or who show growth faltering are referred to the nearest clinic and followed up by the nutrition monitors. Furthermore, in 2003, the South African Heart Foundation (SAHF) launched an educational programme called "Edu-Heart". This initiative was designed to assist schools in offering healthy choices in an attempt to ensure that the foods children consume are suitable. The project is aimed at primary schools throughout South Africa, and was first introduced in the Western Cape Province.

5 Conclusions & Future Investigations

Obesity is a complex multi-factoral disorder prevalent in both developing and developed countries that affects children and adults alike. Even though the problem of childhood obesity has come to light in the past decade, a paucity of information still exists in many countries. This is especially true for middle-income and developing countries such as South Africa, which faces the double burden of infection- and poverty-associated diseases, together with the emerging concerns of chronic diseases. On the other hand, in low-income urban households the coexistence of overweight and obesity may occur simply as the result of rapid changes in the food supply and/or age-specific differences in risks related to obesity vs underweight. It is clear that chronic diseases linked to childhood and adult obesity could retard economic progress in many developing countries unless urgent action is taken. The promotion of healthy eating and regular physical activity is essential for the prevention of future obesity (see [33]) and also for treating those who are already overweight and obese (see [120]). The increasing proportion of fat and energy density of the diet, together with reductions in the level of physical activity and the rise in the level of sedentary behaviour, are thought to be major contributing factors to the rise in the average body weight of populations. Recent large multi-centre trials have shown that significant weight loss is achievable using a contribution of diet and physical activity, and can prevent the onset of type 2 diabetes in subjects at risk (see [87]). Dealing with these issues would appear to be the most effective means of combatting rises in the level of overweight and obesity in the community (see [200]). Finance and trade ministers need to lend their support to health ministers for strategic actions to improve the nutritional welfare of their populations or face huge costs from an epidemic of obesity, type 2 diabetes, heart disease, metabolic syndrome (see [131] and [114]) and other obesity-related health concerns. Other strategies to prevent the development of obesity should include the establishment of regular meal patterns as well as dietary modifications to ensure nutrient intakes in the context of a reduced calorie diet (see [144]). Childhood nutritional stunting, usually an indicator of chronic malnutrition (see [182] and [194]) and undernutrition (see [142] and [193]), has been suggested as a contributory factor to elevated rates of obesity (high weight-for-height) in developing countries.

Subtle differences in nutritional status amongst the diverse populations of South Africa and between the various provinces are evident. Explanations for these differences may be due to the variations in SES (diet and activity level), level of education and perhaps the altitude. Regarding the latter, the study conducted by Jinabhai and co-workers (see [81]) showed a greater increase in overweight/obesity in younger children compared to the study by Mukuddem-Petersen. It could be speculated that the high altitude in the North-West Province of South Africa may have curtailed the prevalence of overweight and obesity in this age group (10 to 15 years) as opposed to the children (8 to 11 years) in Kwazulu Natal who reside at sea level. However, more research is needed regarding the latter.

Generally, the prevention of obesity in childhood is the best strategy to control today's epidemic in adults. The paradox of over- and undernutrition, as well as the range of micronutrient deficiencies of public health significance, requires complementing strategies and an integrated approach to ensure optimal nutrition for all South Africans. The situation is further complicated by the many causes of malnutrition which could be direct factors such as inadequate food intake, or underlying factors such as household food insecurity or even basic factors such as a lack of resources. Future efforts to prevent childhood obesity should explore whether parental education programmes can decrease the prevalence of obesity by encouraging more activity-related home environments for young children. In order to identify the group that is at risk we should be able to categorize the different forms of overweight and stunting in children. Further research is necessary to establish the energy requirements of stunted children and to recommend appropriate nutritional interventions to promote growth but not excess fat deposition. Cross-sectional studies are thus required to establish whether the prevalence of overweight and obesity is increasing in South Africa, and whether there is any link with stunting. Longitudinal and intervention studies are required to establish the trajectory of any possible nutrition transition in terms of geography, culture and socio-economic status, in order to identify and control risk factors and assess the differential impact of stunting and overweight on children. We agree with the limitations identified by other researchers, who recognize that the majority of research into stunting and obesity in children is cross-sectional and thus does not follow the same children through childhood and adolescence. Changes in growth and body composition over time can, thus, only be inferred through implication and not measured within the same children. Consequently, it is imperative that increasing amounts of longitudinal studies needs to be conducted in the future, to elucidate the effects of early growth on body composition in mid- to late childhood (see [90] and [91]).

6 Appendices

In this section, we provide an appendix that includes abbreviations of important terms used in our study. Also, another appendix highlighting important information from investigations discussing childhood obesity, overweight and stunting in South Africa is given.

6.1 Appendix A: Abbreviations of Terms Related to Childhood Obesity, Overweight and Stunting

Obesity Term	Abbreviation
Black Boy:	BB
Black Children:	BC
Black Girl:	BG
Body Mass Index:	BMI
Commercial Farm Children:	CFC
Confidence Interval:	CI
Height-for-Age z-score:	HAZ
Homeostasis Model Assessment:	HOMA
Indian Boy:	IB
Indian Girl:	IG
Medical Research Council:	MRC
Mixed Ancestory Boy:	MAB
Mixed Ancestory Children:	MAC
Mixed Ancestory Girl:	MAG
National Food Consumption Survey:	NFCS
National Health and Nutrition Examination Survey:	NHANES
National Heart, Lung and Blood Institute Growth and Health Study Research Group:	NHLBIGHSRG
Non-Communicable Disease:	NCD
Nutritional Status:	NS
Odds Ratio:	OR
Overfatness:	OF
Primary Health Care:	PHC
Respiratory Quotient:	RQ
Resting Energy Expenditure:	REE
Rural Boy:	RB
Rural Children:	RC
Rural Girl:	RG
Small for Gestational Age:	SGA
Socioeconomic Status:	SES
South Africa Demographic and Health Survey:	SADHS
South African Heart Foundation:	SAHF
South African Heart Foundations Community Childrens Programme:	SAHFCCP
Standard Deviation:	SD
Subscapular Skinfolds:	SSF
Tribal Children:	TC
Tricep Skinfolds:	TSF
United Nations International Children's Education Fund:	UNICEF
Urban Children:	UC
Waist Circumference:	WC
Weight-for-Age z-score:	WAZ
White Boy:	WB
White Girl:	WG
World Health Organization:	WHO

Figure 1: Abbreviations of Terms Related to Childhood Obesity, Overweight and Stunting

6.2 Appendix B: Summary of Information from Studies about Childhood Obesity, Overweight and Stunting in South Africa

Ref.	NS	Age (yrs)	Community	Provincial	National
[21]	% Obesity	3-6	20.1	–	–
[81]	% Obesity	4-5 & 8-11 4-11	1-10 0.9 (girls)	– –	– –
[102]	% Obesity	3	24 (BC)	–	–
[173]	% Obesity	1-9	–	–	3.7
[81]	% Overweight	4-5 & 8-11 4-11	5-24 1.4 (girls)	– –	– –
[102]	% Overweight	3	22 (BC)	–	–
[112]	% Overweight	3-4 3-10	15 (RBs OF) 0-2.5 (boys) 0-4.3 (girls)	– – –	– – –
[113]	% Overweight	10-15	– – – –	14.2 (WGs) 7.1 (BGs) 6.4 (IGs) 2.9 (MAGs)	– – – –
[173]	% Overweight	1-9	–	–	6.7
[149]	% Overweight or Obesity	≥ 15	–	–	56.6 girls
[173]	% Overweight & Obesity	1-9	–	–	10.4
[21]	% Stunting	3-6	27.6	–	–
[26]	% Stunting	≤ 2	–	–	20 (UC)
[81]	% Stunting	4-5 & 8-11	10-25	–	–
[90] & [91]	% Stunting	1-9	–	–	21.6
[102]	% Stunting	3	48 (BC)	–	–
[113]	% Stunting	10-15 10-15 10-15 10-15	– – – –	26.7 (RB) 23.7 (RG) 17.1 (UB) 11.6 (UG)	– – – –
[142]	% Stunting	3-6 & 7-9	–	–	30.6 (BC+MAC)
[173]	% Stunting	1-9 1-3 1-3 1-3 1-3	– – – – –	– – – – –	19.3 24.4 23.8 (RC) 25.6 (CFC) 30.6 (CFC+TC+RC)
[102]	% Stunting & Obesity	3	19 (BC)	–	–

Figure 2: Summary of Information from Studies about Childhood Obesity, Overweight and Stunting in South Africa

References

[1] Adhikari, M; Coovadia, HM. Mid-upper arm circumference in the assessment of growth retardation. *South African Medical Journal*, 1981 59, 2.

[2] Amigo, H; Bustos, P; Leone, C; Radrigan, ME. Growth deficits in Chilean school children. *American Society for Nutritional Sciences*, 2000 1, 251-254.

[3] Aristimuno, GG; Foster, TA; Voors, AW; Srinivasan, SR; Berenson, GS. Influence of persistent obesity in children on cardiovascular risk factors. *Circulation*, 1984 69, 895-904.

[4] Asayama, K; Hayashi, K; Hayashibe, H; Uchida, N; Kodera, K; Nakazawa, S. Relationships between an index of body fat distribution (based on waist and hip circumferences) and stature and biochemical complications in obese children. *International Journal of Obesity and Related Metabolic Disorders*, 1988 22, 1209-1216.

[5] Asayama, K; Hayashibe, H; Dobashi, K; Uchida, N; Kawada, Y; Nakazawa, S. Relationships between biochemical abnormalities and anthropometric indices of overweight, adiposity and body fat distribution in Japanese elementary school children. *International Journal of Obesity and Related Metabolic Disorders*, 1995 19, 253-259.

[6] Asayama, K; Oguni, T; Hayashi, K; Dobashi, K; Fukunaga, Y; Kodera, K; Tamai, H; Nakazawa, S. Critical value for the index of body fat distribution based on waist and hip circumference and stature in obese girls. *International Journal of Obesity and Related Metabolic Disorders*, 2000 24, 1026-1031.

[7] Ashworth, A. Growth rates in children recovering from protein-calorie malnutrition. *British Journal of Nutrition*, 1969 23, 835-845.

[8] Barac-Nicto, M. *Body composition and physical work capacity in undernutrition.* In: White PL, Selvey N, eds. Malnutrition: determinants and consequences. New York: Alan R. Liss; 1984; 165-168.

[9] Barker, DJP. *Fetal and Infant Origins of Adult Disease*. London: British Medical Journal Publishing Group; 1992.

[10] Barsh, GS; Farooqi, IS; OReilly, S. Genetics of body-weight regulation. *Nature*, 2000 404, 644-651.

[11] Bellamy, C. *The state of the world's children 2000*. UNICEF p.71 and Tables 1 and 2.

[12] Bell, AC; Ge, K; Popkin, BM. The road to obesity or the path to prevention ? Motorized transportation and obesity in China. *Obesity Research*, 2002 10, 277-283.

[13] Benefice, E; Garnier, D; Simondon, KB; Malina, RM. Relationship between stunting in infancy and growth and fat distribution during adolescence in Senegalese girls. *European Journal of Clinical Nutrition*, 2001 55, 50-58.

[14] Berenson, GS; Srinivasan, SR; Bao, W; Newman, WP; Tracy, RE; Wattigney, WA. Association between multiple cardiovascular risk factors and atherosclerosis in children and young adults. The Bogalusa Heart Study. *New England Journal of Medicine*, 1998 338, 1650-1656.

[15] Berenson, GS; Srinivasan, SR; Wattigney, WA; Harsha, DW. Obesity and cardiovascular risk in children. *Annals of the New York Academy of Sciences*, 1993 699, 93-103.

[16] Berkman, DS; Lescano, AG; Gilman, RH; Lopez, SL; Black, MM. Effects of stunting, diarrhoeal disease and parasitic infection during infancy on cognition in late childhood: a follow-up study. *Lancet*, 2002 359, 564-571.

[17] Bini, V; Celi, F; Bertioli, MG; Bacosi, ML; Stella, P; Giglio, P; Tosti, L; Falorn, A. Body mass index in children and adolescents according to age and pubertal stage. *European Journal of Clinical Nutrition*, 2000 54, 214-218.

[18] Bonjour, JP; Carrie, AL; Ferrari, S; Clavien, H; Slosman, D; Theintz, G; Rizzoli, R. Calcium-enriched foods and bone mass growth in prepubertal girls: a randomized, double-blind, placebo-controlled trial. *Journal of Clinical Investigations*, 1997 99(6), 1287-1294.

[19] Booth, ML; Macaskill, P; Lazarus, R; Baur, LA. Sociodemographic distribution of measures of body fatness among children and adolescents in New South Wales, Australia. *International Journal of Obesity and Related Metabolic Disorders*, 1999 23, 456-462.

[20] Bourne, LT; Lambert, EV; Steyn, K. Where does the black population of South Africa stand on the nutrition transition ? *Public Health Nutrition*, 2001 5(1A), 157-162.

[21] Bourne, LT; Langenhoven, ML; Steyn, K; Jooste, PL; Laubscher, JA; Bourne, DE. Nutritional status of 3-6 year-old African children in the Cape Peninsula. *East African Medical Journal*, 1994 71(11), 695-702.

[22] Bray, GA; Bouchard, C; James, WPT. *Handbook of Obesity*. New York, Marcel Dekker Inc, 1998.

[23] Brownell, KD; Stunkard, AJ. *Physical activity in the development and control of obesity*. Obesity. Philadelphia: Saunders, 1999, 300-324.

[24] Budlender, D. *Human development*. In: Poverty and Inequality in South Africa: Meeting the Challenge. ed. J May Cape Town: David Philip and Zed Press, 2000, 97-140.

[25] Cameron, N. Catch-up growth increases risk factors for obesity in urban children in South Africa by one year of age. *International Journal of Obesity and Related Metabolic Disorders*, 2001 25 (Suppl 2), S48.

[26] Cameron, N; De Wet, T; Ellison, GTH; Bogin, B. Growth in height and weight of South African urban infants from birth to five years: the Birth To Ten Study. *American Journal of Human Biology*, 1998 10, 495-504.

[27] Cameron, N; Getz, B. Sex differences in the prevalence of obesity in rural African adolescents. *International Journal of Obesity and Related Metabolic Disorders*, 1997 21, 775.

[28] Cameron, N; Wright, MM; Griffiths, PL; Norris, SA; Pettifor, JM. Stunting at 2 Years in Relation to Body Composition at 9 Years in African Urban Children *Obesity Research*, 2005 13(1), 131-136.

[29] Centers for Disease Control and Prevention. *Pediatric nutrition surveillance, 1977 full report.* Atlanta: U.S. Department of Health and Human Services, 1998, 1-23.

[30] Cole, TJ; Bellizzi, MC; Flegal, KM; Dietz, WH. Establishing a standard definition for child overweight and obesity worldwide: international survey. *British Medical Journal*, 2000 320, 1240-1243.

[31] Cole, TJ; Freeman, JV; Preece, MA. Body mass index reference curves for the UK, 1990. *Archives of Disease in Childhood*, 1995 73, 25-29.

[32] Cooper, C; Kuh, D; Egger, P; Wadsworth, M; Barker D. Childhood growth and age at menarche. *British Journal of Obstetrics and Gynaecology*, 1996 103, 814-817.

[33] Crawford, D. Population strategies to prevent obesity. *British Medical Journal*, 2002 325, 728-9.

[34] Cronk, CE; Roche, AF. Race and sex-specific reference data for triceps and subscapular skinfolds and weight/stature. *American Journal of Clinical Nutrition*, 1982 35, 347-354.

[35] Crowther, NJ; Cameron, N; Trusler, J; Gray, IP. Association between poor glucose tolerance and rapid post natal weight gain in seven-year-old children. *Diabetologia*, 1998 41(10), 1163-1167.

[36] Dibley, MJ; Goldsby, JB; Staehling, NW; Trowbridge, FL. Development of normalized curves for the international growth reference: historical and technical considerations. *American Journal of Clinical Nutrition*, 1987 46, 736-748.

[37] Dietz, WH. Critical periods in childhood for the development of obesity. *American Journal of Clinical Nutrition*, 1994 59, 955-959.

[38] Dietz, WH. How to tackle the problem ? The role of education in the prevention of obesity. *International Journal of Obesity and Related Metabolic Disorders*, 1999 23(4) Supplement, S7-S9.

[39] Dietz, WH; Bellizzi, MC. Introduction: the use of body mass index to assess obesity in children. *American Journal of Clinical Nutrition*, 1999 70, 123-125.

[40] Dietz, WH; Gortmaker, SL. Do we fatten our children at the television set ? Obesity and television viewing in children and adolescents. *Pediatrics*, 1985 75, 807-812.

[41] De Onis, M; Blossner, M. Prevalence and trends of overweight among preschool children in developing countries. *American Journal of Clinical Nutrition*, 2000 72, 1032-1039.

[42] Deurenberg, P; Deurenberg-Yap, M. Differences in body-composition assumptions across ethnic groups: practical consequences. *Current Opinion in Clinical Nutrition and Metabolic Care*, 2001 4, 377-383.

[43] Deurenberg-Yap, M; Schmidt, G; van Steveren, WA; Deurenberg P. The paradox of low body mass index and high body fat percentage among Chinese, Malays and Indians in Singapore. *International Journal of Obesity and Related Metabolic Disorders*, 2000 24, 1011-1017.

[44] Deurenberg, P; Yap, M; van Staveren, WA. Body mass index and percent body fat: a meta analysis among different ethnic groups. *International Journal of Obesity and Related Metabolic Disorders*, 1998 22, 1164-1171.

[45] Dipietro, L; Mossenberg, HO; Stunkard, AJ. A 40-year history of overweight children in Stockholm: lifetime overweight, morbidity and mortality. *International Journal of Obesity and Related Metabolic Disorders*, 1994 18, 895-904.

[46] Doak, CM. Large-scale interventions and programmes addressing nutrition-related chronic diseases and obesity: examples from 14 countries. *Public Health Nutrition*, 2002 5(1A), 275-277.

[47] Doak, CM; Adair, L; Bentley, M; Fengying, Z; Popkin, B. The underweight/overweight household: an exploration of household sociodemographic and dietary factors in China. *Public Health Nutrition*, 2002 5, 215221.

[48] Doak, CM; Adair, LS; Bentley, M; Montiero, C; Popkin, BM. The dual burden household and the nutrition transition paradox. *International Journal of Obesity and Related Metabolic Disorders*, 2005 29, 129-136.

[49] Doak, CM; Adair, LS; Montiero, C; Popkin, BM. Overweight and underweight coexist within households in Brazil, China and Russia. *Journal of Nutrition*, 2000 130, 2965-2971.

[50] Doak, CM; Montiero, C; Adair, LS; Bentley, ME; Popkin, BM. Coexisting overweight and underweight within households is related to the nutrition transition. *Federation of American Societies for Experimental Biology (FASEB)*, 2000 14, A792.

[51] Eckhardt, CL; Adair, LS; Caballero, B; Avila, J; Kon, IY; Wang, J; Popkin, BM. Estimating Body Fat from Anthropometry and Isotopic Dilution: A Four-Country Comparison. *Obesity Research*, 2003 11(12), 1553-1562.

[52] Fjeld, CR; Schoeller, DA; Brown, KH. Body composition of children recovering from severe protein-energy malnutrition at two rates of catch-up growth. *American Journal of Clinical Nutrition*, 1989 50, 1266-1275.

[53] Flegal, KM. The obesity epidemic in children and adults: current evidence and research issues. *Medical Science and Sports Exercise*, 1999 31 (Suppl 11), S509-S514.

[54] Flegal, KM; Carroll, MD; Kuczmarski, RJ; Johnson, CL. Overweight and obesity in the United States: prevalence and trends. *International Journal of Obesity and Related Metabolic Disorders*, 1998 22, 39-47.

[55] Florencio, TM; Ferreira, HS; de Franca, AP; Cavalcante, JC; Sawaya, AL. Obesity and undernutrition in a very-low-income population in the city of Maceio, Northeastern Brazil. *Brazil Journal of Nutrition*, 2001 86, 277-284.

[56] Fogel, R. Economic growth, population theory and physiology: the bearing of long-term processes on the making of economic policy. *American Economic Review*, 1994 84, 369-395.

[57] Fogel, R. Health, nutrition and economic growth. *Economic Development and Cultural Change*, 2004 52, 643-660.

[58] French, SA; Story, M; Perry, CL. Self-esteem and obesity in children and adolescents: a literature review. *Obesity Research*, 1995 3, 479-490.

[59] Freedman, DS; Serdula, MK; Srinivasan, SR; Berenson, GS. Relation of circumferences and skinfold thicknesses to lipid and insulin concentrations in children and adolescents: The Bogalusa Heart Study. *American Journal of Clinical Nutrition*, 1999 69, 308–317.

[60] Freedman, DS; Srinivasan, SR; Webber, LS; Burke, GL; Berenson, GS. Black-white differences in serum lipoproteins during sexual maturation: The Bogalusa Heart Study. *Journal of Chronic Diseases*, 1987 40, 309-318.

[61] Frongillo, EA. Symposium: Causes and etiology of stunting. *Journal of Nutrition*, 1999 129(2), S529-S530.

[62] Gallagher, D; Heymsfield, SB; Heo, M; Jebb, SA; Murgatroyd, PR; Sakamoto, Y. Health percentage body fat ranges: an approach for developing guidelines based on body mass index. *American Journal of Clinical Nutrition*, 2000 71, 694-701.

[63] Garn, SM; Bailey, SM; Solomon, MA; Hopkins, PJ. Effect of remaining family members on fatness prediction. *American Journal of Clinical Nutrition*, 1981 34, 148-153.

[64] Garn, SM; Haskell, JA. Fat and growth during childhood. *Science*, 1959 130, 1711-1712.

[65] Garn, SM; Sullivan, TV; Hawthorne, VM. Fatness and obesity of parents of obese individuals. *American Journal of Clinical Nutrition*, 1989 56, 1308-1313.

[66] Garrett, J; Ruel, M. Stunted child-overweight mother pairs: an emerging policy concern ? 17th International Congress of Nutrition. *Annals of Nutrition Metabolism*, 2001 45(1), S404.

[67] Garrow, JS. *Health implications of obesity*. In: Obesity and related diseases. London: Churchill Livingstone, 1988, 1-16.

[68] Ghassemi, H; Harrison, G; Mohammad, K. An accelerated nutrition transition in Iran. *Public Health Nutrition*, 2002 5, 1149-1156.

[69] Griffiths, M; Payne, PR; Stunkard, AJ; Rivers, JPW; Cox, M. Metabolic rate and physical development in children at risk of obesity. *Lancet*, 1990 336, 76.

[70] Grundy, SM. Metabolic complications of obesity. *Endocrine Journal*, 2000 13, 155-165.

[71] Guo, SS; Chumlea, WC. Tracking of body mass index in children in relation to overweight in adulthood. *American Journal of Clinical Nutrition*, 1999 70, S145-S148.

[72] Guo, SS; Huang, C; Maynard, LM; Demerath, E; Towne, B; Chumlea, WC; Siervogel, RM. Body mass index during childhood, adolescence and young adulthood in relation to adult overweight and adiposity: the Fels Longitudinal Study. *International Journal of Obesity and Related Metabolic Disorders*, 2000 24, 1628-1635.

[73] Harris, NS; Crawford, PB; Yangzom, Y; Pinzo, L; Gylatsen, P; Hudes, M. Nutritional and health status of Tibetan children living at high altitudes. *New England Journal of Medicine*, 2001 344(5), 341–347.

[74] Heymsfield, SB; McManus, C; Stevens, V; Smith J. Muscle mass; reliable indicator of protein energy malnutrition severity and outcome. *American Journal of Clinical Nutrition*, 2000 35, 1192-1199.

[75] Himes, JH; Dietz, WH. Guidelines for overweight in adolescent preventive services: recommendations from an expert committee. *American Journal of Clinical Nutrition*, 1994 59, 307-316.

[76] Hoffman, DJ; Roberts, SB; Verreschi, I; Martins, PA; de Nascimento, C; Tucker, KL; Sawaya, AL. Regulation of energy intake may be impaired in nutritionally stunted children from the shantytowns of Sao Paulo, Brazil. *Journal of Nutrition*, 2000 130, 2265-2270.

[77] Hoffman, DJ; Sawaya, AL; Verreschui, I; Tucker, KL; Roberts, SB. Why are nutritionally stunted children at increased risk of obesity ? Studies of metabolic rate of fat oxidation in shantytown children from Sao Paulo, Brazil. *American Journal of Clinical Nutrition*, 2000 72, 702-707.

[78] Hoffman, DJ; Sawaya, AL; Coward, WA; Wright, A; Martins, PA; De Nascimento, C; Tucker, KL; Roberts, SB. Energy expenditure of stunted and nonstunted boys and girls living in the shantytowns of Sao Paulo, Brazil. *American Journal of Clinical Nutrition*, 2000 72, 1025-1031.

[79] James, PT; Leach, R; Kalamara, E; Shayeghi, M. The worldwide obesity epidemic. *Obesity Research*, 2001 9 (Suppl 4), 228S-33.

[80] Jinabhai, CC; Taylor, M; Sullivan, KR. Implications of the prevalence of stunting, overweight and obesity amongst South African primary school children: a possible nutritional transition ? *European Journal of Clinical Nutrition*, 2003 57, 358-365.

[81] Jinabhai, CC; Taylor, M; Sullivan, KR. Changing patterns of under- and over-nutrition in South African children-future risks of non-communicable diseases. *Annals of Tropical Paediatrics*, 2005 25(1), 3-15.

[82] Kain, J; Vio, F; Albala, C. Obesity trends and determinant factors in Latin America. *Cadernos de Saude Publica*, 2003 19(1), S77-S86.

[83] Kikafunda, JK; Walker, AF; Collett, D; Tumwine, JK. Risk factors for early childhood malnutrition in Uganda. *Pediatrics*, 1998 102, E45.

[84] Kim, S; Moon, S; Popkin, BM. The nutrition transition in South Korea. *American Journal of Clinical Nutrition*, 2000 71, 44–53.

[85] Ko, GT; Tang, J; Chan, JC; Sung, R; Wu, MM; Wai, HP; Chen, R. Lower BMI cut-off value to define obesity in Hong Kong Chinese: an analysis based on body fat assessment by bioelectrical impedence. *British Journal of Nutrition*, 2001 85, 239-242.

[86] Kosulwat, V. The nutrition and health transition in Thailand. *Public Health Nutrition*, 2002 5, 183-190.

[87] Kriska, AM; Delahanty, LM; Pettee, KK. Lifestyle intervention for the prevention of type 2 diabetes: translation and future recommendation. *Current Diabetes Reports*, 2004 4, 113-118.

[88] Kruger, HS; Margetts, BM; Vorster, HH. Evidence for relatively greater subcutaneous fat deposition in stunted girls in the North West Province, South Africa, as compared with non-stunted girls. *Nutrition*, 2004 20(6), 564-569.

[89] Kuczmarski, RJ; Flegal, KM; Campbell, SM; Johnson, CL. Increasing prevalence of overweight among US adults: The National Health and Nutrition Examination Surveys, 1960 to 1991. *Journal of the American Medical Association*, 1994 274, 205-211.

[90] Labadarios, D; Maunder, E; Steyn, N; MacIntyre, U; Swart, R; Gericke, G; Nesamvuni, E; Huskisson, J; Vorster, HH; Dannhauser, A. National food consumption survey in children aged 1-9 years: South Africa 1999. *Forum Nutrition*, 2003 56, 106-109.

[91] Labadarios, D (editor); Steyn, NP; Maunder, E; MacIntyre, U; Swart, R; Gericke, G; Huskisson, J; Dannhauser, A; Vorster, HH; Nesamvuni, AE. The National Food Consumption Survey (NFCS): South Africa, 1999. *Public Health Nutrition*, 2005 8(5), 533-543.

[92] Lake, JK; Power, C; Cole, TJ. Child to adult body mass index in the 1958 British Birth cohort: associations with parental obesity. *Archives of Disease in Childhood*, 1997 77, 376-378.

[93] Law, CM; Shiell, AW; Newsome, CA; Syddall, HE; Shinebourne, EA; Fayers, PM; Martyn, CN; de Swiet, M. Fetal, infant, and childhood growth and adult blood pressure: a longitudinal study from birth to 22 years of age. *Circulation*, 2002 105, 1088-1092.

[94] Lawless, JW; Latham, MC; Stephenson, LS; Kinoti, SN; Pertet, AM. Iron supplementation improves appetite and growth in anaemic Kenyan primary school children. *Journal of Nutrition*, 1994 124(5), 645-654.

[95] Lebowitz, SF. Neurochemical-neuroendocrine systems in the brain controlling macronutrient intake and metabolism. *Trends in Neurosciences*, 1992 15, 491-497.

[96] Lloyd, JK; Wolff, MA; Whelen, WS. Childhood obesity: A long-term study of height and weight. *British Medical Journal*, 1961 77(5), 145-148.

[97] Locard, E; Mamelle, N; Billette, A; Miginiac, M; Munoz, F; Rey, S. Risk factors of obesity in a five year-old population. Parental versus environmental factors. *International Journal of Obesity and Related Metabolic Disorders*, 1994 16, 721-729.

[98] Lohman, TG. The use of skinfolds to estimate body fatness on children and youth. *Journal of Physical Education, Recreation and Dance*, 1987 58(9), 98-102, EJ 364 412.

[99] Loveridge, N; Noble, BS. Control of longitudinal growth: the role of nutrition. *European Journal of Clinical Nutrition*, 1994 48, 75-84.

[100] Lustig, RH. The neuroendocrinology of obesity. *Endocrinology and Metabolic Clinics of North America*, 2001 30, 765-785.

[101] Mahoney, LT; Burns, TL; Stanford, W. Coronary risk factors measured in childhood and young adult life are associated with coronary artery calcification in young adults: the Muscatine Study. *Journal of the American College of Cardiology*, 1996 27, 277-284.

[102] Mamabolo, RL; Alberts, M; Steyn, NP; Delemarre-van de Waal, HA; Levitt, NS. Prevalence and determinants of stunting and overweight in 3-year-old black South African children residing in the Central Region of Limpopo Province, South Africa. *Public Health Nutrition*, 2005 8(5), 501-508.

[103] Martorell, R. The role of nutrition in economic development. *Nutrition Reviews*, 1996 54, Supplement: 66S-71S.

[104] Martorell, R; Khan, LK; Schroeder, DG. Reversibility of stunting: epidemiological finding in children from developing countries. *European Journal of Clinical Nutrition*, 1994 48(1), S45-S57.

[105] May, J (ed.) *Poverty and Inequality in South Africa: Meeting the Challenge*. London: David Philip and Zed Press, 2000.

[106] Melanson, KJ; McInnis, KJ; Rippe, JM; Blackburn, G; Wilson, PF. Obesity and cardiovascular disease risk: Research update. *Cardiology Reviews*, 2001 9, 202-207.

[107] Mendez, MA; Adair, LS. Severity and timing of stunting in the first two years of life affect performance on cognitive tests in late childhood. *Journal of Nutrition*, 1999 129, 1555-1562.

[108] Mills, JL; Shiono, PH; Shapiro, LR; Crawford, PB; Rhoads, GG. Early growth predicts timing of puberty in boys: results of a 14-year nutrition and growth study. *Journal of Pediatrics*, 1986 109, 543-547.

[109] Montiero, CA; Conde, WL; Popkin, BM. Is obesity replacing or adding to undernutrition ? Evidence from different social classes in Brazil. *Public Health Nutrition*, 2002 5, 105-112.

[110] Montiero, CA; Mondini, L; Medeiros de Souza, AL; Popkin, BM. The nutrition transition in Brazil. *European Journal of Clinical Nutrition*, 1995 49, 105–113.

[111] Mo-Suwan, L; Lebel, L; Puetpaiboon, A; Junjana, C. School performance and weight status of children and young adolescents in a transitional society in Thailand. *International Journal of Obesity and Related Metabolic Disorders*, 1999 23, 272-277.

[112] Monyeki, KD; van Lenthe, FJ; Steyn, NP. Obesity: does it occur in African children in a rural community in South Africa. *International Journal of Epidemiology*, 1999 28(2), 287-292.

[113] Mukuddem-Petersen, J; Kruger, HS. The association between obesity and stunting among 10 to 15 year-old children in the North-West Province. *International Journal of Obesity and Related Metabolic Disorders*, 2004 28, 842-851.

[114] Mukuddem-Petersen, J; Oosthuizen, W; Jerling, JC. A systematic review of the effects of nuts on blood lipid profiles in humans. *Journal of Nutrition*, 2005 135, 2082-2089.

[115] Musaiger, AO; Gregory, WB. Profile of body composition of school children (6-18 years) in Bahrain. *International Journal of Obesity and Related Metabolic Disorders*, 2000 24, 1093–1096.

[116] Must, A; Dallal, GE; Dietz, WH. Reference data for obesity: 85th and 95th percentiles of body mass index (wt/ht^2) and triceps skinfold thickness. *American Journal of Clinical Nutrition*, 1991 53, 839-846.

[117] Must, A; Jacques, PF; Dallal, GE; Bajema, CJ; Dietz, WH. Long-term morbidity and mortality of overweight adolescents. A follow-up of the Harvard growth study of 1922 to 1935. *New England Journal of Medicine*, 1992 327, 1350-1355.

[118] National Heart, Lung and Blood Institute Growth and Health Study Research Group. Obesity and cardiovascular disease risk factors in black and white girls; the NHLBI growth and health study. *American Journal of Public Health*, 1992 82(12), 1613-1620.

[119] Nakamura, T; Nishiyama, S; Futagoishi Suginohara, Y; Matsuda, I; Higashi, A. Mild to moderate zinc deficiency in short children: effect of zinc supplementation on linear growth velocity. *Journal of Pediatrics*, 1994 124(1), 163-164.

[120] Noel, PH; Pugh, JA. Management of overweight and obese adults. *British Medical Journal*, 2002 325, 757-61.

[121] Norgan, NG. Changes in patterns of growth and nutritional anthropometry in two rural modernizing Papua New Guinea communities. *Annals of Human Biology*, 1995 22, 491-513.

[122] Norgan, NG. Long-term physiological and economic consequences of growth retardation in children and adolescents. *Proceedings of the Nutrition Society*, 2000 59, 245-256.

[123] O'Dea, J; Abrahams, S. Should body mass index be used in young adolescents ? *Lancet*, 1995 345, 657.

[124] Olshansky, SJ; Ault, AB. The fourth stage of the epidemiologic transition: the age of delayed degenerative diseases. *Milbank Memorial Fund Quarterly*, 1986 64, 355–391.

[125] Omran, AR. The epidemiologic transition: a theory of the epidemiology of population change. *Milbank Memorial Fund Quarterly*, 1971 49, 509–538.

[126] Ong, KKL; Ahmed, ML; Emmett, PM; Preece, MA; Dunger, DB. The ALSPAC Study Team (2000). Association between postnatal catch-up growth and obesity in childhood: prospective cohort study. *British Medical Journal*, 2000 320, 967-971.

[127] Ong, KKL; Kratzsch, J; Kiess, W; Dunger, D. The ALSPAC Study Team (2002). Circulating IGF-I levels in childhood are related to both current body composition and early postnatal growth rate. *Journal of Clinical Endocrinology and Metabolism*, 2002 87, 1041-1044.

[128] Penland, JG; Sandstead, HH; Alcock, NW; Dayal, HH; Chen, XC; Li, JS; Zhao, F; Yang, JJ. A preliminary report: effects of zinc and micronutrient repletion on growth and neuropsychological function of urban Chinese children. *Journal of American Colloquial Nutrition*, 1997 16(3), 268-272.

[129] Perusse, L; Bouchard, C. Role of genetic factors in childhood obesity an in susceptibility to dietary variations. *Annals of Medicine*, 1999 31, 19-25.

[130] Perusse, L; Rankinen, T; Zuberi, A; Chagnon, YC; Weisnagel, SJ; Argyropoulos, G; Walts, B; Snyder, EE; Bouchard, C. The human obesity gene map: the 2004 update. *Obesity Research*, 2005 13(3), 381-490.

[131] Pieters, M; Oosthuizen, W; Jerling, JC; Loots, du T; Mukuddem-Petersen, J; Hanekom, SM. Clustering of haemostatic variables and the effect of high cashew and walnut diets on these variables in metabolic syndrome patients. *Blood Coagulation and Fibrinolysis*, 2005 16(6), 429-437.

[132] Popkin, BM. The nutrition transition and its health implications in lower income countries. *Public Health Nutrition*, 1986 1, 5–21.

[133] Popkin, BM. The nutrition transition in low-income countries: an emerging crisis. *Nutrition Reviews*, 1994 52, 285–298.

[134] Popkin, BM. Urbanization, lifestyle changes and the nutrition transition. *World Development*, 1999 27, 1905-1916.

[135] Popkin, BM. The nutrition transition and obesity in the developing world. *Journal of Nutrition*, 2001 131, S871-S873.

[136] Popkin, BM. An overview on the nutrition transition and its health implications: the Bellagio meeting. *Public Health Nutrition*, 2002 5, 93-103.

[137] Popkin, BM. The shift in stages of the nutrition transition in the developing world differs from past experiences. *Public Health Nutrition*, 2002 5, 205-214.

[138] Popkin, BM; Bisgrove, ES. Urbanization and nutrition in low-income countries. *Food Nutrition Bulletin*, 1998 10, 3-23.

[139] Popkin, BM; Doak, CM. The obesity epidemic is a worldwide phenomenon. *Nutrition Reviews*, 1998 56(4), 106-114.

[140] Popkin, BM; Gordon-Larsen, P. The nutrition transition: worldwide obesity dynamics and their determinants. *International Journal of Obesity and Related Metabolic Disorders*, 2004 **28** Suppl 3, S2-9.

[141] Popkin, BM; Paeratakul, S; Zhai, F; Ge, K. A review of dietary and environmental correlates of obesity with emphasis on developing countries. *Obesity Research*, 1995 3, S145.

[142] Popkin, BM; Richards, MK; Montiero, CA. Stunting is associated with overweight in children of four nations that are undergoing the nutrition transition. *Journal of Nutrition*, 1996 126, 3009-3016.

[143] Power, C; Lake, JK; Cole, TJ. Measurement and long-term health risks of child and adolescent fatness. *International Journal of Obesity and Related Metabolic Disorders*, 1997 21, 507-526.

[144] Power, C; Moynihan, C. Measurement and long-term health risks of child and adolescent fatness. *International Journal of Obesity and Related Metabolic Disorders*, 1998 22, 445-453.

[145] Prader, A; Tanner, JM; Von Harnack, GA. Catch-up growth following illness or starvation. *Journal of Paediatrics*, 1963 62, 646-659.

[146] Prasad, AS. Zinc deficiency in women, infants and children. *Journal of American Colloquial Nutrition*, 1996 15(2), 113-120.

[147] Prentice, AM; Jebb, SA. Obesity in Britain; gluttony or sloth ? *British Medical Journal*, 1995 311, 437-439.

[148] Pretoria Stats South Africa. *Living in North West*. Selected findings of the 1995 October household survey. Statistics South Africa: Pretoria; 1997. 7.

[149] Puoane, T; Steyn, K; Bradshaw, D; Laubscher, R; Fourie, J; Lambert, V; Mbananga, N. Obesity in South Africa: the South African demographic and health survey. *Obesity Research*, 2002 10, 1038-1048.

[150] Regional Office for the Western Pacific of the World Health Organization. *The Asia-Pacific perspective: Redefining obesity and its treatment*. The International Association for the Study of Obesity and the International Obesity Task Force. Health Communications, Australia Pty Limited, Sydney, Australia, 2000, 1–56.

[151] Reilly, JJ; Dorosty, AR; Emmett, P. Identification of the obese child: adequacy of the body mass index for clinical practice and epidemiology. *International Journal of Obesity and Related Metabolic Disorders*, 2000 24, 1623-1627.

[152] Rivera, JA; Barquera, S; Campirano, F; Campos, I; Safdie, M; Tovar, V. Epidemiological and nutritional transition in Mexico: rapid increase of non-communicable diseases and obesity. *Public Health Nutrition*, 2002 5, 113-122.

[153] Roche, AF; Siervogel, RM; Chumlea, C; Webb, P. Grading of body fatness from limited anthropometric data. *American Journal of Clinical Nutrition*, 1981 34, 2831-2838.

[154] Ross, J; Chen, CM; He, W; Fu, G; Wang, YY; Fu, ZY; Chen, MX. Effects of malnutrition on economic productivity in China as estimated by PROFILES. *Biomedical and Environmental Science*, 2003 16, 195-205.

[155] Rossow, I; Rise, J. Concordance of parental and adolescent health behaviours. *Social Science Medicine*, 1994 38, 1299-1305.

[156] Satyanarayanna, K; Radihaih, G; Murali-Mohan, R; Thimmayamma, BVS; Pralhad, RN; Narasinga, RBS. The adolescent growth spurt of height among rural Indian boys in relation to childhood nutritional background: an 18 year longitudinal study. *Annals of Human Biology*, 1989 16, 289-300.

[157] Sawaya, AL; Roberts, S. Stunting and future risk of obesity: principal physiological mechanisms. *Cadernos de Saude Publica*, 2003 19(1), S21-S22.

[158] Schroeder, DG; Martorell, R; Flores, R. Infant and child growth and fatness and fat distribution in Guatemalan adults. *American Journal of Epidemiology*, 1999 149, 177-185.

[159] Scrimshaw, NS. The challenge of global malnutrition to the food industry. *Food Technology*, 1993, 60-71.

[160] Sawaya, AL; Dallal, G; Solymos, G. Obesity and malnutrition in a shantytown population in the city of Sao Paulo, Brazil. *Obesity Research*, 1995 3 (Supplement), S107–S115.

[161] Sawaya, AL; Grillo, LP; Verreschi, I; Carlos Da Silva, A; Roberts, SB. Mild stunting is associated with higher susceptibility to the effects of high-fat diets; studies in a shantytown population in the city of Sao Paulo, Brazil. *Journal of Nutrition*, 1998 128 (Supplement), S415–S420.

[162] Schutte, AE; Van Rooyen, JM; Huisman, HW; Mukuddem-Petersen, J; Oosthuizen, W; Hanekom, SM; Jerling, JC. Modulation of baroreflex sensitivity by walnuts versus cashew nuts in metabolic syndrome subjects. *American Journal of Hypertension*, 2006, to appear.

[163] Seidell, JC; Cigolini, M; Deslypere, JP; Charzewska, K; Ellsinger, BM; Cruz, A. Body fat distribution in relation to physical activity and smoking habits in 38 year-old European men. *American Journal of Epidemiology*, 1991 133, 257-265.

[164] Seidell, JC. Obesity: a growing problem. *Acta Paediatrica*, 1999 88, 46-50.

[165] Seidell, JC. Obesity, insulin resistance and diabetes: a worldwide epidemic. *British Journal of Nutrition*, 2000 83 (Suppl 1), S5-S8.

[166] Serdula, MK; Ivery, D; Coates, RJ; Freedman, DS; Williamson, DF; Byers, T. Do obese children become obese adults ? A review of the literature. *Preventative Medicine*, 1993 22, 167-177.

[167] Stark, O; Peckham, CS; Moynihan, C. Weight and age at menarche. *Archives of Diseases in Childhood*, 1989 64, 383-387.

[168] Statistics South Africa. *Stats in brief 2000*. Department of Statistics, Pretoria; 2000.

[169] Stephens, T; Jacobs, DR; White, CC. A descriptive epidemiology of leisure time physical activity. *Public Health Report*, 1985 100, 147-158.

[170] Steyn, K; Bourne, L; Jooste, P; Fourie, JM; Rossouw, K; Lombard, C. Anthropometric profile of a black population of the Cape Peninsula in South Africa. *East African Medical Journal*, 1998 75, 35-40.

[171] Steyn, NP; Senekal, M; Brits, S; Alberts, M; Mashego, T; Nel, JH. Weight and health status of black female students. *South African Medical Journal*, 2000 90, 146-152.

[172] Steyn, NP; Senekal, M; Brits, S; Nel, JH. Urban and rural differences in dietary intake, weight status and nutrition knowledge of black female students. *Asia-Pacific Journal of Clinical Nutrition*, 2000 9, 53-59.

[173] Steyn, NP; Labadarios, D; Maunder, E; Nel, J; Lombard, C. Secondary anthropometric data analysis of the National Food Consumption Survey in South Africa: double burden. *Nutrition*, 2005 21, 4-13.

[174] Steyn, NP; Wicht, CL; Rossouw, JE; Van Wyk Kotze, TJ; Van Eck, M. Nutritional status of 11-year-old children in the Western Cape II. Anthropometry. *South African Journal of Food Science Nutrition*, 1989 1, 21-27.

[175] Tanner, JM. Growth and maturation during adolescence. *Nutrition Reviews*, 1981 39, 43-55.

[176] Tanner, JM. *Growth as a target-seeking function: catch-up and catch-down growth in man*. Falkner, F eds. *Human Growth: A Comprehensive Treatise*, Plenum New York, 1986, 167-179.

[177] Tanner, JM. Growth from birth to two: a critical review. *Acta Med Auxol (Milano)*, 1994 26, 7-45.

[178] Tomkins, A. Malnutrition, morbidity and mortality in children and their mothers. *Proceedings of Nutrition Society*, 2000 59, 135-146.

[179] Torun, B; Viteri, FE. Influence of exercise on linear growth. *European Journal of Clinical Nutrition*, 1994 48(1) Supplement, S186-S190.

[180] Tremblay, A; Despres, J-P; Le Blanc, C; Craig, CL; Ferris, B; Stephens, T; Bouchard, C. Effect of intensity of physical activity on body fatness and fat distribution. *American Journal of Clinical Nutrition*, 1990 51, 153-157.

[181] Troiano, RP; Flegal, KM; Kuczmarski, RJ; Campbell, SM; Johnson, CL. Overweight prevalence and trends for children and adolescents. The National Health and Nutrition Examination Surveys, 1963 to 1991. *Archives of Pediatric Adolescent Medicine*, 1995 149, 1085-1091.

[182] Trowbridge, FL; Marks, JS; Romana, GL; Mandrid, S; Boutton, TW; Klein, PD. Body composition of Peruvian children with short stature and high weight-for-height II. Implications for the interpretation for weight-for-height as an indicator of nutritional status. *American Journal of Clinical Nutrition*, 1987 45, 513–525.

[183] Verhoef, H; West, CE; Veenemans, J; Beguin, Y; Kok, FJ. Stunting may determine the severity of malaria-associated anemia in African children. *Pediatrics*, 2002 110, e48.

[184] Villalpando, S; Lopez-Alarcon, M. Growth faltering is prevented by breastfeeding in underprivileged infants from Mexico City. *Journal of Nutrition*, 2000 130, 546-552.

[185] Vorster, HH; Wissing, MP; Venter, CS; Kruger, HS; Kruger, A; Malan, NT; de Ridder, JH; Veldman, FJ; Steyn, HS, Margetts, BM; MacIntyre, U. The impact of urbanization on physical, physiological and mental health of Africans in the North West Province of South Africa: the THUSA study. *South African Journal of Science*, 2000 96, 505.

[186] Van Lethe, FJ; Kemper, CG; van Mechelan, W. Rapid maturation in adolescence results in greater obesity in adulthood. The Amsterdam Growth and Health Study. *American Journal of Clinical Nutrition*, 1996 64, 18-24.

[187] Van Lethe, FJ; Kemper, CG; van Mechelan, W; Post, GB; Twisk, DC; Snel, J. Biological maturation and the distribution of subcutaneous fat from adolescence to adulthood: the Amsterdam Growth and Health Study. *International Journal of Obesity and Related Metabolic Disorders*, 1996 20, 121-129.

[188] Visscher, TL; Seidell, JC. The public health impact of obesity. *Annual Review of Public Health*, 2001 22, 355-375.

[189] Walker, SP; Forrester, TE; Grantham-McGregor, SM. Early linear growth retardation and later blood pressure. *European Journal of Clinical Nutrition*, 2000 54, 563-567.

[190] Walker, SP; Gaskin, P; Powell, CA; Bennett, FI; Forrester, TE; Grantham-McGregor, S. The effects of birth weight and postnatal linear growth retardation on blood pressure at age 11-12 years. *Journal of Epidemiology and Community Health*, 2001 55, 394-398.

[191] Walker, AR; Walker, BF. Weight, height and triceps skinfold in South African black, Indian and white school pupils of 18 years. *Journal of Tropical Medicine and Hygiene*, 1977 80(6), 119-125.

[192] Wang, Y; Montiero, C; Popkin, BM. Trends of overweight and underweight in children and adolescents in the United States, Brazil, China and Russia. *American Journal of Clinical Nutrition*, 2002 75, 971-977.

[193] Waterlow, JC. *Protein Energy Malnutrition*. Edward Arnold: London; 1992. 407.

[194] Waterlow, JC. Causes and mechanisms of linear growth retardation (stunting). *European Journal of Clinical Nutrition*, 1994 481, S1–S4.

[195] Whitaker, RC; Wright, JA; Pepe, MS; Seidel, KD; Dietz, WH. Predicting obesity in young adulthood from childhood and parental obesity. *New England Journal of Medicine*, 1997 337, 869-873.

[196] Wolf, AM; Gortmaker, SL; Cheung, L; Gray, H; Herzog, DB; Colditz, GA. Activity, inactivity and obesity: Racial, ethnic and age differences among schoolgirls. *American Journal of Public Health*, 1993 83(11), 1625-1627.

[197] World Cancer Research Fund (in association with the American Institute for Cancer Research). *Food, nutrition and the prevention of cancer: a global perspective 1997*. American Institute for Cancer Research, Washington, D.C.

[198] World Health Organization Expert Committee (1995). *Physical status, the use and interpretation of anthropometry*. WHO Technical Report Series No. 854, World Health Organization Geneva, Switzerland.

[199] WHO/UNICEF/ORSTOM/University of California at Davis. *Complementary feeding of young children in developing countries: a review of current scientific knowledge*. Geneva, World Health Organization, 1998 (WHO/NUT/98.1).

[200] Report of a WHO consultation. *Obesity: Preventing and managing the global epidemic*. World Health Organization: Geneva. World Health Organization Technical Report Series, 2000; 894: i-xii, 1-253.

[201] Report of a Joint WHO/FAO Expert Consultation. *Diet, nutrition and the prevention of chronic diseases.* World Health Organization: Geneva. World Health Organization Technical Report Series, 2003; 916:i-viii, 1-149.

[202] Zere, E; McIntyre, D. Inequities in under-five child malnutrition in South Africa. *International Journal of Equity Health*, 2003 11 2(1), 7.

[203] Zheng, BJ; Lo, SKF; Tam, JS. Prospective study of community-acquired rotavirus infection. *Journal of Clinical Microbiology*, 1989 27, 2083-2090.

In: Global Dimensions of Childhood Obesity
Editor: Richard K. Flamenbaum, pp. 51-68
ISBN: 1-60021-037-6

Chapter 2

CHILD OBESITY IN GLOBAL PERSPECTIVE. EMERGENT RISKS RELATED TO SOCIAL STATUS, URBANISM, AND POVERTY

***Alexandra Brewis*[a*] *and Mary C. Meyer*[b**]**

[a] School of Human Evolution and Social Change, Arizona State University, Tempe, AZ 85287-2402, USA

[b] Department of Statistics, University of Georgia, Athens, Georgia 30602, USA

Abstract

Very little is known currently about the pattern of risk for early childhood overweight and obesity in the least developed countries, where child under-nutrition remains very common and a pressing concern. We use standardized anthropometric and interview data pertaining to seventeen nationally-representative samples of 37,714 children aged between 30 and 60 months to model that risk. We particularly consider the possible roles of changing social and economic status of households and urban residence, and take into account such factors as variations in family size, in maternal nutritional status, and children's histories of under-nutrition (observed as growth stunting). The relationships among these variables are quite different across world regions except for mothers' overweight status, which was a strong predictor in all. In sub-Saharan Africa, overweight children are extremely rare and the only strong predictor is having a mother who is overweight. In Northern Africa urban residence is a risk factor. In the Americas, increasing wealth and social status of households raises risk substantially. Stunting places children in Africa, but not the Americas, at significantly increased risk of being overweight, and in northern Africa this effect is particularly pronounced in cities. We find every indication in these trends that child obesity and overweight might very quickly emerge as the modal nutritional status of children worldwide. The model suggests that childhood overweight in many ways embodies relative poverty as national wealth rises, just as child stunting reflects the conditions of absolute poverty. As economic growth accelerates in the poorer countries, the least advantaged sectors of their populations can remain absolutely poor while their relative poverty also increases. This eans that risk for childhood obesity will grow, and probably rapidly, and it will increasingly co-exist with and so be intensified by under-nutrition.

* E-mail address: alex.brewis@asu.
** E-mail address: mmeyer@stat.uga.edu

Introduction

Child overweight and obesity have been growing rapidly in the U.S. over the last several decades, and the shifts from normal to overweight are occurring at increasingly young ages (Ogden et al. 1997). According to analyses of National Health and Nutrition Examination Survey data (NHANES), by 2002 some 23 percent of children aged 2-5 years were overweight or obese (Hedley et al. 2004). The general patterns and proximal causes of these increases of early childhood overweight and obesity in the U.S. and other wealthy nations has been both a subject of mounting policy concern and increasing research attention. We know considerably less about childhood overweight and obesity (hereafter 'overweight') beyond the industrialized world: perhaps the least is known about preschool-age children in developing countries (Martorell et al. 2000) who are our focus here. The lack of research might be explained in part by the understanding that the rates of child overweight and obesity in the developing world remain comparatively low and are seemingly stable (e.g., Monteiro et al., 2004a, 2004b, Martorell 2000:966). The underlying presumption of our chapter is that this is likely to change, and soon. Especially in middle-income developing countries, and most particularly among women, adult obesity is rising extremely rapidly, at earlier levels of economic development, and a pace much greater than that observed historically in industrialized countries (Popkin 2004). If mothers are overweight, then some of the causal mechanisms that proximally underwrite child overweight risk are likely already present.

Drawing any global picture of how and why risk of early childhood obesity is distributed in the poorer developing world has also been difficult because of methodological inconsistencies in the conduct and reporting of national studies (Shetty 1999, WHO 1998, Wang 2001). Here we use very large and comparable datasets from seventeen developing countries to model where and how young children are most at risk of being overweight. We are well able to model regional and global patterns because our samples are large enough to capture a sufficient number of cases (N=1,455 overweight children, representing 3.4 percent of the total sample) and because the individual country samples we use were all collected using standardized sampling, measurement, and interview procedures, and designed to be nationally representative. The countries range from some of the poorest to lower middle income nations, and in all the risk of being underweight greatly exceeds the risk of being overweight in early childhood (see Table 1). The rates of early childhood overweight vary from less than one percent in Haiti and Ethiopia to a high of nine percent in Egypt.

In developing the model we focus on how early childhood overweight risk is patterned across countries in relation to three core proximate factors: (1) urban-rural residence, (2) the social status of households, and (3) the economic status of households. We also consider (4) whether there might be regional effects, particularly how the relationships among these other variables might be distinct in different world regions. One of the main questions we ask here is: Is the risk of child obesity in developing countries predominantly an urban phenomenon, and if so, is this mainly explained by differences in socioeconomic status of households in urban settings compared to rural? Urbanism, social status (education and occupation), and household wealth all may certainly interact in vitally important ways to explain children's obesity risk, and need to be disassociated statistically if we are to unravel the relative influence of each. For example, urbanism and household assets are highly positively associated variables, and the relationship between poverty and overweight risk may be more relative than absolute, a product of the interaction between household and broader economic conditions. The use of a very large sample combined with careful choice of the right model allows us to distinguish the effects of these, while also taking into account a variety of other potentially confounding micro-level, familial, and life history factors, such as child's gender, growth stunting of the child, breastfeeding history, number of other children in the household, and the weight status of their mothers.

The Possible Roles of Urbanism and Socio-economics in Early Childhood Overweight in Developing Countries

What do we currently know about the likely relationship between child obesity and the related processes of urbanism and socio-economic shifts in developing countries? While some localized studies in low and middle income countries have shown a positive association between urban residence and childhood obesity risk, across-country studies have not identified any clear or consistent pattern (Wang 2001). The findings are clearer for adult women, who tend to obesity in urban areas; certainly national women's obesity rates are highest in the developing countries with the highest proportion of their population in urban centers (Mendez and Popkin 2004). Children's *under*-nutritional risk is lower in cities in the developing world, and it is suggested that this is mainly a product of an overall improvement in socioeconomic conditions in urban areas relative to rural (Smith et al. 2004). While studies with U.S. samples have concluded that once you take into account such factors as ethnicity, income, and education, the urban-rural differences in adult and child obesity shrink considerably, it is unclear at this time if this is also the case for developing countries because conclusive studies are absent. It is, however, possible that - even careful control for such aspects of social and economic status (SES) - that the distinctions between the rural and urban lifeways in developing countries might be much more differentiated than they are in the U.S. (with very different food systems, food economies, and food availability, as well as educational, occupational, and cash economy constraints and opportunities (Brody 2002)) and thus might create quite different geographies of risk. Here we test both possibilities.

SES and adult obesity is conventionally understood to have a negative relationship among adults in developed countries (Ball and Crawford 2005). Children in lower SES groups in the U.S. are at increased risk of being overweight (e.g., Crooks 1995), just as is the case for adults in the U.S. and other high income countries such as Britain, Australia, and in Europe (Jebb et al. 2003, Livingstone 2000, Margery et al. 2001). The relationship between SES and obesity in developing countries, by contrast, is considered inverted, whereby the greatest risk of being overweight in poorer countries is among the relatively wealthy. This view derives substantively from a review of the studies in developing countries conducted prior to 1989 showing that in most cases higher SES was associated with greater risk of obesity (Sobal and Stunkard 1989). Notably, although the association was quite clear and robust for women, it was less consistent for men and children. Subsequently, studies have shown the advantaged sectors of developing countries can have child overweight rates that are extremely high (e.g., Brewis 2003). And, among the very poor living in subsistence conditions, the realities of food shortages and manual labor continue to make it difficult to exceed energy balance chronically in such a way as to create any real risk of being overweight (Caballero 2005).

Studies conducted at the national level have shown that national income has found to be a strong predictor of adult obesity risk. For example, in very low GNP countries low SES has been found highly protective against adult obesity (Monteiro et al 2004a, b). But, in the middle income developing countries, where wealth is increasing rapidly, the pattern appears to be shifting. Recently the burden of adult (especially women's) obesity in middle GNP countries (defined as those with above US $2500) appears to have moved into the shifted to lower SES groups, a process that appears to be accelerating as the wealth of countries increases (Popkin 2004, Monteiro et al 2004a, b).

It is important to recognize that different measures of SES, such as household assets versus educational level, can differently predict obesity risk (Ball and Crawford 2005). Many studies that consider SES-obesity relationships in developing countries use singular measures that clump social and economic variation into a single dimension, making it more difficult to interpret findings. In our analyses, we are careful to distinguish as much as possible different aspects of the social and economic status of children proximate (household) and national circumstances, allowing improved understanding of how these might influence risk. This includes a need to differentiate how absolute and relative social and economic standing relate to risk of childhood obesity. Here we model these in relation to each other across and within regional and country contexts. By absolute wealth, we mean empirical economic and social assets (such as if you have running water, electricity, permanent flooring, a television, or car, or your educational and occupational standing). By relative wealth, we mean the relativity of the household's absolute wealth to that of others in the some country and region. That is, the absolute wealth (material assets or educational levels) in a household in the poorest sector of a higher income country could match that of a household in the wealthiest sector of a very poor country, but the relative wealth of each is completely different (low in the former versus high in the latter). Based on what has been observed in adult women's patterns in developing countries, we could predict that child overweight would be linked to relative rather than absolute wealth, That is, risk of child obesity might not necessarily increase with household wealth per se., but rather as GNP rises the greater the effect of relatively lower SES should be on young children's risk of being overweight.

The Country Samples

The seventeen country samples were based on Demographic and Health Surveys (Measure DHS+) studies conducted between 1998 and 2004 in Africa and the Americas. We selected those country surveys where anthropometric (height and weight) data was available for children aged 36-60 months and for their mothers. This provided a sample of 41,343 children. (We also originally planned to include a Bangladesh dataset as a South Asian case, which qualified based on these criteria, but the rate of child overweight was so very low that there was an insufficient basis to model risk. So we removed it from the study.) We then removed any cases where data were not available for all the variables of interest, and where the mother was more than three months pregnant (because it would affect the accuracy of their body weight measures), resulting in a final sample for analysis of 37,714. The DHS+ survey procedures are designed to be identical across countries: the standardized data collection procedures, including anthropometric measurement, interview schedules, and sampling

Table 1 : Sample sizes, survey dates, and some descriptive statistics for the seventeen individual country samples.

Country	GNI in 2002	Survey Dates	Sample Size[a]	Percent Urban[b]	Percent homes with television [c]	Percent children overweight[d]	Percent children stunted[e]	Percent children underweight[e]	Percent mothers overweight[c]	Breastfeeding duration [b, f]	Percentage of mothers with no formal education[b]
NORTH AFRICA											
Egypt	1470	2000	3998	40.7	85.6	9.0	18.7	4	70.4	3.6	43.2
Morocco	1170	2003-2004	2236	43.6	56.3	4.9	18.2	10.2	44.4	2.0	50
SUB-SAHARAN AFRICA											
Benin	380	2001	1239	32.7	17.3	1.0	30.4	22.8	19.1	2.9	64.1
Burkina Faso	250	2003	3195	16.8	9.5	2.2	38.6	37.6	7.6	7.2	80.3
Ethiopia	100	2000	3440	16.2	3.3	0.3	51.2	47.1	3.8	4.2	75.2
Ghana	270	2003	1148	25.4	14.2	2.1	29.4	21.8	23.2	5	28.2
Kenya	350	2003	1696	21.9	16.8	1.4	30.6	19.8	21.2	0.9	12.7
Malawi	160	2000	3136	18	2	2.9	49	25.4	13.4	2.7	27
Nigeria	300	2003	1535	36.1	29	2.2	38.5	28.7	21.8	3.7	41.6
Uganda	240	2000-2001	1796	20.8	6.2	1.4	38.6	22.5	15.1	3.8	21.9
Zambia	340	2001-2002	1897	25.6	15.6	1.6	46.8	28.2	11.2	3.7	12.1
The AMERICAS											
Bolivia	920	2003	3836	54	55.9	4.2	26.4	7.4	52.2	3.8	6.2
Colombia	1810	2000	1590	67.6	81.9	2.8	13.5	6.7	44.8	1.6	3.3
Guatemala	1750	1998-1999	1492	24.1	34.9	2.2	46.4	24.2	44.8	1.3	25.3
Haiti	440	2000	2044	26.8	11.6	0.9	21.9	16.8	24.4	1.5	28.9
Nicaragua	730	2001	2277	43.2	41.2	5.6	20.1	9.7	49.1	1.5	14.4
Peru	2020	2000??	4773	46.8	54.7	5.6	25.4	7.1	48.5	4.4	5.1

a. Based on number of children included in the samples used to build our model: country survey samples were much larger.
b. Based on total country sample (estimates provided by country at www..measuredhs.com).
c. Based on the limited samples used to build our model.
d. Based on total country survey sample aged 0-60 months, using >2 SD. Source: www.meaduredhs.com.
e. Based on total country survey sample, aged 0-60 months, using <2 SD. Source: www.meaduredhs.com
f. Median duration, in months.

frames can be found at the Marco International website (www.measuredhs.com). The basic sampling strategy is to produce a nationally-representative sample of households through a multiple-stage cluster design that begins with a selection of primary sampling units then randomly selects household within each (ORC Macro 1996). The primary participants in the surveys are all women aged 15-49 in the selected households, with all their children under five years then also targeted for anthropometric data collection. The sample size and collection dates for the included country surveys, along with some basic descriptive statistics, are presented in Table One.

The Variables and Model

A logistic regression model was employed to determine which of the predictors were significantly associated with the overweight status of the child. Because the relationships proved to vary substantially by region, we modeled each separately. In the final models for each region, all predictors and two-way interactions were considered; standard model-building techniques were employed to construct the "best" model, i.e., all predictors that remained significant ($p<0.01$) in the presence of other predictors, and there was no lack-of-fit as determined by the Hosmer-Lemeshow statistic. The dependent variable of interest was children's overweight status, which was derived from their weight-for-height measures, following World Health Organization recommendations (World Health Organization 1995). This was dichotomously coded based on whether weight-for-height was (1) or was not (0) more than two standard deviations (>2 SD) above the CDC growth reference curves derived from the NCHS/FELS/CDC reference populations. The predictor (independent) variables were:

A. Absolute household assets/wealth. The DHS surveys collect categorical information on selected household amenities, such as water source, toilet type, housing materials, and ownership of durable goods. In other studies considering health-socioeconomic relationships using DHS data it has been proposed that these variables can, via scoring of items followed by a factor analysis, be used to create a "wealth index" that is a reasonable and usable proxy for expressing summary household variation in income and expenditure (Rutstein and Johnson 2004, Filmer and Prichett 2001). Factor analysis is generally applicable for variables with values on a continuous scale, creating a smaller set of variables that are also on a continuous scale. Using a continuous variable in logistic regression is often leads to lack of fit because a very specific functional form for the probability curve is assumed. Categorical predictors are much less subject to lack of fit. Thus, we created an absolute household wealth variable with three levels: (1) bare floors, no electricity, and no flush toilet available (66.75% of the households of sample children in sub-Saharan Africa, 36.19% in the Americas and 5.47% in Northern Africa), (3) homes with flush toilet, electricity, finished floors, and either a television and/or a car (2.73% in sub-Saharan Africa, 21.07% in the Americas, and 60.20% in North Africa), and (2) all other households (i.e., the middle wealth category). This seemed a reasonable categorization, given that over half of children's households had essentially no basic services (that is, were classifiable as level 1). It is thus important to also note that being classified in the more affluent category in this sample in fact simply indicates a relative absence of poverty. The inclusion of a household social status variable (below) was intended to capture some different aspects of the variation in income beyond this.

B. Household social status. This variable was based on parental occupation and education. For the same reasons we outlined in considering household wealth, we found that creation of a standardized index based on factor analysis was not justifiable. Instead we identified six levels of the variable, which is feasible given the very large size of the sample. Paternal education and occupation tends to display far more heterogeneity than that of women (Fotso and Kuate-Defo 2005), so we built categories of social status with this in mind. The categorizations also recognize that many households, especially in the Americas, are female-headed, so that social status was assigned on the basis of either husband or wife's education and/or occupation (husband or dual-headed households) or wife's status alone (female headed-households). The six levels were:

(1) Professionals: Woman or her partner works in professional, technical, or managerial position or either has some tertiary education.
(2) Educated agricultural self-employed: Woman or her partner is self-employed in the agricultural sector, and either completed primary school.
(3) Educated service employed: Woman or her partner works in sales, clerical, skilled manual, or services industry, and at least one attended primary school.
(4) Educated unskilled laborer: Either woman or husband completed primary school and is employed as domestic, unskilled, or agricultural laborer.
(5) Unschooled agricultural self-employed: Woman or partner is agricultural self-employed and neither completed primary school.
(6) All others: unskilled labor or agricultural employment where either woman or partner did not attend school, or both the woman and partner are unemployed or the women does not have a partner and is unemployed.

C. Region. Separate logistic regression models were developed for each region. We categorized countries into the following regions: Northern Africa (Morocco and Egypt), Sub-Saharan Africa (including Ethiopia), and the Americas (including Haiti). See Table 1.

D. Urban-rural residence. This was entered into the model as a two-level variable based on women's de facto residence at the time she was interviewed. A strict urban/rural distinction can hide much heterogeneity in living conditions and so in related risk factors; particularly there can be important differences between living in an urban core versus the peri-urban surrounds of large cities versus a rural town and the countryside (McDade and Adair 2001). For most of the cases (N=37,071) we had data further distinguished into four categories: capital city or city over one million people, small cities (population over 50,000), town, or the countryside. When we ran the model based on these cases, we found the results were essentially the same (i.e., the differences were between small town/countryside and small/large city). We thus completed the model using the two level urban/rural categories.

E. Mother's weight status. This was classified based on mother's body mass index (BMI = kg/m^2), whereby overweight was BMI of greater than 25, underweight was BMI of less than

18.5, and normal weight was anything between these. Overweight entered into the model as 3, normal weight as 2, and underweight as 1.

F. Mother's (a) age and (b) total number of other children in the household. Mother's risk of overweight tends to increase both with her age and parity, so these were also entered into the model. The number of other young children in the household (highly associated with maternal parity) should also directly impact the availability of food to the target child, especially under extreme poverty conditions. Mother's age was entered into the model in the following three categories: 15-24 years, 25-34 years, and 35-49 years. The number of siblings under age five currently living in the household was entered into the model in following categories: no other children, 1-2 others, or more than 2 others.

G. Child's breastfeeding history. This was based on mother's reports of age in months at weaning and was categorized as follows: target child was breastfed for 0-11 months, 12-35 months, or 36 or more months.

H. Growth stunting (very low height-for-age) has been observed to place developing country children at increased risk of overweight, especially in middle income nations (e.g., Popkin et al., 1996, Sawaya et al., 1998), so was included in the model. This was entered as a dummy variable categorized on the basis of whether the child was below two standard deviations (<-2 SD) of height-for-age (1) or not (0), based on comparison with reference curves derived from the NCHS/FELS/CDC reference populations. Of the total sample, 37.6 percent of children were classified as stunted: the range was from 14.5 percent in Colombia to almost 60 percent in Guatemala. Stunting was more common than overweight in all the country samples, although some children in all regions were affected by both (see Table 2).

I. Other Variables: We intended to enter country wealth (per-capita gross national income [GNI]) into our model. The per-capita GNI of countries in our sample ranged from $100 to $2,020 (Table 1), which is classified by the World Bank as very low to lower-middle income (World Bank 2005). We found that because most of the countries we are sampling are very low income or low income, the range was fairly narrow and the levels in wealth were distinguished mostly by region; region and country wealth are thus strong proxies for each other in the model. Children's gender was not a significant predictor of overweight status either as a main effect in combination with other variables; it was removed from the model. We also had available birth weight data for a subset of the children (N=14,847). Based on analyses of these children, we found low birth weight (<2500 grams) did not predict overweight status, and thus could reasonably be removed.

Table 2: Percentage of Children Stunted and Overweight by Region

	Overweight	**Stunted**	**Both Overweight and Stunted**		
			Total	Urban only	Rural only
Sub-Saharan Africa	1.7%	47.3%	.9%	0.5%	1.0%
Northern Africa	7.7%	17.4%	2.2%	2.2%	2.2%
The Americas	4.2%	31.5%	.9%	0.7%	1.1%

Results

We find that that absolute household wealth, household social status, mother's overweight status, breastfeeding, and urbanism have different effects for early childhood overweight risk in different world regions. Particularly, the patterns in the Americas are generally distinct from those observed for Africa, so the associations between household wealth, social status, and urban status in predicting child overweight risk need to be considered particular to each. The results of the logistic regression are presented in Tables 3, 4, and 5, differentiated by region. The first three figures illustrate the differences in risk of overweight for children in each region, and the plots show different patterns of overweight by some of the major predictors. North Africa has the highest prevalence of overweight children, and sub-Saharan Africa the lowest. Note that in reporting of the regional patterns, we do not discuss variables that proved to have no interactional or independent effect on children's overweight risk once other variables were taken into account.

Table 3: Results for the Model for Sub-Saharan Africa. All comparisons for household social status were made against the final category (6), which represented those households with the under or unemployed and least educated parents.

Predictor	Odds Ratio	95% Confidence Interval	p-value
Overweight mother	2.08	(1.47,2.96)	<0.0001
Household social status (category 1 versus 6)	2.46	(1.32,4.58)	0.0003
(2 versus 6)	2.64	(1.55,4.48)	
(3 versus 6)	3.09	(1.91,4.97)	
(4 versus 6)	1.81	(0.86,3.08)	
(5 versus 6)	2.13	(1.16,3.91)	
Stunted	1.46	(1.12,1.91)	0.0025

Table 4: Results for the Model for the Americas. All comparisons for household social status were made against the final category (6), which represented those households with the under or unemployed and least educated parents. Urban residence results are compared to rural with the same household wealth categories.

Predictor	Odds Ratio	95% Confidence Interval	p-value
Overweight mother	2.05	(1.72,2.44)	<0.0001
Small family	1.42	(1.18,1.70)	0.0001
Household Social Status (category 1 versus 6)	1.48	(1.10,2.00)	0.0003
(2 versus 6)	1.86	(1.35,2.55)	
(3 versus 6)	1.78	(1.26,2.52)	
(4 versus 6)	1.11	(0.80,1.54)	
(5 versus 6)	1.21	(0.89,1.64)	
Urban and lowest household wealth	0.30	(0.11,0.80)	<0.0001
Urban and middle household wealth	1.49	(1.17,1.90)	
Urban and highest household wealth	1.96	(1.52,2.53)	
Breastfeeding 12 -35 months	0.76	(0.64,0.91)	0.0025

Table 5. Results of the Model for Northern Africa. All noted categories report significantly different odds than their comparison categories.

Predictor	Odds Ratio	95% Confidence Interval	p-value
Overweight mother	2.44	(1.91,3.12)	<0.0001
Highest household wealth category	1.53	(1.20,1.95)	0.0007
Urban residence and breastfeed 12 -35 months	0.59	(0.45,0.76)	<0.0001
Stunted, rural residence	1.79	(1.34,2.38)	<0.0001
Stunted, urban residence	3.74	(2.63,5.33)	<0.0001

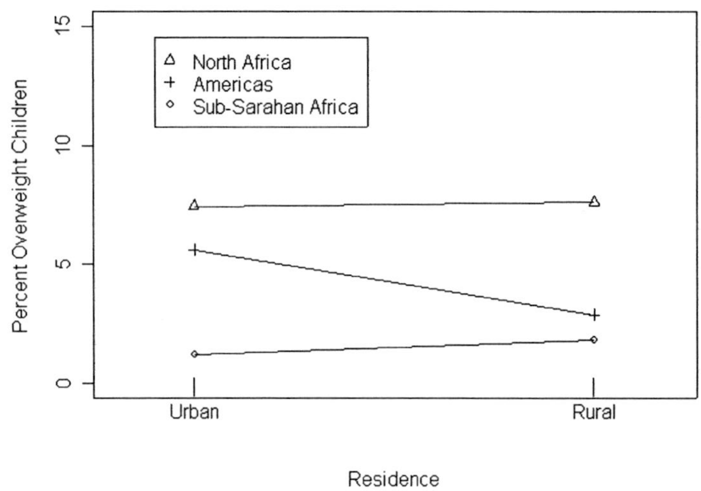

Figure 1: Percentage of Overweight Children by Urban/Rural Residence by Developing Country Region. The lines on all the figures are for visual purposes only.

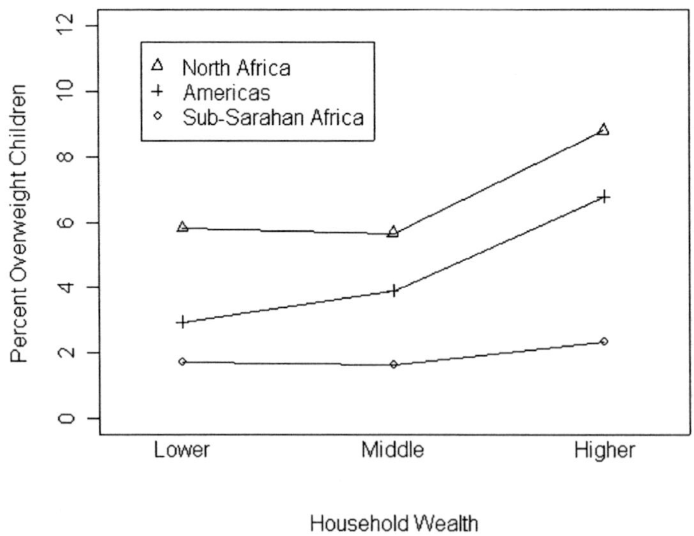

Figure 2: Percentage of Overweight Children by Level of Household Wealth by Developing Country Region.

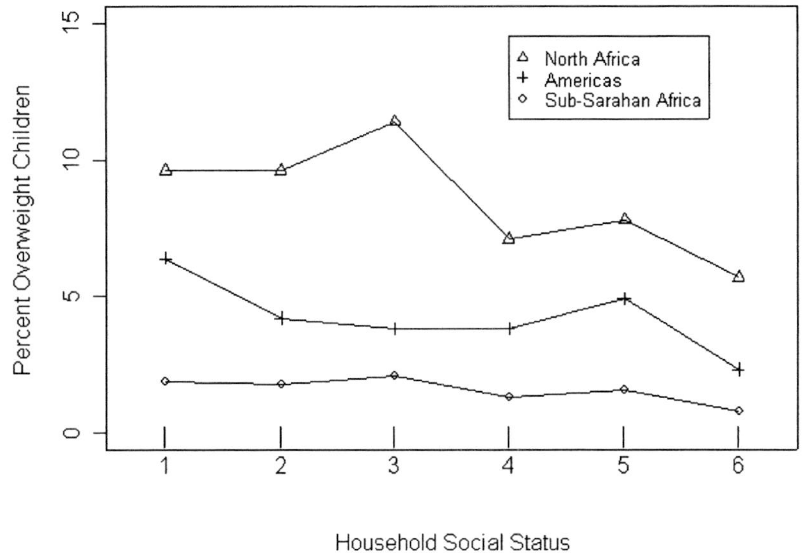

Figure 3: Percentage of Overweight Children by Household Status (based on parental education and occupation) by Developing Country Region. Note: the categories are not necessarily ordered, although group 6 is definitely the lowest status (mostly unemployed or unskilled with no education) and group 1 the highest (at least one parent is professionally employed and better educated).

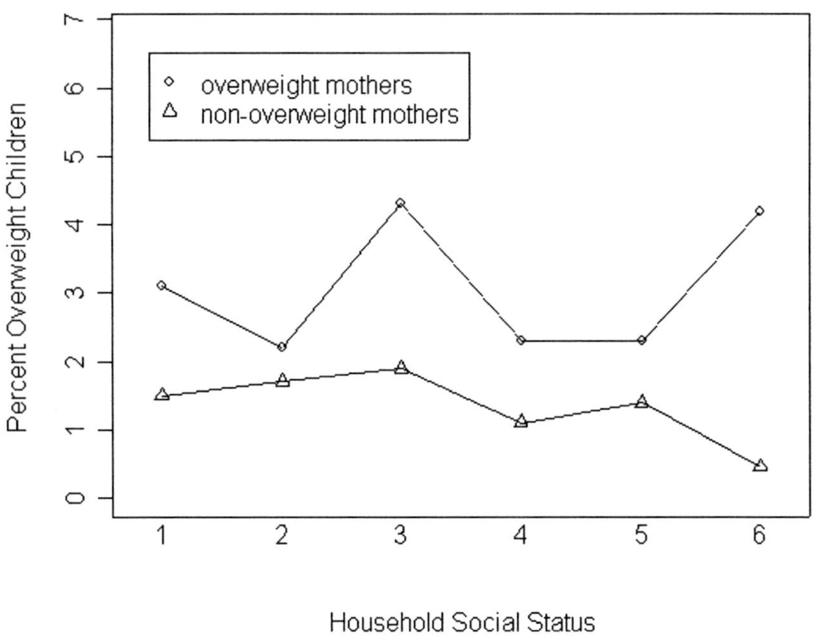

Figure 4: Percentage of Overweight Children by Household Social Status and Overweight Status of Mothers in Sub-Saharan Africa. See the Figure 3 legend regarding the social status categories.

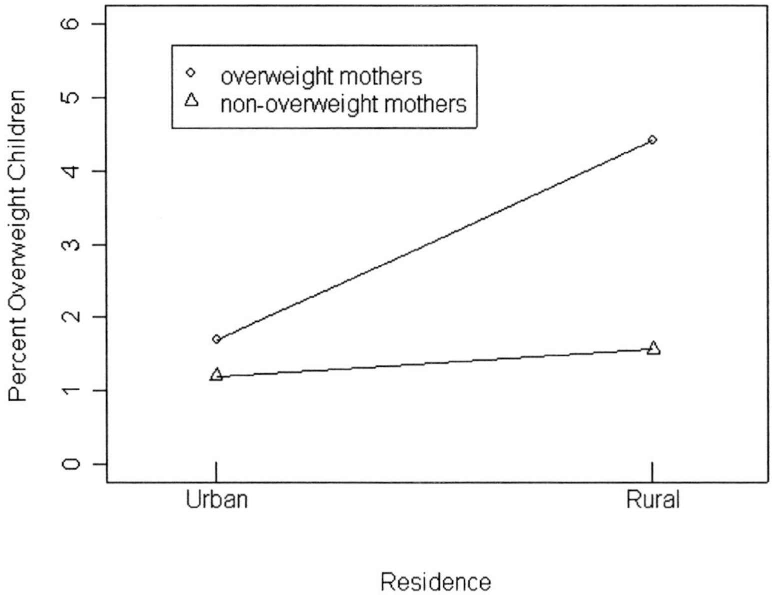

Figure 5: Percentage of Overweight Children by Household Wealth Level and Overweight Status of Mothers in Sub-Saharan Africa.

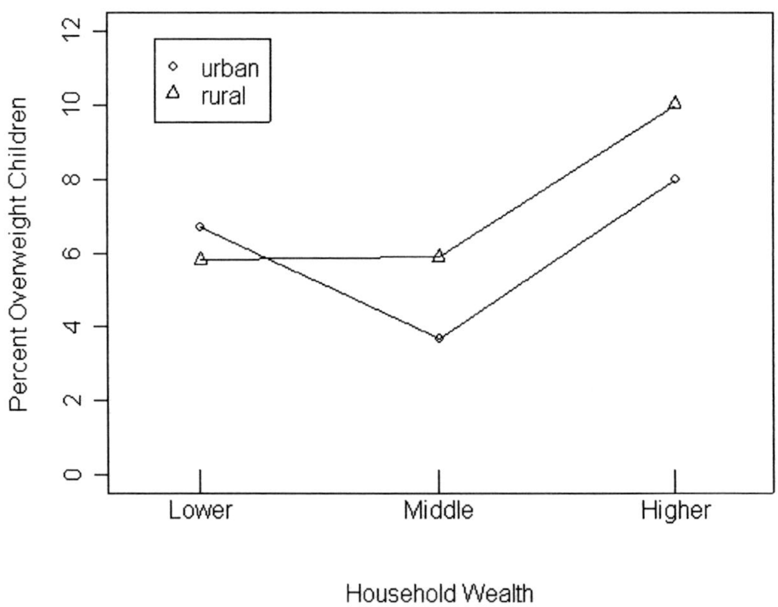

Figure 6: Percentage of Overweight Children by Urban/Rural Residence and Overweight Status of Mothers in Northern Africa.

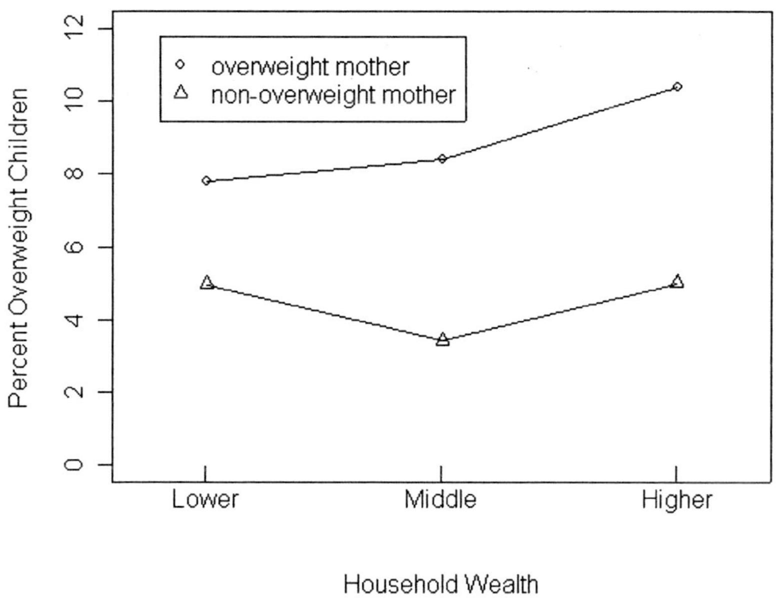

Figure 7: Percentage of Overweight Children by Household Wealth and Overweight Status of Mothers in Northern Africa.

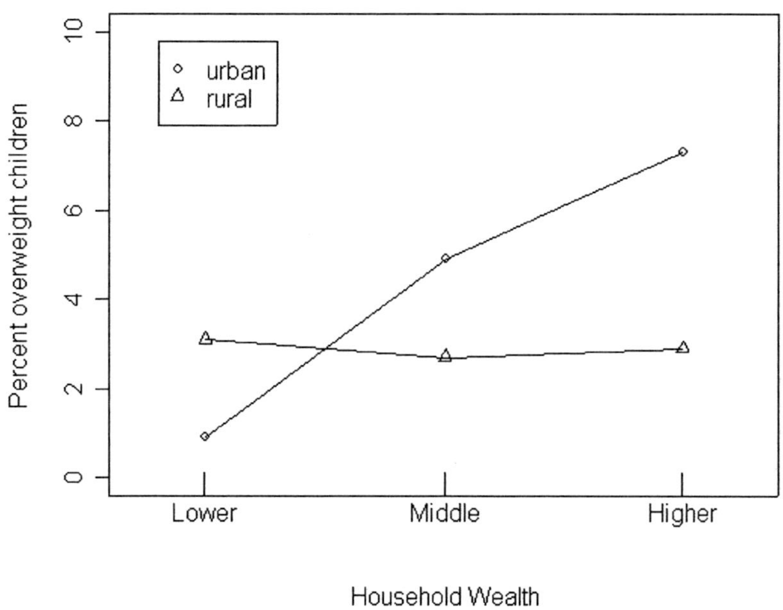

Figure 8: Percentage of Overweight Children by Rural/Urban Residence and Household Wealth in the Americas.

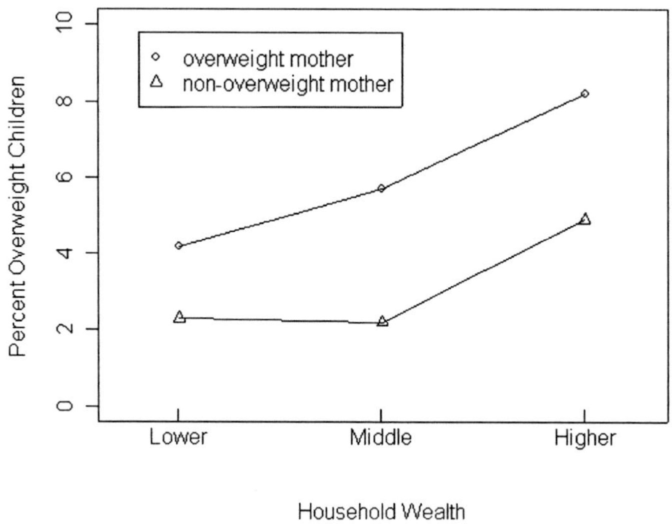

Figure 9: Percentage of Overweight Children by Household Wealth and Overweight Status of Mothers in the Americas.

The Pattern in Sub-Saharan Africa. Rates of overweight in early childhood are very low in all the sub-Saharan African countries. The strongest predictor of child overweight is the overweight status of the mother. The logistic regression model results (see Table 3) indicate that the odds of child being overweight is slightly more than two times higher for children of overweight mothers compared to children of mothers who are not overweight. Of course, this may be a surrogate for household social and economic conditions, as presumably these are predictors of mother's overweight, but the number of overweight children in the sample is too small to be able to detect any more precision if this is the case. Stunting (representing prior chronic under-nutrition) also places Sub-Saharan children at increased risk: stunted children have odds of overweight about 1.5 times higher than those who are not stunted. The household social status is a significant predictor of child overweight, with the first five categories having higher odds of overweight than the sixth. In particular, categories 1-3 have odds of overweight at least 2.5 times higher than category 6, and these differences are highly statistically significant.

The Pattern in Northern Africa. The strongest predictors of child overweight in the two Northern African countries are the mother's overweight status, whether the child's home is urban or rural, and whether the child is stunted. We see a 144% increased odds of child overweight if the mother is overweight. The type of residence strongly interacts with stunting and with long breastfeeding. The effect of stunting on risk of overweight in North Africa is different for urban and rural children. Urban children's odds of overweight are 3.7 times higher if the child is stunted, and rural children's odds of overweight are 1.8 times higher if the child is stunted. If the child is not stunted, the risk of overweight is not significantly different by type of residence (Figure 6). If the child's household wealth is of the highest level, the child has 53% larger odds of overweight compared with children in the less affluent categories (Figure 7). Finally, if an urban child is breastfed for at least 36 months, the odds of overweight are 41% lower than otherwise, but there is no breastfeeding effect for rural children.

The Pattern in the Americas. There are many highly significant predictors of child overweight in the developing countries of the Americas. Social and wealth status of the child's household are strong predictors, with wealth interacting strongly with the urban/rural location of the residence. The interaction effect is illustrated in Figure 8: we see that for urban children there is a strong relationship between family wealth and risk of overweight, with children from more wealthy families showing higher probability of overweight. For rural children, the risk of overweight does not vary significantly with family wealth. The logistic regression output (Table 5) allows us to quantify the risk of overweight by family affluence and on the urban/rural residence indicator. Because risk of overweight for rural children does not vary significantly by family affluence, we compare urban affluence groups to rural. Children in the urban, poor group have 70% lower odds of being overweight compared with rural children, while children in the urban, middle wealth group have 49% higher odds, and children in the urban, affluent group have 96% higher odds, compared with rural children. Family size is a predictor of overweight, with children from smaller families having larger risk of overweight. Specifically, the odds of overweight for children with zero or one sibling is 42% higher than the odds for children with 2 or more siblings. Children with parents with the lowest education and occupational status (category 6) have the lowest risk of child overweight. Compared to this group, children in groups 1, 2 and 3 (children of professionals, and educated skilled workers and self-employed agriculturalists) have significantly higher risk: odds are 48%, 86%, and 78% higher, respectively. The risk of overweight for children in groups 4 and 5 (children with less skilled and less educated parents) do not vary significantly from those in group 6 (the least skilled and educated). Breastfeeding duration is found to be associated with risk of overweight, with children that were breastfed for a year or more having 24% smaller odds of overweight, compared with children that were breastfed less than a year. Notably, stunting did not predict any increased risk of a child also being overweight.

The "Global" Pattern. Placing the regional patterns in the context of each other we find that controlling for household social and wealth categories, it is rural children in the Africas who are more at risk of overweight (although the effect is not a particularly strong one) and it is urban children in the Americas. In the Americas, rural children show no difference in overweight risk based on household wealth, but in urban contexts this has a substantial effect – whereby, the more affluent the household, the higher the risk of being overweight. In all regions, children are more likely to be overweight if their mothers are overweight: in sum, it is the strongest predictor of all. In sub-Saharan Africa, where almost all the households are in the very poor category, mother's overweight status is the only very strong significant predictor of child overweight risk. In this situation, it is likely that mother's nutritional status is a proxy for some aspects of household wealth and/or social status factors we have failed to capture, but we cannot observe this variation because the number of overweight children is so few (even with this very large sample size). For Northern Africa, the predictors are much the same, but there is a much higher prevalence rate of child overweight overall, and children from most affluent households are more likely to be overweight, controlling for differences in household social status. In the Americas, we observe that household social status exerts an influence on child overweight risk that was independent of household wealth (and vice versa).

That is, in rural households risk of being overweight varies by social status but not with wealth, but in urban households it varies by wealth even once social status is controlled for. Breastfeeding only predicts overweight status in the Americas, in which case it is protective: where children are breastfed for at least one year they are more likely to be overweight once household location, wealth, and social status are taken into account. Overweight risk was also higher where there are not other young siblings in the home. The finding that child stunting increases the risk of child overweight, at least in Africa, and that this effect is strongest in urban settings (at least in Northern Africa, where child obesity was much more common), is consistent with what has been observed in the few studies that have been done in middle income developing countries (e.g., Sawaya 1998). It is particularly important to note that the risk of child stunting in this sample, if we run it as an outcome variable, is very strongly predicted by household wealth: meaning that it is in the poorer households that we can observe stunting emerging as a critical predictor of childhood overweight risk, even at these very young ages.

Conclusion

Once we control for social status, household wealth, and such factors as children's prior under-nutrition (stunting) and maternal weight status, urbanism plays a limited role in constructing children's risk of being overweight. Household economics do have a significant role: the wealthiest families in Africa, and the wealthiest urban families in the Americas have the greatest risk of early childhood overweight. As low income countries continue a trajectory of economic growth, however, rising rates of child overweight are predicted. Stunting, which is much more common in this sample of developing country children than overweight, does place children in both sub-Saharan and North Africa (but not the Americas) at an elevated risk of potentially unhealthy levels of weight gain, even when you control for such other factors as income and even mother's weight status. However, we also detected an interaction between urban residence and stunting, in that children in urban settings have considerably greater risk of being overweight if they are stunted, compared to their stunted rural counterparts. Overall, however, it is the weight status of mothers independent of all these other factors that appears to best predict young children's risk of being overweight.

What implications does this have as we consider emerging risks for child obesity in the poorer developing countries? First, the model suggests that women's obesity rates are the harbingers of an emerging risk of early childhood obesity, indicating both the possible scale and where it is most likely to occur. It also suggests that increases the absolute wealth of households among the very poor, tied to the economic development of countries, will increase children's risk of over-nutrition, possibly very rapidly. Given the prevalence of stunting in many of these populations and ongoing urbanization, it means that childhood overweight and stunting will likely increasingly course together to amplify risk – perhaps most especially in Africa. Thus, child obesity may well emerge as an embodiment of relative poverty, just as stunting reflects the manifestation of absolute poverty. Moreover, the goal of a healthy 'normal' weight could prove as elusive and transitory for many of the world's least affluent, children, just as it now increasingly appears to be for their mothers.

References

Ball, K. & Crawford, D., (2005). Socioeconomic status and weight change in adults: A review. *Social Science and Medicine* **60**, 1817-2010.

Brewis, A. (2003). Biocultural aspects of obesity in young Mexican schoolchildren, *American Journal of Human Biology,* **15**, 446-60.

Brody, J. (2002). The global epidemic of childhood obesity: Poverty, urbanization, and the nutrition transition. *Nutrition Bytes*, **8**, Article 1. http://repositories.cdlib.org/uclabiolchem/nutritionbytes/vol8/iss2/art1

Caballero, B. (2005). A nutrition paradox – underweight and obesity in developing countries. *New England Journal of Medicine* **352**:1514-1516.

Crooks, D. L. (1995). American children at risk: Poverty and its consequences for growth, health and school achievement. *Yearbook of Physical Anthropology*, **38**,57-86.

Darnton-Hill, I. & Coyne, E. (1998). Feast and famine: Socioeconomic disparities in global nutrition and health. *Public Health Nutrition* **1**, 23-31.

Filmer, D. & Pritchett, L. (2001). Estimating wealth effects without expenditure data—or tears: An application to educational enrollments in states in India. *Demography*, **38**, 115-132.

Fotso, J-C., & Kuate-Defo, B., (2005). Household and community socioeconomic influences on early childhood malnutrition in Africa. *Journal of Biosocial Science*, **38**, 289-313.

Hedley, A., Ogden, C., Johnson, C., Carroll, M., Curtin, M., & Flegal, K. (2004). Prevlance of overweight and obesity among US children, adolescents, and adults, 1999-2002. *Journal of the American Medical Association*, **291**, 2847-2850.

Jebb, S., Rennie, K., & Cole, T. (2003). Prevlance of overweight and obesity among young people in Great Britain. *Public Health Nutrition*, **7**, 461-465.

Livingstone, M. (2000). Epidemiology of childhood obesity in Europe. *European Journal of Pediatrics*, **195**, S14-S34.

McDade, T. & Adair, L. (2001). Defining the "urban" in urbanization and health: A factor analysis approach. *Social Science & Medicine*, **53**, 55-70.

ORC Macro (1996) Sampling Manual. *DHS-III Basic Documentation*, No. **6.** Calverton, Maryland.

Magarey A.M., Daniels L.A., & Boulton T.J.(2001) Prevalence of overweight and obesity in Australian children and adolescents: reassessment of 1985 and 1995 data against new standard international definitions. *Medical Journal of Australia*, **174**, 561-565.

Martorell, R., Kettel Khan, L., Hughes, M.L., & Grummer-Strawn, L.M. (2000). Overweight and obesity in preschool children from developing countries. *International Journal of Obesity*, **24**, 959-967.

Mendez, M.A. & Popkin, B. (2004). Globalization, urbanization, and nutritional change in the developing world. *Journal of Agricultural and Development Economics*. **1**, 220-241.

Monteiro, C., Conde, W.L., Lu, B., & Popkin, B. (2004a). Obesity and inequities in health in the developing world. *International Journal of Obesity*, **28**, 1181-1186.

Monteiro, C., Moura, E., Conde, W., & Popkin, B. (2004b). Socioeconomic status and obesity in adult populations of developing countries: a review. *Bulletin of the World Health Organization*, **82**, 940-946.

Ogden, C., Troiano, R., Briefel, R., Kuczmarski, R., Flegal, K., & Johnson, C. (1997). Prevalence of overweight among preschool children in the United States, 1971 through 1994. *Pediatrics* **99**, e1.

Popkin, B. (2004). The nutrition transition: Patterns of Change. *Nutrition Reviews*, **62**, S140-143.

Popkin, B., Richards, M., & Monteiro, C. (1996). Stunting is associated with overweight in children of four nations that are undergoing the nutrition transition. *Journal of Nutrition*, **126**, 3009-3016.

Rutstein, S., & Johnson, K. (2004) The DHS Wealth Index. *DHS Comparative Reports* No. **6**. ORC Macro, Calverton, Maryland.

Sawaya, A.L., Grillo, L., Verreschi, I., da Silva, A.C., & Roberts, S. (1998). Mild stunting is associated with higher susceptibility to the effects of high fat diets: Studies in a shantytown population in São Paulo, Brazil. *Journal of Nutrition* **128**, 415S-420S.

Shetty P. S. (1999). Obesity in children in developing societies: indicator of economic progress or a prelude to a health disaster [editorial]. *Indian Pediatrics*, **36**, 11-15.

Sobal, J. & Stunkard, A.J. (1989). Socioeconomic status and obesity: A review of the literature. *Psychological Bulletin*, **105**, 260-275.

Wang, Y. (2001), Cross-national comparison of childhood obesity: The epidemic and the relationship between obesity and socioeconomic status. *International Journal of epidemiology*, **30**, 1129-1136.

World Bank, (2005). World Development Indicators 2005. World Bank, Washington, DC.

World Health Organization [WHO], (1998). Obesity: preventing and managing the global epidemic. *Report of a WHO consultation on obesity*. WHO, Geneva.

World Health Organization [WHO], (1995). Physical Status: The Use and Interpretation of Anthropometry. *WHO Technical Report* 1995:854.

In: Global Dimensions of Childhood Obesity
Editor: Richard K. Flamenbaum, pp. 69-87

ISBN: 1-60021-037-6

Chapter 3

CHILDHOOD OBESITY IN THE EASTERN MEDITERRANEAN REGION

Roya Kelishadi*
Preventive Pediatric Cardiology, Isfahan Cardiovascular Research Center,
Isfahan University of Medical Sciences, Iran

Abstract

The potential increase in non-communicable disease (NCD) is escalating much more rapidly in developing than industrialized countries. In this regard, a potential emerging public health concerning developing countries may be the increasing incidence of childhood obesity and as a result , an enormous socioeconomic and public health burden for poorer nations in the near future. However, little is known about its prevalence because of limited number of national studies, various definitions used and different age groups studied that make the comparisons difficult.

In the last decades, the countries located in the Eastern Mediterranean region (EMR) have experienced a transition from a traditional to a Westernized lifestyle and has undergone a rapidly occurring epidemiologic transition. The Middle- East located in this region has the highest dietary energy surplus of the developing countries. As a result, a rapid rise in NCD risk factors is according in different age groups, but very limited data exists about children living in this part of the world.

Through a systematic review, the present study compares surveys on the prevalence of overweight and obesity among children and adolescents living in the EMR, not only to review the differences, but also to assess the quality of methodologies, to explore the most important environmental influences, and to scrutinize the variations among sub-groups of the population.

The prevalence of overweight (based on WHO definition) among preschool children varies from near 3% in United Arab Emirates (UAE), Iran and Pakistan to 8.6% in Egypt. Among older children and adolescents (6-18y), the prevalence of overweight among girls ranges between 6.3% in Bahrain to 31.8% in Kuwait; among boys, it ranges between 4.9% in Saudi Arabia to 30% in Kuwait. The prevalence of obesity in girls is reported from near 3% in UAE and Iran to 35.1% in Bahrain; among boys, it ranges from 2.1% in Iran to 21% in Bahrain and 14.7% in Kuwait.

---

* E-mail address: kroya@aap.net , kelishadi@med.mui.ac.ir, Tel: +98 311 33771-8,Fax:+98 311 3373435, Address: PO.Box81465-1148, Isfahan,Iran

Overall, the prevalence of childhood overweight and obesity in Iran is reported much lower than in Arab countries of the EMR that is suggested to be because of underlying genetic and lifestyle differences. However, the recent national survey in Iran found a higher prevalence of obesity among the younger than older children, and is alarming for the rapid increase in childhood obesity.

Few studies performed in the EMR have assessed the environmental influences on childhood obesity, but the few studies addressing this matter emphasized that sedentary lifestyle, especially in girls and in urban residents, along with low nutrient but energy dense foods consumed, as well as the public belief considering fatness as a sign for health and beauty are the major factors in the high prevalence of obesity in this region.

It should be acknowledged that many of reviewed studies do not reflect national data, and include various age groups with different cutoffs used for overweight, making the comparison difficult.

Nevertheless, in spite of these limitations, the findings of the present study provide alarming evidence-based data for health professionals and policy makers about the considerable prevalence of childhood obesity in the EMR countries, many of them still grappling with the public health effects of malnutrition and micronutrient deficiencies.

Introduction

The developing world is experiencing an upcoming epidemic of childhood obesity but little is known about its prevalence because of limited national studies, and different definitions used that make the comparisons difficult.[1] According to the World Health organization (WHO) estimates, by the year 2020, non-communicable diseases (NCD) will account for approximately three-quarters of all death in the developing world[2]. In this regard, a potential emerging public health concerning developing countries may be the increasing incidence of childhood obesity and as a result , new cases of children with the metabolic syndrome, which in turn is likely to create an enormous socioeconomic and public health burden for poorer nations in the near future. [3]

Childhood obesity is becoming as an increasing public-health problem of different developed and developing countries [4-5]. The tracking of obesity from childhood to adulthood and its contribution to adult obesity-related morbidity and mortality is of great health significance [6-7]. Given difficulties in changing established eating and exercise behaviors, identifying the modifiable environmental factors is of great concern to prevent obesity during development.

In Western countries, the incidence of childhood obesity has more than doubled over the past generation.[8] A similar pattern is now emerging in developing countries, but has been largely ignored in health strategies developed at national and international levels.[9] This is partly because generally, the prevalence of this medical condition is not recognized and the different cut-offs used make the geographical comparisons difficult.

Data bases used for electronic search of literatures to find relevant studies were as follows:

1. AMED (Allied and Complementary Medicine) 1985 to 2005
2. CINAHL (Cumulative Index to Nursing & Allied Health Literature) 1982 to 2005
3. EMBASE (1980 to 2005)
4. Ovid MEDLINE(R) (1966 to present with daily update)
5. Ovid MEDLINE(R) in process and other non-indexed citations (2005)

6. Ovid OLDMEDLINE(R) (1950 to 1965)
7. CAB Abstracts (1973 to 2005)
8. Global Health (1973 to 2005)

Childhood Obesity Comorbidities

Obesity is a chronic disorder that has multiple causes.Overweight and obesity in childhood have significant impact on both physical and psychological health. Childhood obesity is multisystem disease with potentially devastating consequences [10], most of these complications warrant special attention.

As with adults, obesity in childhood causes hypertension, dyslipidemia, chronic inflammation, increased blood clotting tendency, endothelial dysfunction and hyperinsulinemia[11].This risk factor of chronic disease is known as metabolic syndrome or insulin resistance syndrome, and has been identified in children as young as 5 years of age.[12] Among adolescents and young adults who died of traumatic causes, the presence of such risk factors correlated with asymptomatic coronary atherosclerosis and lesions, and were more advanced in obese individuals.[13]Furthermore, in a British cohort, overweight in children increased the risk of death from ischemic heart disease in adulthood by two fold over 57years. [14]

Clinically significant obesity related morbidities are rare in children and are generally restricted to severely obese children. Such morbidities include Pick-Wickian syndrome, orthopedic disorders like genu varum and respiratory disorders like upper respiratory obstruction.[15] The most prevalent immediate consequence of obesity in children are social isolation and peer problem.[16] Type2 diabetes, once virtually unrecognized in adolescents, now account for as many as half of all new diagnoses of diabetes in some populations.[17] This condition is virtually entirely attributable to the pediatric obesity epidemic, though heredity and lifestyle factors affect individual risk.[18]Of greater concern, a peripatetic condition, consisting of glucose intolerance and insulin resistance, seem to be highly prevalent among severely obese children irrespective of ethnic group, even before formal diagnostic criteria for diabetes have bee met.[19]The emergence of type 2 diabetes in children represent an ominous development, in the view of the macro- vascular(heart disease,stroke,limb amputation) and microvascular(kidney failure, blindness) sequelae.

Frequent pulmonary complications include sleep disordered breathing (sleep apnea) [20], asthma[21] and exercise intolerance[22]development of asthma or exercise intolerance in an obese child can limit physical activity and consequently further weight gain. Moreover serious hepatic, renal, musculoskeletal ad neurological complications have been increasingly recognized.[24-27]

Findings of many studies indicate substantial psychosocial consequences of childhood obesity. obese children are stereotyped as unhealthy ,academically unsuccessful, socially inept, unhygienic and lazy.[28] Healthcare providers with expertise in obesity treatment share these stereotypes to some degree.[29] Overweight children as young as 5 years can develop a negative self-image[30] and obese adolescents show declining degrees of self-esteem associated with sadness,loneliness,nervousness,and high risk behaviors.[31]

Risks of obesity-related complications differ by ethnic region and as a result of cultural factors.[32-33] However obesity only explains part of this raised disease risks, since fasting serum insulin concentration and prevalence of insulin resistance syndrome remain much higher in minority youths after statistical adjustment for body mass index or adiposity.[34-35] By contrast, adverse psychosocial effects are often more severe in white children particularly girls, than in other ethnic groups.[36] Researchers have shown an association between childhood obesity and high prevalence of blood pressure[37], diabetes[38], respiratory disease[39] and orthopedic and psychosocial disorders. [40]Of greater concern though is the tracking of obesity from childhood to adulthood and its contribution to adult obesity related morbidity and mortality.[40]The risk of adult morbidity and mortality that may follow childhood obesity is potentially of great public health significance, therefore signifying the importance community based health strategies designed upon a firm, accurate and reliable data base.

Etiology of Childhood Obesity

Although the mechanism of childhood obesity is not fully understood, it is well documented that obesity occurs when energy intake exceeds energy expenditure. Since there are multiple etiologies for this imbalance, the rising prevalence of obesity cannot be explained by a single etiology. Body weight is regulated by numerous physiological mechanisms that maintain the balance between energy intake and energy expenditure.[41] Genetic factors can have a great effect on individual predisposition; however, rising prevalence rates among genetically stable population s indicate that environmental and possibly, perinatal factors must underline the childhood obesity epidemic. Obviously overweight in any population is the result of a long-term positive energy balance. Energy balance in human beings must follow the rules of thermodyamics. The general equation for energy balance in men can be stated as follows: energy intake=energy expenditure+energy stored. Excessive storage in adipose tissue (obesity) is the final result of four general mechanisms:

1. An increase in energy intake without proportionate increase in energy expenditure
2. A decrease in energy expenditure without a decrease in intake
3. A combination of 1 and 2
4. Greater decrease in energy expenditure than in intake. diverging trends in energy intake(falling)and obesity prevalence(rising) in both united states and Europe, suggested that there must be a dramatic decrease in total energy expenditure exceeding the decrease in total energy intake(4th mechanism).[42-43]

Our previous study comparing the differences in energy intake and expenditure of obese and non-obese siblings revealed that the obese children had both lower energy intake and lower energy expenditure than their non-obese sibling.[44]

However energy intake data are by no means concordant .The main components of energy expenditure are resting metabolic rate (60-70%), thermic effect of food (10-15%) and thermic effect of physical activity. while the former two components are relatively constant, thermic effect of physical activity is the most variable of all and may comprise from 0%(total inactivity) to 50%(elite athletes) of total energy expenditure in humans. Therefore it was suggested that decreased physical activity is probably the main factor accounting for reduction of total energy expenditure leading to positive energy balance and decreased prevalence of obesity. In 1997 two severely obese Pakistani children of consanguineous parents were found to have leptin gene mutations.[45] Leptin is produced by adipose tissue and its quantity is related to the amount of body fat[46] Up to now five genetic mutations that cause obesity during childhood have been identified[47] ,additionally, many candidate alleles, such as those in variable nucleotide tandem repeat region of the insulin gene, have been discovered that seem to affect risk of early-onset obesity.[48] Although genetic loci of some obesity syndromes like Prader-Willi, Bardet-Biedel, Cohen and Astrom syndrome have been mapped, molecular base of these syndromes are not as clear.[49]

However small gene defects account for only a small proportion of human obesity, conversely, predisposition to obesity seems to be caused by a complex interaction between over 250 obesity-associated genes and perhaps perinatal factors.[50]

Whitaker and Dietz advanced the intriguing hypothesis that prenatal over-nutrition might affect lifelong risk of obesity. [50] According to this hypothesis, maternal obesity increases the transfer of nutrients across the placenta and induces permanent changes in appetite, neuro-endocrine functioning or energy metabolism. Observational studies revealed a direct relation between maternal obesity, birth weight and obesity later in life; however, the relative contribution of shared maternal genes versus intrauterine factors are difficult to differentiate studies in animals have shown the possible long-term consequences of maternal obesity. It can be concluded that the obesity epidemic could accelerate through successive generations independent of further genetic or environmental factors[51]. However under nutrition in some important stages of fetal development can also lead to permanent physiological changes that may induce obesity[52],therefore, nutrition transition described by Popkin could lace children of developing countries at higher risk of obesity.[53] According to these findings, the best time for prevention of obesity may be before conception. There are some other risk factors such as bottle feeding, probably because of some physiological changes related to unknown intrinsic characteristics of human milk during early childhood[54]. BMI normally decreases until age 5-6 years and then increase, which is termed adiposity rebound.[55] It is shown that children with early adiposity rebound, is associated with increased risk of obesity, later in life[56-57], however biological and clinical value of this finding is not clear[58]

Some studies have revealed that obese children have less moderate to vigorous physical activity than their non-obese counterparts[59].Another study revealed association of low vigorous physical activity and TV watching with obesity. [60]

Familial environment and parental habits can have influence in this regard. Parents provide both the genes and eating environment for their children, familial patterns of adiposity are the result of gene-environment interactions.[61]In our previous study, we found a significant inverse relationship was found between the education level of both parents, as well as maternal employment and obesity in their children. Overall, 72.3% of mothers and 39.5% of fathers reported that before their children become fat, they believed that an obese child is healthier than low- or normal weight peers; 79.2% of mothers reported a history of using pressure in child feeding. The BMI of mother was associated with food habits of their daughters and sons, and the BMI of fathers had significant association with the frequency of activities of their sons. [62] These finding emphasize that in addition to community-based lifestyle modification, culturally relevant family-based interventions especially focusing on mothers' beliefs and behavior are needed to prevent and/or to treat childhood obesity and its long-term consequences; special emphasis should be directed at families that are affected and/or concerned with obesity. As suggested by the review of published data, effective interventions for prevention and treatment of overweight should be approached from a health-centered rather than a weight- centered perspective, with the parents as central agents of change. [63]

➢ ***Prevalence of childhood obesity in developing countries***

There is strong evidence that childhood obesity is becoming increasingly prevalent in developing countries[64-65]. In such societies, the rapid progress of urbanization and demographic trends is associated with a cluster of NCD and unhealthy lifestyle described as the "Lifestyle Syndrome" or the "New World Syndrome". This is suggested as the most important etiology for the very high rates of obesity and its consequent morbidity and mortality in developing nations. In addition, in such communities, childhood obesity still is considered as a sign of healthiness and high social class. Among developing countries, the prevalence of childhood obesity is highest in the Middle East, Central and Eastern Europe[66].

The analysis of one hundred sixty nationally representative surveys from 94 developing countries showed an increasing prevalence of overweight and obesity from childhood to adulthood, although rates of early childhood malnutrition remained relatively high[67].

The study of Mia and colleagues showed a high clustering of risk factors of chronic diseases including obesity among Indian adolescents with a possible genetic and dietary interaction as causative factor.[68]A study performed in Turkey revealed that 47.7% of school children, ages 7-18 had at least one of these risk factors and 11.7% of them exhibited two or more risk factors.[69]

➢ ***Prevalence of childhood obesity in the Mediterranean region***

In a representative sample of adolescents living in urban and rural area of central Edrine, Turkey, data concerning the height and weight of 989 adolescents, aged between 12 and 17 years were collected. The prevalence of overweight and obesity were based on the cut off points of the IOTF values. The prevalence of overweight and obesity among adolescent girls was 10.6% and 2.1%, respectively, while it was 11.3% and 1.6% for adolescent boys. In the urban area the prevalence of overweight and obesity among adolescent girls was 10.3% and 2.1%, while it was 11.6% and 1.6% for boys, respectively. In the rural area; the prevalence of overweight and obesity among adolescent girls was 12.4% and 2.2%, while it was 9.6% and 1.2% for boys, respectively. Analyses of data collected during these studies support that adolescents living in Turkey carry relatively lower further risk of overweight and obesity than adolescents in other countries do[70].

In Greece, data concerning the height and weight of 2,458 schoolchildren aged 6 to 17 years (1,226 6-10 years, 1,232 11-17 years) of 27 primary and secondary public schools were collected. . In the analyses, the estimations of the prevalence of overweight and obesity are based on recently established international BMI percentile curves and cut-off points from 2-18 years. To investigate the secular trends in obesity in Greece, data of schoolchildren from four successive surveys were used. In the younger group (6-10 yr), the prevalence of overweight and obesity were 25.3% and 5.6%, while for adolescents (11-17 yr) they were 19.0% and 2.6%, respectively. The prevalence was 25.9% and 5.1% for all males, and 19.1% and 3.2% for all females, respectively. As far as trends are concerned, an increase of BMI was found among males when the results of our survey were compared with those of the previous three. However, the trends for girls are different. An increase was found when the results of our study were compared with 1942. A decrease of BMI at most ages was found when the results of our study were compared with those of the 1982 survey, while an increase was recorded only for younger girls below 13 years compared to the 1984-5 study. This study demonstrates that the prevalence of overweight and obesity among schoolchildren is 22.2% and 4.1%, respectively, and has been increasing in the last decades, especially among boys[71].

Another study, which was part of the Health Behavior in School Aged Children (HBSC) study, was to provide national estimates for overweight and obesity in Greek school-aged children and adolescents. A total of4299 student, 51.3% girls and 48.7% boys, aged 11.5, 13.5 and 15.5 y consisted of. Self-reported weight and height data were used. According to the body mass index cutoff points adopted by the International Obesity Task Force (IOTF), 9.1% of girls and 21.7% of boys were classified as overweight, and 1.2% of girls and 2.5% of boys as obese. Corresponding values using CDC growth charts were 8.1% of girls and 18.8% of boys for overweight, and 1.7% of girls and 5.8% of boys for obese. Compared to most other western countries, the prevalence of obesity is lower in Greek children aged 11-16 years[72].

➢ ***Prevalence of childhood obesity in the Eastern Mediterranean region(EMR)***

According to the divisions of the World Health Organization, in addition to some Asian countries, the Eastern Mediterranean region (WHO/EMRO) includes some African countries, as well. As every large scale preventive strategy needs valid and strong data-base, we studied a number of researches in the Eastern Mediterranean region. Studies performed in this region are limited in this regard, but show a high prevalence of risk factors of chronic diseases notably obesity in children and adolescents. In Tunisia- as one of these countries with a rapid epidemiological transition- a high prevalence of NCD risk factors is demonstrated in urban population of school children.[73] Hakeem et al. have evaluated the prevalence of certain NCD risk factors in 10-12 year old school children living at different levels of urbanization and have compared the Pakistani; British Pakistani, British Indian and British Caucasian children and found that the proportion of children having high NCD risk increased with urbanization rank. They have suggested that in addition to genetic predisposition, the environmental factors like undernourishment in early life, adoption of urbanized lifestyle or a combination of both could be the major determinants of this high NCD rate.[74] The study of Baddrudin et al. in Pakistan found a high prevalence of NCD risk factors among school children from low and middle- income families.[75]

As the Middle East has the highest dietary energy surplus of the developing countries, and considering the rapid changes in the demographic characteristics of the region, large shifts in dietary and physical activity patterns, a rapid rise in NCD risk factors especially obesity is according.[76] Most of the surveys in this region are performed in adult population; in addition, the cut-offs used and the age groups studied differ between studies, making comparison difficult; however, the few studies evaluating obesity among youth living in these countries have shown considerably high prevalence especially among adolescents. The prevalence of obesity in Kuwait is among the highest in the Arab Peninsula.[77] The recent study performed among 10-14 year old adolescents in this country revealed a very high prevalence of overweight (31.8% of girls and 30% of boys) and obesity (13.1% of girls and 14.7% of boys)[78]. A review on data extracted from the Ministry of Health annual health report, as well as, the 1981 and 1991 censuses in Bahrain revealed a high prevalence of obesity among different age groups[79]. The recent study among 506 Bahraini school students found that according to the IOTF criteria, the overall prevalence of obesity was 15% in boys and 18% in girls[80]. A study among 898 adolescent girls in the United Arab Emirates revealed that 14% of subjects were overweight and 9% were obese according to the CDC criteria.[81]A survey in Saudi Arabian male school children, aged between 6 to 18 showed a prevalence of 11% of overweight and 15.8% of obesity.[82] This finding a higher prevalence of obesity than overweight is contrary to most other studies.

The prevalence of overweight and associated characteristics has been assessed in a representative sample of pre-pubertal children in Lebanon. A total of 234 children aged 6-8 years including 131 boys and 103 girls were tested. Prevalence of overweight and obesity was based on the international cut-off points for body mass index (BMI) by age and gender proposed by the International Obesity Task Force. Prevalence of overweight and obesity was 26% and 7% respectively in boys, 25% and 6% in girls. Overweight was significantly associated with low physical activity and mother's BMI. This study identified a high proportion of overweight in 6- to 8-year-old children in Lebanon[83].

A cross-sectional survey of a representative sample of 2104 individuals, 3 years of age and older was performed in Lebanon. Overweight and obesity (classes I to III) were defined according to internationally standardized criteria for classification of BMI. For children 3 to 19 years of age, prevalence rates of overweight and obesity were higher overall for boys than girls (22.5% vs. 16.1% and 7.5% vs. 3.2%, respectively). For adult men and women (age > or = 20 years), the prevalence of overweight was 57.7% and 49.4%, respectively. In contrast, obesity (BMI > or = 30 kg/m(2)) was higher overall among women (18.8%) than men (14.3%), a trend that became more evident with increasing obesity class. BMI, percentage of body fat, and waist circumference increased to middle age and declined thereafter. Whereas lack of exercise associated significantly with obesity among children, obesity in older adults was more prevalent among the least educated, nonsmokers, and those reporting a family history of obesity. The results showed high prevalence rates of overweight and obesity comparable with those observed in developed countries such as the United States[84].

A total of 12,701 children (6,281 boys and 6,420 girls) with ages ranging from 1 to 18 years were enrolled during a household screening program in different provinces of Saudi Arabia. The overall prevalence of overweight was 10.68 and 12.7 percent and that of obesity was 5.98 and 6.74 per cent in the boys and girls, respectively. In the different provinces the prevalence of overweight ranged from 8.8 to 27.4 percent and from 9.3 to 27.6 percent and obesity ranged from 4.7 to 10.4 per cent and from 4.3 to 13.8 percent in the boys and girls, respectively. In general, girls have a higher prevalence of both overweight and obesity compared with boys. When grouped according to age, overweight and obesity tended to increase with age.[85]

The study conducted in 1996 in Saudi Arabia assessed 9061 male school children, attending public schools. Their ages ranged from 6-18 y and covered the entire 12 grade levels of school. The percentage of body mass index (BMI) of expected BMI at the 50th percentile for each age group was computed. The 50th percentile of The National Center for Health Statistics/Center for Disease Control reference population was used as the expected standard population values for defining childhood overweight and obesity. The overall prevalence of overweight was 11.7% and obesity 15.8%. There was a statistically significant variation in the regional distribution of overweight and obesity ($P < 0.01$).[86]

The prevalence of overweight and obesity and its correlates among Saudi male adolescents in Riyadh was studied during a 5-month period, September 2001-January 2002. A sample of 894 Saudi male adolescents (age 12-20 years) was selected through the multi-stage sampling technique. Adolescents with a BMI age-specific percentile of > or = 85th-< 95th were considered overweight and > or = 95th were considered obese. RESULTS: The prevalence of overweight was 13.8% and obesity was 20.5%. Family history (odds ratio, 2.49; 95% confidence interval, 1.72-3.61) and lack of physical activity (odds ratio, 1.63; 95% confidence interval, 1.01-2.62) were associated with adolescent obesity. Twenty percent of overweight participants did not think they were overweight.[87]

A cross-sectional study was to assess the levels of overweight and obesity among Kuwaiti intermediate school adolescents aged 10-14 y. The study comprised a multistage stratified random sample of 14659 adolescents (7205 males and 7454 females), which constitutes approximately 17% of the target population of this school level. Overweight and obesity were defined as BMI >85th and >95th centiles, respectively, of the National Center for Health Statistics (NCHS) reference data. The overall prevalence of overweight and obesity among males were 30.0 and 14.7%, respectively (P<0.001). The overall prevalence of overweight and obesity among females were 31.8 and 13.1%, respectively (P<0.001 and P<0.01). There was no consistent rise or decline in overweight and obesity in both genders with respect to age. However, the overall prevalence of overweight was lower in males than in females but obesity was higher in males than in females. When compared to the NCHS reference population, the BMI of Kuwaiti adolescents exceeded that of the Americans in each centile category > or = 50th centile.[88]

A cross-sectional sample of 3473 3to5 year old Kuwaiti pupils (1748 boys and 1725 girls) was selected for the other study from kindergartens using a multi-stage random sampling technique. Overweight and obesity were defined as weight-for-height (W/H) > or = 90th-< 95th and > or = 95th centiles of the NCHS/CDC reference population, respectively. Factors that were found to be significantly associated with overweight and obesity were gender, age, region (governorate), parents' education, birth order, dental status, eating regular meals and SES. Factors that were significantly associated with overweight and obesity males were age, governorate eating regular meals, number of persons living at home and SES. Among females these factors were governorate, dental status, number of servants and SES. The logistic regression analysis showed that the same factors shared by both genders significantly contributed to the development of overweight and obesity except father's education. This study concludes that ecological factors play an important role in the development of overweight and obesity, especially those related to affluence; Kuwait has been undergoing modernization and increasing affluence and changes to sedentary lifestyle and increased food consumption may have contributed to changes in overweight and obesity among the children.[89]

Another Cross-sectional prevalence study was conducted in intermediate and secondary schools of Bahrain and included a population-representative sample of 506 Bahraini students (249 males and 257 females) between 12 and 17 y of age. The overall prevalence of obesity among Bahraini boys and girls was high, especially in girls. Obesity was highest (21% in males and 35% in females) when the WHO recommended criteria of BMI for age and skinfolds for age percentiles were applied and lowest (15% in boys and 18% in girls) when the age and sex specific BMI cut-off values of Cole et al were used. This study revealed a much higher prevalence rate of obesity in the Bahraini adolescent population than was previously reported, especially among girls. [90]

Another study conducted in 2005assessed the national prevalence of obesity among schoolchildren in the United Arab Emirates (UAE).A stratified 10% random sample of 16,391 children was drawn from 145,492 pupils in the UAE. BMIs for UAE were compared to international standards. Comparison of BMIs to international reference data revealed that UAE children are at increased risk for overweight (>25 kg/m^2 and $\geq$30 kg/ m/^{2}) and obesity ($\geq$30 kg /m^2). For instance, 10-year-old male UAE children had 1.7 times the rate of overweight compared to international standards and 1.9 times at 18 years. Similarly, female UAE children have 1.8 times the rate of overweight compared to international standards at 10 and 18 years of age. Obesity was 2.3-fold higher among UAE males at 14 years compared to international standards, and increased to 3.6 times at 18 years of age. Among UAE female children, obesity was same as males at 14 years, 2.3 times than the international standards. At 18 years of age, UAE female obesity was 1.9-fold higher than the international standard, nearly one-half the rate of obesity among UAE males at the same age. The frequency of obesity among UAE youth is two to three times greater than the recently published international standard.[91]

➢ ***Prevalence of childhood obesity in African countries of the EMR***

A study compiled about the prevalence of obesity and its determinants in Morocco and Tunisia. Results from the authors' two surveys on nutrition-related disease among reproductive-age women (sample size: 2800) and their children (1200 children under 5 y and 500 adolescents) were combined with data from four national income and expenditure surveys (dating from 1980) to assess obesity trends and development in Morocco and Tunisia. Overall levels of obesity, identified by body mass index (BMI) $\geq$ 30 kg/m(2), were 12.2% in Morocco and 14.4% in Tunisia. Obesity is significantly higher among women than among men in both countries (22.7% vs. 6.7% in Tunisia and 18% vs. 5.7% in Morocco) and prevalence among women has tripled over the past 20 y. Half of all women are overweight or obese (BMI > 25) with 50.9% in Tunisia and 51.3% in Morocco. Overweight increases with age and seems to take hold in adolescence, particularly among girls. In Tunisia, 9.1% of adolescent girls are at risk for being overweight (BMI/age > or = 85th percentile). Prevalence of overweight and obesity are greater for women in urban areas and with lower education levels. Obese women in both countries take in significantly more calories and macronutrients than normal-weight women. The percentage contribution to calories from fat, protein and carbohydrates seems to be within normal limits, whereas fat intake is high (31%) in Tunisia and carbohydrate intake (65-67%) is high in Morocco.[92]

In Tunisia,a survey based on a representative sample of 1569 urban schoolchildren of Sousse in Tunisia was conducted. The main results showed that girls had significantly higher levels of body mass index (BMI), diastolic blood pressure (DBP), total cholesterol, low-density lipoprotein (LDL) cholesterol and high-density lipoprotein (HDL) cholesterol than boys, who however had significantly higher levels of systolic blood pressure (SBP). Total cholesterol was significantly correlated to BMI and decreased with age. Obesity (BMI = 27) was found in 7.9% of the study population and was significantly higher in girls than in boys (9.7% vs, 6%, P=0.01). Overweight (BMI = 25) was also significantly higher among girls than in boys (16% vs,11.1%, P = 0.004).[73]

In a study among female adolescents in Egypt,35% of the girls were overweight and 13% were obese. Overweight was more prevalent in urban than rural girls and in those with higher socio-economic status than in lower socio-economic status girls.[93]

➢ ***Prevalence of childhood obesity in Iran***

Similar with many other developing countries, Iran is rapidly moving along epidemiologic, demographic and nutrition transitions, that is suggested to be secondary to the rapid change in fertility and mortality patterns and to urbanization which have led to a considerable imbalance in food consumption with low nutrient density characterizing diets, over-consumption evident among more than a third of households.9[94-95] The other suggested underlying factor for the increasing rate of childhood obesity in Iran is that still in our community; plumpness is considered as a sign of the child healthiness.Limited regional studies have been performed in Iran. The study performed in Kerman (South-East) among 1000 high school female students, ages 14-21, found a prevalence of 4.6% for overweight and 0.7% for obesity.[96]A study among 1516 female students, aged 14-20 year, in Tabriz (North-West) showed that 10.1% and 3.9% of the subjects were overweight and obese, respectively.[97]The study performed on 3-18 year-old children and adolescents in Tehran(capital city) showed that 5.1% of subjects were obese.[98] Another study among 2321 students aged 11-16 years in Tehran showed that according to the CDC criteria, 21.1% of subjects were overweight and 7.8% were obese.[99] Our previous study among 2000 students aged between 11 to 18, living in three counties in central Iran showed that according to CDC cut-offs, 10.7% of girls and 7.4% of boys were overweight and 2.2% of girls and 1.9% of boys were overweight.[100] Our study evaluating the trend of overweight among 2-18 year old children and adolescents ,according to the NCHS criteria revealed a double fold increase in the prevalence of overweight from 4% in 1993 to 8% in 1999.[101]The differences between the age groups studied, the subjects' living area (urban/rural) as well as the BMI cut-offs used make the comparisons difficult. In general, these studies show that the prevalence of childhood obesity in Iran is much lower than Arab countries in the region, which is suggested to be due to both genetic and lifestyle differences between Iranian and Arab nations.

The only national survey performed for assessment of the risk behaviors and risk factors of chronic diseases among Iranian children and adolescents was performed in 2003-2004 as the baseline survey for implementation of a school-based surveillance system entitled: "Childhood & Adolescence Surveillance and PreventIon of Adult Non-communicable disease": CASPIAN[1]* Study.

This multi-centric study was performed among 21,111 school students (96% participation rate), aged 6-to-18 years, living in urban and rural areas of 23 provinces in Iran (Fig1).

The samples were selected as a representative sample of near 16,000,000 Iranian school-students (from near 67,000,000 total population of the country)with different ethnicities (Persian 51%, Azeri 24%, Gilaki and Mazandarani 8%, Kurd 7%, Arab 3%, Lur 2%, Baloch 2%, Turkmen 2%, other 1%). The mean (±SD) age of students was 12.2± 3.3 years, 84.6% of them were from urban and 15.4% from rural areas and 90% were from public and 10% from private schools. The prevalence of underweight was 13.9% (8.1% of boys and 5.7% of girls) according to the CDC[11] percentiles, and 5 % (2.6% of boys and 2.4% of girls) according to the obtained percentiles. The prevalence of normal weight was 72.7% (36.6% of boys and

*- Caspian is the name of the world largest lake in North Iran

36.2% of girls) according to the CDC percentiles, and 80.1% (41.3% of boys and 38.9% of girls) according to the obtained percentiles (Fig 2).

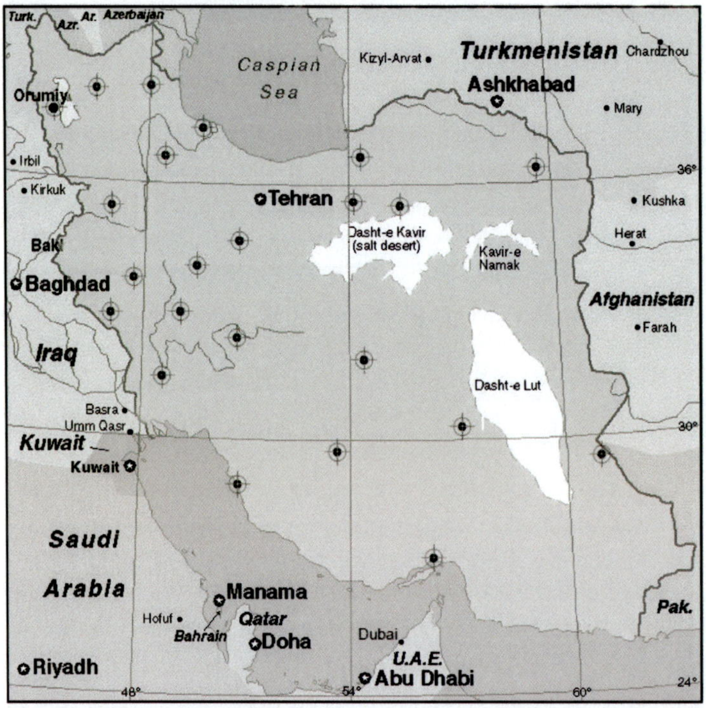

Figure 1. The counties studied by the CASPIAN Study in Iran

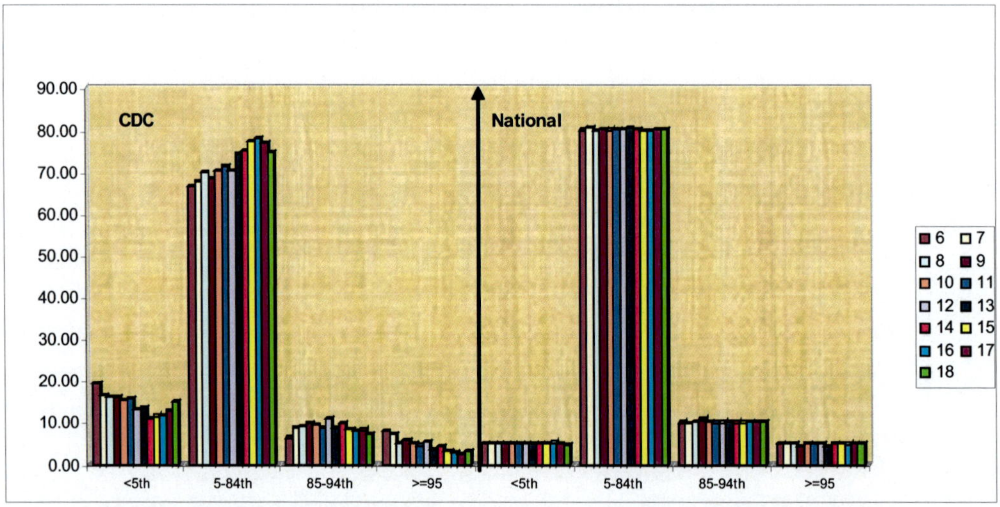

Fig 2. Distribution of different BMI categories according to the percentiles of CDC and the percentiles obtained from a national sample of 6-18 year-old Iranian children and adolescents (n=21,111): CASPIAN Study

According to the CDC, IOTF and national cut-offs, the prevalence of overweight was 8.82%, 11.3% and 10.1%, respectively; and the prevalence of obesity was 4.5%, 2.9% and

4.79%, respectively.Significant difference was found between various counties, the lowest prevalence (according to CDC criteria) being in Zahedan (3.1% overweight and 0.6% obesity), and Shahrekord (6.2% overweight and 2.3% obesity), respectively, and the highest prevalence being in Rasht (18.8% overweight and 7.4% obesity) and Qom (18.4% overweight and 7.3% obesity), respectively.[102]

Based on the extrapolation of our findings, it can be estimated that among the approximate 16 million school students in Iran, over 2 million currently are overweight and obese, illustrating the necessity of an enormous effort to educate the general population and health professionals will to identify and properly control this large number of cases.

The prevalence of childhood obesity in some countries located in the EMR (with available data among boys and girls) is presented in Figure 3.

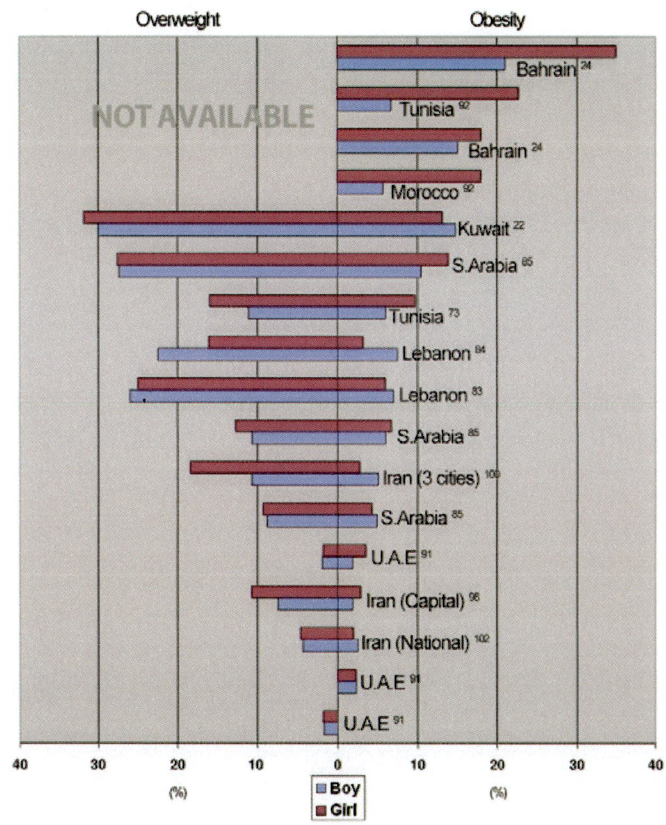

Fig3.Comparison of the prevalence (%) of childhood obesity in some countries in the Eastern Mediterranean region

Conclusion

Childhood obesity is becoming as an emerging health problem in the Eastern Mediterranean region. Till now, in this region most national public health programs and policies, as well as national-level researches on children and adolescents focused on under-nutrition and its effects on survival, mortality and development of mothers and children. The findings of recent studies in this region provide alarming evidence-based data for health professionals and policy makers about the considerable prevalence of childhood overweight and obesity in our and other countries still grappling with the public health effects of malnutrition and micronutrient deficiencies. This also warrants the necessity of paying special attention to the elevated future risk of chronic diseases, and to establish a surveillance system for monitoring the time-trends in child obesity based on uniform definitions, as well as to design programs to prevent and control associated factors in an action-oriented manner.

References

[1] Ebbeling CB,Pawlak DB, Ludwig DS.Childhood obesity:public-health crisis, common sense cure. *Lancet* 2002; 360: 473-482

[2] Onis M. The use of anthropometry in the prevention of childhood overweight . *Int J Obes Relat Metab Disord.* 2004 ;28 Suppl 3:S81-5

[3] Freedman DS, Khan LK, Dietz WH, Srinivasan SR, Berenson GS. Relationship of childhood obesity to coronary heart disease risk factors in adulthood: the Bogalusa *Heart Study. Pediatrics* 2001; 100: 712-718.

[4] Strauss RS, Pollack HA. Epidemic increase in childhood overweight, 1986-1998. *JAMA* 2001; 286(22): 2845-8.

[5] Onis M, Blossner M. Prevalence and trends of overweight among preschool children in developing countries. *Am J Clin Nutr* 2000; 72: 1032-9.

[6] Must A, Jacques PF, Dallal GE, Bajema CJ, Dietz WH. Long-term morbidity and mortality of overweight adolescents. A follow-up of the Harvard Growth Study of 1922 to 1935. *N Engl J Med* 1992; 327: 1350-5.

[7] Gunnell DJ, Frankel SJ, Nanchakal K, Peters TJ, Davey Smith G. Childhood obesity and adult cardiovascular mortality: A 57-year follow up study based on the Boyd Orr cohort. *Am J Clin Nutr* 1998; 67: 1111-5.

[8] Dietz WH, Robinson TN. Overweight Children and Adolescents. *N Engl J Med* 2005;352:2100-2109.

[9] Obesity: Preventing and managing the global epidemic. Report of a WHO Consultation on Obesity. Geneva, 3-5 June 1997 (1st ed.) Geneva: World Health Organization, 1998 *WHO/NUT/NCD/98.***1**

[10] Must A, Strauss RS. Risks and consequences of childhood and adolescent obesity. *Int J Obesity* 1999; 23 (suppl): S2-S11.

[11] Ford ES, Galuska DA, Gillespie C, Will JC, Giles WH, Dietz WH. C-reactive protein and body mass index in children: findings from the Third National Health and Nutrition Examination Survey, 1988–1994. *J Pediatr* 2001; 138: 486-92.

[12] Strong JP, Malcom GT, McMahan CA, et al. Prevalence and extent of atherosclerosis in adolescents and young adults: implications for prevention from the Pathobiological Determinants of Atherosclerosis in Youth Study. *JAMA* 1999; 281: 727-35.

[13] McGill HC, McMahan A, Zieske AW, et al. Association of coronary heart disease risk factors with microscopic qualities of coronary atherosclerosis in youth. *Circulation* 2000; 102: 374-9.

[14] Gunnell DJ, Frankel SJ, Nanchahal K, Peters TJ, Smith GD. Childhood obesity and adult cardiovascular mortality: a 57-y follow-up study based on the Boyd Orr cohort. *Am J Clin Nutr* 1998; 67: 1111-8.

[15] Must A. Morbidity and mortality associated with elevated body weight in children and adolescents.*Am J Clin Nutr* 1996; 6(suppl):445S-7S.

[16] Dietz WH. Health consequences of obesity in youth: childhood predictors of adult disease. *Pediatrics* 1998; 101(suppl):518-25.

[17] Fagot-Campagna A, Pettitt DJ, Engelgau MM, et al. Type 2 diabetes among North American children and adolescents: an epidemiologic review and a public health perspective. *J Pediatr* 2000; 136: 664-72.

[18] Loder RT, Aronson DD, Greenfield ML. The epidemiology of bilateral slipped capital femoral epiphysis. *J Bone Joint Surg* 1993; 75: 1141-7.

[19] Sinha R, Fisch G, Teague B, et al. Prevalence of impaired glucose tolerance among children and adolescents with marked obesity. *N Engl J Med* 2002; 346: 802-10.

[20] Redline S, Tishler PV, Schluchter M, Aylor J, Clark K, Graham G. Risk factors for sleep-disordered breathing in children: associations with obesity, race, and respiratory problems. *Am J Respir Crit Care Med* 1999; 159: 1527-32.

[21] Figueroa-Munoz JI, Chinn S, Rona RJ. Association between obesity and asthma in 4–11 year old children in the UK. *Thorax* 2001; 56: 133-7.

[22] Reybrouck T, Mertens L, Schepers D, Vinckx J, ewilling M. Assessment of cardiovascular exercise function in obese children and adolescents by body mass-independent parameters. *Eur J Appl Physiol* 1997; 75: 478-83.

[23] Balcer LJ, Liu GT, Forman S, et al. Idiopathic intracranial hypertension: relation oge and obesity in children. *Neurology* 1999; 52: 870-2.

[24] Strauss RS, Barlow SE, Dietz WH. Prevalence of abnormal serum aminotransferase values in overweight and obese adolescents. *J Pediatr* 2000; 136: 727-33.

[25] Castro-Magana M. Hypogonadism and obesity. *Pediatr nn* 1984; 13: 494-7.

[26] Adelman RD, Restaino IR, Alon US, Blowey DL. Proteinuria and focal segmental glomerulosclerosis in severely obese adolescents. *J Pediatr* 2001; 138: 481-5.

[27] Goulding A, Jones IE, Taylor RW, Williams SM, Manning PJ. Bone mineral density and body composition in boys with distal forearm fractures: a dual-energy X-ray absorptiometry study. *J Pediatr* 2001; 139: 509-15.

[28] Hill AJ, Silver EK. Fat, friendless and unhealthy: 9-year old children's perception of body shape stereotypes. *Int J Obesity* 1995; 19: 423-30.

[29] Teachman BA, Brownell KD. Implicit anti-fat bias among health professionals: is anyone immune?. *Int J Obesity* 2001; 25: 1525-31.

[30] Davison KK, Birch LL. Weight status, parent reaction, and self-concept in five-year-old girls. *Pediatrics* 2001; 107: 46-53.

[31] Strauss RS. Childhood obesity and self-steem. *Pediatrics* 2000; 105: e15.

[32] Fagot-Campagna A, Pettitt DJ, Engelgau MM, et al. Type 2 diabetes among North American children and adolescents: an epidemiologic review and a public health perspective. *J Pediatr* 2000; 136: 664-72.

[33] Winkleby MA, Robinson TN, Sundquist J, Kraemer H. Ethnic variation in cardiovascular disease risk factors among children and young adults: findings from the Third National Health and Nutrition Examination Survey, 1988–1994. *JAMA* 1999; 281: 1006-13.

[34] Gower BA, Nagy TR, Trowbridge CA, Dezenberg C, Goran MI. Fat distribution and insulin response in prepubertal African American and white children. *Am J Clin Nutr* 1998; 67: 821-7.
[35] Reaven P, Nader PR, Berry C, Hoy T. Cardiovascular disease insulin risk in Mexican-American and Anglo-American children and mothers. *Pediatrics* 1998; 101: e12.
[36] Kimm SY, Barton BA, Berhane K, Ross JW, Payne GH, Schreiber GB. Self-esteem and adiposity in black and white girls: the NHLBI Growth and Health Study. Ann *Epidemiol* 1997; 7: 550-60.
[37] Tracey VV, De NC, Harper JR. Obesity and respiratory infection in infants and young children.*Br Med J* 1991;1:16-8.
[38] Dietz WH Jr, Gross WL, Kirkpatrick JA Jr.Blount disease(tibia vara):another skeletal disorder associated with childhood obesity.*J Pediatr* 1982;101:7335-7.
[39] .Mossberg HO. 40-year-follow up of overweight children. *Lancet* 1989;2:491-3.
[40] Nieto FJ, Szklo M, Comstock G. Childhood weight and growth rate as predictors of adult mortality. *Am J Epidemiol* 1992; 16: 201-13.
[41] Lustig RH. The neuroendocrinology of childhood obesity. *Pediatr Clin North Am* 2001; 48: 909-30.
[42] Schlicker SA,Borra ST, Regan C. The weight and fitness status of United States children.*Nutr Rev* 1994;52:11-7.
[43] Sunnegardh J, Bratteby LE, Hagman U, Samuelson G, Sjolin S. Physical activity in relation to energy intake and body fat in 8-and 13-year-old children in Sweden. *Acta Paediatr Scand* 1986:955-63.
[44] Kelishadi R. Energy intake and expenditure in obese and normal weight siblings. The 2nd World Congress of Pediatric *Gastroenterology Hepatology and Nutrition*, Paris, France, July 2004.
[45] Montague CT, Farooqi IS, Whitehead JP, et al. Congenital leptin deficiency is associated with severe early-onset obesity in humans. *Nature* 1997; 387: 903-8.
[46] Zhang Y, Proenca R, Maffei M, Barone M, Leopold L, Friedman JM. Positional cloning of the mouse *obese* gene and its human homologue. *Nature* 1994; 372: 425-32.
[47] Farooqi IS, O'Rahilly S. Recent advances in the genetics of severe obesity. *Arch Dis Child* 2000; 83: 31-4.
[48] LeStunff C, Fallin D, Bougneres P. Paternal transmission of the very common class I *INS* VNTR alleles predisposes to childhood obesity. *Nat Genet* 2001; 29: 96-9.
[49] Rankinen T, Perusse L, Weisnagel SJ, Snyder EE, Chagnon YC, Bouchard C. The human obesity gene map: the 2001 update. *Obes Res* 2002; 10: 196-243.
[50] Whitaker RC, Dietz WH. Role of the prenatal environment in the development of obesity. *J Pediatr* 1998; 132: 768-76.
[51] Levin BE, Govek E. Gestational obesity accentuates obesity in obesity-prone progeny. *Am J Physiol* 1998; 275: R1374-9.
[52] Ravelli GP, Stein ZA, Susser MW. Obesity in young men after famine exposure in utero and early infancy. *N Engl J Med* 1976; 295: 349-53.
[53] Popkin BM. The nutrition transition and its health implications in lower income countries. *Public Health Nutr* 1998; 1: 5-21.
[54] Gillman MW, Rifas-Shiman SL, Camargo CA, et al. Risk of overweight among adolescents who were breastfed as infants. *JAMA* 2001; 285: 2461-2467.

[55] Rolland-Cachera M-F, Deheeger M, Bellisle F, Sempe M, Guillound-Bataille M, Patois E. Adiposity rebound in children: a simple indicator for predicting obesity. *Am J Clin Nutr* 1984; 39: 129-35.

[56] Whitaker RC, Pepe MS, Wright JA, Seidel KD, Dietz WH. Early adiposity rebound and the risk of adult obesity. *Pediatrics* 1998; 101: e5.

[57] Wisemandle W, Maynard M, Guo SS, Siervogel RM. Childhood weight, stature, and body mass index among never overweight, early-onset overweight, and late-onset overweight groups. *Pediatrics* 2000; 106: e14.

[58] Freedman DS, Kettel Khan L, Serdula MK, Srinivasan SR, Berenson GS. BMI rebound, childhood height and obesity among adults: the Bogalusa Heart Study. *Int J Obes* 2001; 25: 543-9.

[59] Trost SG, Kerr LM, Ward DS, Pate RR. Physical activity and determinants of physical activity in obese and non-obese children. *Int J Obes Relat Metab Disord* 2001; 25: 822-9.

[60] Andersen RE, Crespo CJ, Bartlett SJ, Cheskin LJ, Pratt M. Relationship of physical activity and television watching with body weight and level of fatness among children: results from the Third National Health and Nutrition Examination Survey. *JAMA* 1998; 279: 938-42.

[61] Whitaker RC, Deeks CM, Baughcum AE, Specker BL. The relationship of childhood adiposity to parent body mass index and eating behavior. *Obesity Research* 2000; 8(3): 234-40.

[62] Kelishadi R, Hashemipour M, Sadeghi M, Roohafza HR, Tavasoli AA, Khosravi A, et al. The Impact of Familial Factors on Obesity in Iranian Children and Adolescents. *J Ped Neonat* 2005; 2(2): 16-23.

[63] Golan M, Crow S. Parents are key players in the prevention and treatment of weight-related problems.*Nutr Rev* 2004;62(1):39-50.

[64] Monteiro CA, Conde WL, Popkin BM. Is obesity replacing to undernutrition? Evidence from different social classes in Brazil. *Public Health Nutr* 2002; 5: 105–112.

[65] Monteiro CA, Conde WL, Lu B , Popkin BM. Obesity and inequities in health in the developing world. *Int J Obes* 2004; 28:1181–1186.

[66] James PT. Obesity: The worldwide epidemic. *Clinics in Dermatology* 2004, 22:276-80.

[67] Onis M, Blossner M. Prevalence and trends of Overweight among preschool children in developing countries. *Am J Clin Nutr* 2000; 72:1032-1039.

[68] Mia FB, Vorster HH. Coronary heart disease risk factors in Indian adolescents the role of diet. *Cardiovasc J S Afr* 2000; 11(2): 68-75.

[69] Ucar B, Kilic Z, Colak O, Oner S, Kalyoncu C. Coronary risk factors in Turkish schoolchildren: Randomized cross-sectional study. *Ped Int* 2000; (42): 259-67.

[70] Oner N, Vatansever U, Sari A, Ekuklu E, Guzel A, Karasalihoglu S, Boris NW. Prevalence of underweight, overweight and obesity in Turkish adolescents. *Swiss Med Wkly* 2004;134(35-36):529-33.

[71] Krassas GE, Tzotzas T, Tsametis C, Konstantinidis T.Prevalence and trends in overweight and obesity among children and adolescents in Thessaloniki, Greece. *J Pediatr Endocrinol Metab* 2001;14 Suppl 5:1319-26

[72] Karayiannis D, Yannakoulia M, Terzidou M, Sidossis LS, Kokkevi A. Prevalence of overweight and obesity in Greek school-aged children and adolescents.*Eur J Clin Nutr*. 2003 Sep;57(9):1189-92.

[73] Ghannem H, Darioli R, Harrabi I, Gaha R, Trabelsi L, Fredj AH, et al. Epidmiology of cardiovascular risk factors among schoolchildren in Sousse, Tunisia. *J Cardiovasc Risk* 2001; 8(2): 87-91.

[74] Hakeem R, Thomas J, Badruddin SH. Urbanisation and coronary heart disease risk factors in South Asian Children. *J Pak Med Assoc* 2001; 51(1): 22-8.

[75] Badruddin SH, Molla A, Khurshid M, Vaz S, Hassanali S. Cardiovascular risk factors in school children from low middle income families in Karachi, Pakistan. *J Pak Med Assoc* 1994; 44(5): 106-12.

[76] Galal O. Nutrition-related health patterns in the Middle East. Asia Pac J Clin Nutr 2003; 12: 337-343.

[77] Moussa MA, Shaltout AA, Nkansa-Dwamena D, Mourad M, Alsheikh N, Agha N, Galal DO. Factors associated with obesity in Kuwaiti children. *Eur J Epidemiol* 1999; 15: 41-9.

[78] Al-Isa AN. Body mass index, overweight and obesity among Kuwaiti intermediate school adolescents aged 10-14 years. *Eur J Clin Nutr* 2004; 58: 1273-1277.

[79] Hamadeh RR. Noncommunicable diseases among the Bahraini population: a review. *East Mediterr Health J* 2000; 6: 1091-1097.

[80] Al-Sendi AM, Shetty P, Musaiger AO. Prevalence of overweight and obesity among Bahraini adolescents: a comparison between three different sets of criteria. *Eur J Clin Nutr* 2003; 57: 471-474.

[81] Al-Hourani HM, Henry CJ, Lightowler HJ. Prevalence of overweight among adolescent females in the United Arab Emirate. *Am J Hum Biol* 2003; 15: 758-64.

[82] Al-Nuaim AR, Bamgboye EA, Al-Herbish A. The pattern of growth and obesity in Saudi Arabian male school children. *Int J Obes Relat Metab Disord* 1996; 20: 1000-5.

[83] Jabre P, Sikias P, Khater-Menassa B, Baddoura R, Awada H.Overweight children in Beirut: prevalence estimates and characteristics. *Child Care Health Dev* 2005; 31(2): 159-65

[84] Sibai AM, Hwalla N, Adra N, Rahal B. Prevalence and covariates of obesity in Lebanon: findings from the first epidemiological study. *Obes Res* 2003; 11(11) 1353-61.

[85] El-Hazmi MA, Warsy AS.A comparative study of prevalence of overweight and obesity in children in different provinces of Saudi Arabia. *J Trop Pediatr*. 2002; 48(3):172-7.

[86] al-Nuaim AR, Bamgboye EA, al-Herbish A.The pattern of growth and obesity in Saudi Arabian male school children. *Int J Obes Relat Metab Disord* 1996; 20(11): 1000-5.

[87] Al-Rukban MO. Obesity among Saudi male adolescents in Riyadh, Saudi Arabia. *Saudi Med J*. 2003; 24(1):27-33.

[88] Al-Isa AN.Body mass index, overweight and obesity among Kuwaiti intermediate school adolescents aged 10-14 years. *Eur J Clin Nutr* 2004; 58(9):1273-7.

[89] al-Isa AN, Moussa MA. Factors associated with overweight and obesity among Kuwaiti kindergarten children aged 3-5 years. *Nutr Health* 1999; 13(3):125-39.

[90] Al-Sendi AM,Shetty P, Musaiger AO.Prevalence of overweight and obesity among Bahraini adolescents: a comparison between three different sets of criteria.*Eur J Clin Nutr* 2003; 57(3):471-4.

[91] Al-Haddad FH, Little BB, Abdul Ghafoor AG. Childhood obesity in United Arab Emirates schoolchildren: a national study.*Ann Hum Biol.* 2005 ;32(1):72-9.

[92] Mokhtar N, Elati J, Chabir R, Bour A, Elkari K, Schlossman NP, Caballero B, Aguenaou H. Diet culture and obesity in northern *Africa J Nutr* 2001;131(3): 887S-892S.

[93] Jackson RT, Rashed M, Saad-Eldin R. Rural urban differences in weight, body image, and dieting behavior among adolescent Egyptian schoolgirls. *Int J Food Sci Nutr.*2003;54(1):1-11.

[94] Ghassemi H, Harrison G, Mohammad K. An accelerated nutrition transition in Iran. *Public Health Nutr* 2002; 5: 149-55.

[95] Sheikholeslam R, Mohamad A, Mohammad K, Vaseghi S. Non-communicable disease risk factors in Iran. *Asia Pac J Clin Nutr* 2004; 13(Suppl):S100

[96] Janghorbani M, Parvin F. Prevalence of overweight and thinness in high-school girls in Kerman, Iran. *Int J Obes Relat Metab Disord* 1998; 22:629-33.

[97] Gargari BP, Behzad MH, Ghassabpour S, Ayat A. Prevalence of overweight and obesity among high-school girls in Tabriz, Iran, in 2001. *Food Nutr Bull* 2004; 25: 288-91.

[98] Azizi F, Rahmani M, Emami H, Mirmiran P, Hajipour R, Madjid M, et al. Cardiovascular risk factors in an Iranian urban population: Tehran lipid and glucose study (phase 1). *Soz Praventivmed* 2002; 47:408-26.

[99] Mohammadpour-Ahranjani B, Rashidi A, Karandish M, Eshraghian MR, Kalantari N.Prevalence of overweight and obesity in adolescent Tehrani students, 2000-2001: an epidemic health problem. *Public Health Nutr* 2004; 7(5):645-8.

[100] Kelishadi R, Hashemipour M, Sarraf-Zadegan N, Sadry Gh, Ansari R, Alikhassy H, Bashardoust N. Obesity and associated modifiable risk factors in Iranian adolescents: IHHP-HHPC *Int Ped* 2003; 45: 435-42.

[101] Kelishadi R, Hashemipour M, Sarraf-Zadegan N, Amiri M. Trend of atherosclerosis risk factors in children of Isfahan. *Asian Cardiovascular & Throracic Annals* 2001; 9: 36-40.

[102] Kelishadi R, Ardalan G, Gheiratmand R. *Report on WHO Grant TSA03/11*;2004.

In: Global Dimensions of Childhood Obesity
Editor: Richard K. Flamenbaum, pp. 89-98

ISBN: 1-60021-037-6

Chapter 4

ADOLESCENT OBESITY: AN INCREASING PROBLEM. TURKEY AND OTHER COUNTRIES' STATUS

Naci Öner*

Trakya University Faculty of Medicine, Department of Pediatrics, Turkey

Abstract

Introduction: Obesity is currently regarded as a chronic and recurring disorder and it is closely associated with various chronic disorders such as cardiovascular diseases, metabolic syndrome, anxiety and mood abnormalities. Adolescence appears to be high risk period for the development of obesity and obesity in this period is more likely to track into adulthood. The prevalence of childhood and adolescence obesity in Europe and the USA has doubled during the last 10 to 15 years. There are only a few conducted studies related to adolescent obesity in Turkey, therefore, we tried to evaluate the features that represents our region. We also aimed to evaluate the last obesity and overweight prevalence status of the adolescents throughout Europe and the world.

Methods: This was a cross-sectional study, including a representative sample of 928 adolescent girls and 1004 adolescent boys in rural and urban area of Edirne, Turkey. For this study, the body weight and height of adolescents were measured using standard procedures. BMI (kg/m^2) was calculated as the ratio of the body weight to square body height. Prevalence of obesity and overweight was defined as age and gender specific BMI in excess of the 95th and 85th percentiles, respectively.

Results: The prevalence of overweight and obesity among adolescent girls of in our region was found to be 9.6 % and 3.8 %, respectively, while it was 7.8 % and 0.7 % among adolescent boys. Adolescent obesity prevalence was found to be higher in girls than in boys ($p<0.05$), although there was no gender difference in overweight prevalences between adolescent girls and boys. In the urban area, the prevalence of overweight and obesity among adolescent girls was 9.3 % and 0.9 %, while it was 8.6 % and 0.6% among boys, respectively. In the rural area; among adolescent girls, overweight and obesity prevalence was 9.9 % and 3.4 %, while it was 6.0 % and 0.6 % among boys, respectively.

Conclusions: This study has showed that obesity prevalence of our adolescent population was lower than European adolescents and this difference is even higher when it was compared to the adolescents in the USA. The reason for the lower rate of obesity among our adolescents

* E-mail address: nacioner@yahoo.com, nacioner@trakya.edu.tr, Fax: 090 284 235 23 38, Fatih Mahallesi, 28. Sokak, Karcan Sitesi B Blok, Daire: 7, 22030, Edirne, Turkey, Tel: 090 532 257 25 32

are largely unknown. However, one of them may be Mediterranean type of diet which contains more vegetables and less meat and carbohydrate.

Key words: prevalence, overweight, obesity, adolescents, BMI

Introduction

Children and adolescents are needed urgently to provide information on the long-term effects of childhood obesity. Because, overweight and obesity during childhood and adolescence is associated with overweight and obesity during adulthood and those adults are at increased risk for morbidity and mortality associated with many medical conditions, including hypertension, dyslipidemia, coronary heart disease, diabetes mellitus, gallbladder disease, respiratory disease, some types of cancer, gout and arthritis and has been associated with increased use of medical services [1-5].However, most of these medical complications do not become clinically apparent for decades. Rarely, severe childhood obesity is associated with immediate morbidity result from conditions such as slipped capital femoral epiphysis, steatohepatitis and sleep apnea syndrome [6-8]. Besides the wide number of later medical complications which lead to increased morbidity and mortality, obesity is associated with labeling and negative consequences in psychosocial areas, e.g. social marginalization, decreased self-esteem and decreased quality of life [9]. For this reason, every effort should be made effectively to deal with this problem.

Recent concerns have been raised regarding to the increasing prevalence of overweight and obesity in children and adolescents in the higher income countries [10,11]. However, overweight and obesity as a worldwide phenomena, affecting the rich and middle income countries in similar manners and also affecting countries to be poor [12-15].

Until the last years, there has been limited availability of data for Turkish population, especially for adolescents, which allows to evaluate a local and national prevalences of overweight and obesity. Edirne is in the north-west corner of Turkey where the three Thracian nations, Turkey, Greece and Bulgaria meet and is a bridge between Asia and Europe. The aim of this study was to determine the overweight and obesity prevalence in a representative sample of adolescents living in urban and rural areas of Edirne. We also aimed to evaluate the latest obesity and overweight prevalence status of the adolescents throughout Europe and the world.

Methods

Data were derived from current studies, namely "The Prevalence of Anemia Among the Adolescent Girls Living in Edirne" and " Evaluation of the nutritional status of adolescent boys living in rural and urban areas of Edirne, Turkey" in which height and weight were measured simultaneously as blood samples and questionnaires were collected. These cross-sectional studies covered representative samples of the 12–17 years old Turkish (Edirne) adolescents. Written informed consent was obtained and a questionnaire to get demographic data was sent to the parents a day before the measurements. The participation was voluntary and consents from both the parents and the adolescents were obtained. These two studies were approved by the local Ethics Committee of the University of Trakya, Faculty of Medicine.

Adolescents were selected with the cooperation of the Public Health Department of the University of Trakya, Faculty of Medicine. The data were obtained from all the primary, secondary and high schools of urban and rural areas of the Edirne. At the end of the year 2000, the entire population of the Edirne was determined to be 380000, with 30000 adolescents (49% girls, 51% boys) aged between 12 and 17 years [16]. The percentage of adolescents, aged between 12 and 17 years, attending schools was 91.4% for girls and 91.6% for boys. In both studies, the sample size was determined by the following weighing steps. First, the number of adolescents in the different age groups was determined according to their percentages in the whole population. Second, the number of subjects living in rural and urban areas was determined (while 17.4% of them lived in rural areas, 82.6% lived in urban areas). The number of students that were selected from each school was determined according to the total number of the student population of each school. Finally, the classrooms were chosen in systematic random basis, and each adolescent was determined randomly from the selected classrooms. In these studies, we selected substitutes that represented half of the selected adolescents in each classroom and those individuals were used in case of non-participation of the main list members.

Anthropometric Measurements

The measurements of body height and weight were carried out by two trained pediatricians in the morning when the adolescents were in fasting state. Body weight (in kilograms) was measured to the nearest 0.1 kg with an electronic scale (SECA 762; Vogel and Hakle, Hamburg, Germany). Body height was measured to the nearest 0.5 cm as the adolescents stood erect against a vertical wall mounted scale with heels, buttocks, and occiput in the Frankfort plane with anthropometric square. The adolescents were dressed with light underclothing and wore no shoes throughout the measurements. BMI (kg/m2) was calculated as the ratio of the body weight to the square of body height.

Statistical Analysis

Descriptive statistics on BMI, weight and height measurements were performed. The estimations of the prevalence of overweight and obesity were based on the cut off points of International Obesity Task Force (IOTF) values (in excess of the 85th and 95th percentiles, respectively) [17]. Qui square test was used to compare overweight and obesity prevalence between adolescent girls and boys, between adolescents living in rural area and urban area and between adolescents with and without smoking habits. All statistical analysis was performed using Minitab Release 13, reference number: wcp 1331.00197 (Trakya University, Faculty of Medicine, Data Processing Center).

Results

The sample, representing adolescents aged between 12 and 17 years, consisted of 2029 subjects (991 girls, 1038 boys, 6.7% of the target population). From these records, 92 of them (60 girls, 32 boys) were excluded because of lack of important demographic data such as date of birth. We also excluded 3 adolescents (2 girls, 1 boy) who had growth disturbances due to primary diseases (renal failure, diabetes and malignancy) and 2 adolescents (1 girl, 1 boy) who were receiving high dose steroid therapy for severe asthma. The final sample of this study included 1932 adolescents, representing 95.2% of the original sample (928 of them were girls, 1004 of them were boys) and 6.4% of the target population. While 36.1% of the 1932 adolescents lived in rural area, 63.9% lived in urban area.

In the adolescent girls, the prevalence of overweight and obesity were found to be 9.6% and 3.8%, respectively, while those were 7.8% and 0.7% for adolescent boys, respectively. Overweight and obesity prevalence for different ages of Turkish adolescents are shown in Table 1.

Table 1. Underweight, overweight and obesity prevalence for different ages of Turkish adolescents

	Adolescent girls		**Adolescent boys**	
Age (years)	**Overweight**	**Obesity**	**Overweight**	**Obesity**
12	24 (9.1%)	2 (0.8 %)	19 (10.1%)	0
13	25 (12.4%)	14 (6.9 %)	0	1 (0.6 %)
14	14 (7.8%)	8 (4.4 %)	17 (10.4%)	3 (1.8 %)
15	13 (10.5 %)	4 (3.2 %)	16 (10.7 %)	1 (0.7 %)
16	7 (8.0 %)	5 (5.7 %)	13 (8.4 %)	0
17	6 (8.6 %)	2 (1.9 %)	13 (7.6 %)	2 (1.2 %)
Total	89 (9.6 %)	35 (3.8 %)	78 (7.8 %)	7 (0.7 %)

Table 2. Overweight and obesity prevalence among Turkish adolescents with respect to living areas

	Adolescent girls		**Adolescent boys**	
	Overweight prevalence	**Obesity prevalence**	**Overweight prevalence**	**Obesity prevalence**
Urban	9.3 %	0.9 %	8.6 %	0.6 %
Rural	9.9 %	3.4 %	6.0 %	0.6 %
Total	9.6 %	3.8 %	7.8 %	0.7 %

In our study, adolescent obesity prevalence was found to be higher in girls than in boys ($p<0.05$), although there was no gender difference of overweight prevalence between adolescent girls and boys. In the urban area, the prevalence of overweight and obesity among adolescent girls was 9.3% and 0.9%, while it was 8.6% and 0.6% among boys, respectively. In the rural area; the prevalence of overweight and obesity among adolescent girls was 9.9 % and 3.4 %, while it was 6.0 % and 0.6 % among boys, respectively. Overweight and obesity prevalence among Turkish adolescents with respect to living areas are shown in Table 2.

Smoking habit was not found to be different adolescents with and without obesity or with and without overweight ($p>0.05$ for both).

Discussion

Obesity is currently described as one of the major health problems for all ages [18]. Adolescents, appears to be high risk period for the development of obesity, particularly in girls. Moreover, adolescent obesity is associated with increased morbidity and is more likely to track into adulthood [2,3]. Approximately 10-15% of all obese people were obese during their adolescent period [18]. In the past 10-15 years, the prevalence of overweight and obesity in European and US children has doubled, consequently, it is expected that the prevalence of overweight and obese people will increase up during the next coming years [10,11]. Therefore, prevention and treatment of these co-morbid disorders in adolescence represent a considerable workload for the health system and addressing this public health problem requires intervention at international, national and, local levels [1].

The results of this study indicate that adolescents living in this region of Turkey, have lower obesity prevalence rate than other countries' adolescents have. The reasons for the lower prevalence of obesity among our adolescents are largely unknown. However, it may be mainly due to the genetic factors. Mediterranean type diet which contains more vegetables and less meat and carbohydrate may also contribute these hopeful results.

The prevalence of overweight and obesity in children and adolescents have recently been investigated in different countries. However, there are only a few studies, concerning the prevalence in Turkish adolescents, most published in Turkish Medical Journals. Obesity prevalence was similarly reported to be 0.9 % in adolescent boys and 3.8 % in adolescent girls, in Elazıg, Middle East of Turkey and 6.7% and 2.6, respectively, in Ankara, central Turkey [20,21]. Contrary to these low prevalence rates, Neyzi et al. [22] found higher obesity prevalence such as 11.2 % in adolescent boys, and 9.4 % in adolescent girls in 9-17 years old school children in Istanbul, northwest of Turkey.

The obesity prevalence of children and adolescents in Europe increase gradually when traced towards east and south [11]. Dutch, Belgium and Swedish adolescents are slimmer than Middle and Eastern European adolescent populations [10,23]. On the other hand, Hungarian, Austrian, Croatian adolescents have higher overweight and obesity prevalence [24,25]. Bellizzi et al. [26] compared prevalence of overweight and obesity in 15-year-old boys and girls in different Asian and European countries. Among these populations, the prevalence of total overweight (obesity and overweight) in boys ranged from 5.8% (in the Netherlands) to 30.5% (in Taiwan), and in girls from 6.3% (in Hong Kong) to 21.1% (in Taiwan). In Asia, higher obesity prevalence were found among the Taipei and Saudi Arabian adolescents [4,15]. The prevalence of overweight and obesity in Saudi Arabia among 15-20 years of age subjects were 12% and 7% for boys and 15% ad 9% for girls [4]. In Taiwan, Chu et al. [15] investigated 1366 children, aged 12-15 years and they reported that the prevalence of overweight and obesity were 11.8% and 16.3% for boys and 10.3% and 11.8 for girls, respectively. Similar to our data, the prevalence of overweight and obesity among 17-year-old Israeli conscripts was reported as 11.4% and 3.3% for females and 12.4%, 4.1% for males, respectively [27]. However, their study was performed in the Israel army and it did not have Arabic and orthodox adolescents.

Data from the most recent prevalence studies show that large proportions of the adolescent populations of the America continent are highly overweight or obese and overall, the prevalence of overweight and obesity in American adolescents is relatively high compared to European adolescents [10,11]. The prevalence of overweight in a low-income Mexican American adolescents was reported as high as 40% [28]. In a later study, American National Heath and Nutrition Examination Survey III was determined that 16.3% of the Black, 14% of Hispanic and 9.6% of White, Non-Hispanic adolescent girls are obese. In the same survey, the obese proportion of the US adolescent boys are 15%, 12.5%, 11.6% for Hispanic, Black and Whites, respectively [10]. These high values showed that serious precautions against obesity have to be taken in the USA. In another report, Neutzling et al. from Brazil [5] determined that overweight and obesity prevalence were 6.5% and 1.2% among all adolescents in America continent. He also reported that total overweight prevalence was found to be 10.4% among adolescent girls while 4.8% among adolescent boys. The estimated prevalence of overweight among Australian children and adolescents was also reported to be very high (20%) [29].

Some countries showed significant gender differences in overweight and obesity prevalence of adolescents. In particular, some studies which were performed in Asia and Europe (Taiwan, Finland, Austria and Greece), showed higher rates among adolescent boys than girls [15,23,24,30]. On the other hand, Saudi Arabian and Brazilian adolescents have been demonstrated to have the opposite trend [4,5]. We observed higher obesity prevalence in adolescent girls vs. adolescent boys, like Saudi Arabian and Brazilian adolescents. During puberty, the adolescent girls gain fat storage even during the growth spurt in height. The adolescent boys probably lose fat during the fast pubertal growth. The gender differences for the obesity prevalence in our study could be explained by the more prominent increase of body fat storage in our adolescent girls than in adolescent boys. Differences regarding physical activities may also explain the variation in the prevalence of obesity between the sexes. Longitudinal studies in Europe demonstrated that physical activities drop by 50% between the ages of 12 and 18, when the boys are consistently more active than the girls [31]. A similar decrease occurred in the prevalence of regular, vigorous activity among US adolescents [32].

Recent studies in India and other countries revealed that obesity is becoming a big trouble, especially in urban children and adolescents [27,33,34]. Mamalakis et al. [35] revealed that one reason for the high overweight and obesity prevalence in children and adolescents throughout the world may be attributed to ''post-World War II overfeeding syndrome''. Starvation during the World War II created of the model of the overprotected mother who overfeeds her child. Decreased the physical activity and increased of passive entertainment such as television and computers, contribute to their immobility and this results in obesity.

As overweight and obesity are increasing worldwide, it is important that countries should monitor weight status of their children and adolescents. The critical issue is which definition is used? Although, BMI is a measure of relative weight rather than adiposity, it is recommended widely to determine overweight and obesity among children and adolescents and currently it is preferred by many scientists [36-42]. IOTF recommended the use of BMI percentiles, which have been supplied by the results of the studies conducted on the children 2-18 years old in four continents (Asia, Europe, North and South America), with the aim of bringing an international definition for obesity into use [17]. In the international community, the standard definition was introduced firstly by Cole et al. [17]. It is the most accepted definition and increasingly used by other scientists in the prevalence based studies. Krassas et al. [30] from Thessalonica which is very close to Edirne, used also IOTF standards and he reported high overweight and low obesity results, primarily in adolescent boys. However, there are some suspicions about IOTF standards. Ramachandran et al. [43] reported that the criteria of Cole et al. [17] are not appropriate for determining overweight in Asian-Indian adolescent populations.

Our study emphasize that the prevalence rate of the adolescent obesity throughout the world was alarming. This finding indicates that there is a need for defined strategies and additional resources for obesity management in adolescent clinics. A possible decrease in obesity prevalence among adolescents would depend on two main modifications in food intake and physical activity [44]. Educational programs of intervention aimed to adolescents should encourage regular physical activity and adequate dietary habits. Increased access to fast food habit, high fat and low fiber foods should be restricted.

This article provides descriptive information on the current prevalence of overweight or obese adolescents in the city of Edirne, Turkey. However, it had some limitations. This study was performed cross-sectional and the measurements of the subjects could be performed only once. Therefore, it has not been provided direct indication of the chronology of overweight and obesity development. Despite the limitations, the data described in this study still provides a valuable profile for the physical characteristics of a major segment of the adolescent population of Edirne. New longitudinal studies are needed for better estimation of adolescents' body fat status in the future.

Acknowledgement

I would like to acknowledge the contributions of Professor Serap Karasalihoğlu, Asistant Professor Ülfet Vatansever, Asistant Professor Hakan Erbaş, Dr. Çağrı Turan, Dr. Hülya Tuğrul Beyzadeoğlu, Dr. Sebahattin Şit, Dr. Güner Emel Yolsal, Dr. Hülya Karaca, Dr. Evrim Seçkin, Dr. Sema Can, Dr. Güler Ateş in regional data collection and handling.

References

[1] Barlow SE, Dietz WH. Obesity evaluation and treatment: Expert Committee recommendations. The Maternal and Child Health Bureau, Health Resources and Services Administration and the Department of Health and Human Services. *Pediatrics* 1998; 102:E29.

[2] Bandini LG. Natural history of obesity. *Nestle Nutrition Workshop Series Pediatric Program* 2001; 49:20-22.

[3] Must A, Strauss RS. Risk and consequences of childhood and adolescent obesity. *Int J Obes 1999*; 23 Supp 2:S2-11.

[4] al-Nuaim AR, al-Rubeaan, al-Mazrou, al-Attas O, al-Gaghari N, Khoja T. High prevalence of overweight and obesity in Saudi Arabia. *Int J Obes Relat Metab Disord* 1996; 20:547-552.

[5] Neutzling MB, Taddei JA, Rodrigues EM, Sigulem DM. Overweight and obesity in Brazilian adolescents. *Int J Obes Relat Metab Disord* 2000; 24:869-874.

[6] Kelsey JL. Epidemiology of slipped capital femoral epiphysis: a review of the literature. *Pediatrics* 1973;51:1042-1050.

[7] Franseze A, Vajro P, Argenziano A, Puzziello A, Iannucci MP, Saviano MC, Brunetti F, Rubino A. Liver involvement in obese children. Ultrasonography and liver enzyme levels at diagnosis and during follow-up in an Italian population. *Dig Dis Sci* 1997;42:1428-1432.

[8] Mallory GB Jr, Fiser DH, Jackson R. Sleep-associated breathing disorders in morbidity obese children and adolescents. *J Pediatr* 1989;115:892-897.

[9] Whithlock EP, Williams SB, Gold R, Smith PR, Shipman PR. Screening and interventions for childhood overweight: a summary of evidence for the US preventive services task force. *Pediatrics* 2005;116:e125-144.

[10] Troiano RP, Flegal KM, Kuczmarski RJ, Campbell SM, Johnson CL. Overweight prevalence and trends for children and adolescents. The National Health and Nutrition Examination Surveys, 1963 to 1991. *Arch Pediatr Adolesc Med* 1995; 149:1085-1091.

[11] Wabitsch M. Overweight and obesity in the European Children and adolescents, *Eur J Pediatr* 2000; 159 Suppl 1: S5-7.

[12] de Onis M, Blössner M. Prevalence and trends of overweight among preschool children in developing countries. *Am J Clin Nutr* 2000; 72:1032-1039.

[13] Martorell R, Kettel Khan L, Hughes ML, Grummer-Strawn LM. Overweight and obesity in preschool children from developing countries. *Int J Obes Relat Metab Disord* 2000; 24:959-967.

[14] Kelishadi R, Pour MH, Sarraf-Zadegan N et al. Obesity and associated modifiable environmental factors in Iranian adolescents: Isfahan Health Heart Program- Heart Health Promotion from Childhood. *Pediatr Intern* 2002; 45:435-442.

[15] Chu NF. Prevalence and trends of obesity among children in Taiwan –the Taipei Children Heart Study. *Int J Obes Relat Metab Disord* 2001; 25:170-176.

[16] 2000 Turkey Census of Population. State Institute of Statistics Prime Ministry Republic of Turkey, Printing Division, Ankara, 2002.

[17] Cole TJ, Bellizzi MC, Flegal KM, Dietz WH. Establishing a standard definition for child overweight and obesity worldwide: international survey. *BMJ* 2000; 320: 1270-1273.

[18] Maffeis C, Talamini G, Tato L. Influence of diet, physical activity, and parent's obesity on children's adiposity: a four year longitudinal study. *Int J Obes* 1998;22: 758-64.

[19] Ackard DM, Neumark-Sztainer D, Story M, Perry C. Overeating among adolescents: prevalence and associations with weight-related characteristics and psychological health. *Pediatrics* 2003;111:67-74.

[20] Aygün D, Akarsu S, Yenioğlu H, Kocabay K, Güvenç H. Elazığ il merkezinde adolesan çağda obezite prevalansı. Fırat Tıp Dergisi 1997; 1:1167-1170.

[21] Giray M, Tarım Ö, Kınık E. Adolesansta obesite. *Çocuk Sağlığı ve Hastalıkları Dergisi* 1992;35:1-10.

[22] Neyzi O, Saner G, Alp H et al.. Relationships between bodyweight in infancy and weight in later childhood and adolescence. In: Z. Laron, editor. Pediatric and Adolescent Endocrinology. Vol 1. *Basel, Karger*, 1976, 89-93.

[23] Livingstone B. Epidemiology of childhood obesity in Europe. *Eur J Pediatr* 2000; 159 Suppl 1: S14-34.

[24] Elmadfa I, Godina-Zarfl B, Konig J, Dichtl M, Faist V. Prevalence of overweight and plasma lipids in 7-18 year old Austrian children and adolescents. *Int J Obes Relat Metab Disord* 1993; 17 Suppl 2:35.

[25] Prebeg Z, Juresa V, Kujundzig M. Secular growth changes in Zagreb schoolchildren over four decades, 1951-91. *Ann Hum Biol* 1995; 22:99-110.

[26] Bellizzi MC, Horgan GW, Guillaume M, Dietz WH. Prevalence of childhood and adolescent overweight and obesity in Asian and European countries. *Nestle Nutrition Workshop Series Pediatric Program* Volume 49; 2001:4-6.

[27] Dayan YB, Elishkevits K, Grotto I, Goldstein L, Goldberg A, Shvarts S, Levin A, Ohana N, Onn E, Levi Y, Dayan YB. The prevalence of obesity and associated morbidity among 17-year-old Israeli conscript. *Public Health* 2005;119:385-389.

[28] Lacar ES, Soto X, Riley WJ. Adolescent obesity in a low-income Mexican American district in south Texas. *Arch Pediatr Adolesc Med* 2000;154:837-840.

[29] Booth ML, Chey T, Wake M, Norton K, Hesketh K, Dollman J, Robertson I. Change in the prevalence of overweight an obesity among young Australians, 1996-1997. *Am J Clin Nutr* 2003;77:29-36.

[30] Krassas GE, Tzotzas T, Tsametis C, Konstantinidis T. Prevalence and trends in overweight and obesity among children and adolescents in Thessalonica, Greece. *J Pediatr Endocrinol Metab* 2001 Suppl 5:S1327-1333.

[31] Meredith CN, Dwyer JT. Nutrition and exercise: effects on adolescent health. *A Rev Public Health* 1991;12:309-333.

[32] CDC. Vigorous physical activity among high school students-United States, 1990. *Morbid Mortal Weekly Rep* 1992;41:33-35.

[33] Callahan ST, Mansfield MJ. Type 2 diabetes mellitus in adolescents. *Curr Opin Pediatr* 2000;12:310-315.

[34] Acton KJ, Burrows NR, Moore K, Querec L, Geiss LS, Engelgau MM. Trends in diabetes prevalence among American Indian and Alaska native children, adolescents, and young adults. *Am J Public Health* 2002;92:1485-1490.

[35] Mamalakis G, Kafatos A. Prevalance of obesity in Greece. *Int J Obes Relat Metab Disord* 1996;20:488-492.

[36] Dietz WH, Bellizzi MC: Introduction: the use of body mass index to assess obesity in children. *Am J Clin Nutr* 1999; 70:123S-125S.

[37] Rosner B, Prineas P, Loggie J, Daniels SR. Percentiles for body mass index in U.S. children 5 to 17 years of age. *J Pediatr* 1998; 132:211-222.

[38] Hosseini M, Carpenter RG, Mohammad K, Jones ME. Standardized percentile curves of body mass index of Iranian children compared to the US population reference. *Int J Obes Relat Metab Disord* 1999; 23:783-787.

[39] He Q, Albertson-Wikland K, Karlherg I. Population-based body mass index reference values from Gothenburg, Sweden: birth to 18 years of age. *Acta Paediatr* 2000; 89: 582-592.

[40] Savva SC, Kourides Y, Tornaritis M, Epiphaniou-Savva M, Tafouna P, Kafatos A. Reference growth curves for Cypriot children 6 to 17 years of age. *Obes Res* 2001; 9:754-762.

[41] Must A, Dallal GE, Dietz WH. Reference data for obesity: 85th and 95th percentiles of body mass index (wt/ht^2) and triceps skin fold thickness. *Am J Clin Nutr* 1991; 53: 839-846.

[42] Cole TJ, Freeman JV, Preece MA. Body mass index reference curves for the UK 1990. *Arch Dis Child* 1991; 73:25-29.

[43] Ramachandran A, Snehalatha C, Vinitha R et al. Prevalence of overweight in urban Indian adolescent school children. *Diabetes Research and Clinical Practice* 2002; 57:185-190.

[44] Munsch S, Biedert E, Keller U. Evaluation of a lifestyle change programme for the treatment of obesity in general practice. *Swiss Med Wkly* 2003;133:148-154.

In: Global Dimensions of Childhood Obesity
Editor: Richard K. Flamenbaum, pp. 99-126
ISBN: 1-60021-037-6

Chapter 5

MAGNITUDE AND POSSIBLE CONTRIBUTORS OF CHILDHOOD OBESITY IN IRAN: IMPLICATION FOR ACTION

***Behnoush Mohammadpour-Ahranjani*[1], *Arash Rashidi*[1], *Majid Karandish*[2], *Mohammad-Reza Vafa*[1]**
[1]National Nutrition and Food Technology Research Institute, Shaheed Beheshti University of Medical Sciences and Health Services, Tehran, Iran
[2]Faculty of Paramedical Sciences, Ahwaz Jondi-Shapour University of Medical Sciences and Health Services, Ahwaz, Iran

Abstract

This chapter is intended to propose potential strategies and programmes based on the magnitude of overweight and obesity problem among Iranian children as well as an analysis of its possible contributing factors. The chapter includes four sections. In section one, we present international and (sub) national evidence on the prevalence of overweight and obesity in children and adolescents. This will allow us 1) to show the magnitude and trend of the problem; 2) to conduct a comparative study between current figures and the corresponding results reported from other countries (both developing and developed); 3) to make comparison between Iranian children and the reference population; and 4) to draw a geographical map of childhood overweight in Iran. In section two a brief discussion on possible contributing factors of overweight and obesity found by different studies is presented. In the third section, based on the facts and findings presented in the section two as well as available studies and statistics on biological and socio-economic variables and characteristics in Iran, an analysis towards determination of the most relevant contributing factors for overweight and obesity among Iranian children is discussed. Finally in the last section, we briefly suggest potential strategies and programmes aiming at prevention of childhood and adolescence obesity.

Introduction

Overweight/obesity, as one of the main features of epidemiological transition, has emerged as a serious health problem first in developed and nowadays in developing countries during recent decades. This phenomenon, whether simply considered as a pathologic condition and/or a normal physiologic response to a pathologic environment, can not only increase the incidence and prevalence of many common chronic non-communicable patho-physiological as well as patho-psychological conditions (see below), but also can significantly result in economic consequences, including lower productivity (through decreased work capacity and increased work absenteeism), and increased ill health- and therapeutic-related expenditures [Wang G & Dietz WH, 2002; Anderson et al., 2003; Andreyeva et al., 2004; Raebel et al., 2004; Wee et al., 2005].

Available evidence suggests that increased prevalence of obesity has been a major factor in decreasing the onset age of type 2 diabetes mellitus and therefore its increasing burden on children. In addition, a vast number of studies show that diabetes has the biggest share in increased prevalence of CVD in both developed and developing societies. Similarly, many investigators have shown that the risk of asthma, stroke, hypertension, dislipidemias and some types of cancers are significantly increased by obesity [Dietz, 1998; Young et al., 2001; Eisenstein et al., 2002; Sorof & Daniels, 2002; Goran et al., 2003; Caterson et al., 2004; AIHW/NHFA, 2004; Hope et al., 2005]. Psychological problems such as shame and depression caused by discrimination and stigmatisation of obese individuals should also be added to this list [Puhl & Brownell, 2001; Sjöberg et al., 2005].

Finally it could be concluded that the problem of obesity and its complications in a developed country like US are so serious that can threaten all health achievements in terms of quality of life and life expectancy in recent decades [Olshansky et al., 2005].

1 Prevalence of Childhood Overweight and Obesity in the World

An estimated 17.6 million children under five are overweight worldwide. The prevalence of obese children aged 6 to 11 years old has more than doubled since the 1960s [WHO/FAO, 2003]. It has been appeared that the number of overweight and obesity among children living in less-industrialised world, due to their population, is a main component of the above-mentioned figure. Causes of this epidemic will be discussed in detail later in this chapter. In the present section, results obtained from a few representing countries have been mentioned to discuss more in detail the extent and trends of overweight and obesity problem among children living in developed as well as developing countries and Iran.

1.1 Industrialised Countries

The United States is the unique example of a country where has been geared in a massive overweight epidemic among its children. Trend studies show that the number of 6-11 yr children and adolescents who are overweight has more than doubled and tripled, respectively, in the past 20 years (Table 1) [Ogden et al., 2002]. It has been appeared that boys and girls are equally affected.

Table 1. Trend of overweight prevalence in the U.S. children/adolescents

Age group (yr)	Prevalence of overweight		
	1976-1980	1984-1988	1999-2000
2-5	na	7.0	10.5
6-11	6.5	11.5	15.5
12-19	5.0	10.5	15.7

na: not available

Overweight is more common among ethnic minorities in the United States. Prevalence proportions in 2-5, 6-11 and 12-19 yr African-American children are 8.4, 19.5 and 23.6%, respectively. Among Mexican American children, the corresponding values are 11.1, 23.7 and 23.4%, respectively. African-Americans and Mexican Americans have experienced more dramatic increases in the prevalence of obesity during the last 20 years than white Americans [Anjali, 2004; Chopra et al., 2002].

The same phenomenon, however milder than that is seen among the American children, has occurred over the last 20 years in European countries. In the majority of these countries, the prevalence of obesity increased by 10-40% between 1980 and late 1990s. Current prevalence of obesity in European countries is in the range of 10-20 and 10-25% among male and female population, respectively. The United Kingdom has had the fastest growth of obesity in Europe [Anjali, 2004; Garrow et al., 2002].

Since increase in the prevalence of overweight among children mirrors the pattern in adults, these general observations provide equal concern for the younger generation [Chinn et al., 1994]. For example, a study among under-five children in the UK showed a significant increase in childhood obesity within 10 years (1989-98). There was a 60 and 70% increase in the prevalence of overweight and obesity (defined respectively as BMI above the 85th and 95th percentiles of reference population) among British children aged 3 to 4 years. It was found that the proportion of children who were overweight increased from 15% in 1989 to 24% in 1998; the corresponding figures for obese children were 5 and 9%, respectively [Bundred et al. 2001].

Different studies from 1980s onwards conducted in European countries have shown that prevalence of overweight is higher among the populations living in southern countries (e.g. Hungry, Italy, and Greece), especially those outside the former eastern bloc [Biró, 1993; Beccaria et al., 2000; Kafatos et al., 1981; Elmadfa et al., 1993; De Spiegelaere et al., 1998; Power et al., 1997]. The formerly non-eastern bloc countries surrounding the Mediterranean show prevalence proportion of childhood overweight in the range of 20–40%, while those in northern areas are in the range of 10–20% [Anonymous, 2002; Lobstein & Frelut, 2003].

The number of children affected by overweight and obesity is now rising at more than 400,000 a year across the EU, including accession countries in 2002. The prevalence of 24% in 2002 is already higher than the predictions for the year 2010. Presently it is estimated that 14 million children are overweight [IOTF, 2004].

In Australia, between 1985 and 1997, the prevalence of overweight and obesity was doubled among young people [Booth et al., 2003].

1.2 Developing Countries

No longer confined to well-fed, high-income countries, the epidemic of obesity is spreading rapidly among developing nations [Friedrich, 2002]. Consistent data have shown the increasing prevalence of childhood overweight and obesity in almost all developing countries in the Latin America, Asia and Africa.

de Onis and Blössner reviewed 160 nationally representative cross-sectional surveys on overweight and obesity from 94 countries. The global prevalence of overweight was 3.3%. Some countries and regions (e.g., northern and southern Africa and South America; Qatar, Uzbekistan, South Africa, Kuwait, Morocco, Malawi, Egypt, Costa Rica, Bahrain and Armenia) had considerably higher rates. Overweight was shown to increase in 16 of 38 countries with trend data [de Onis & Blössner, 2000].

Martorell et al. using national surveys conducted in 13 Latin American countries during 1980s and 1990s showed that the prevalence of overweight (defined as >1SD of mean weight-for-height) among 1-5 yr children ranged from 6 (Haiti) to 24% (Peru), with higher prevalence among urban and richer households [Martorell et al, 1998].

A recent survey in Cuba has shown that overweight in preschool children is the most frequent nutritional problem within the country, with a prevalence of 5.2 % (Pařízková & Hills, 2001).

In Chile, Kain et al. have shown that the prevalence of obesity ($\geq 95^{th}$ percentile of BMI; CDC Reference) among 6 years old male and female children increased, respectively, from 5.1 to 14.7% and 4.0 to 15.8% between 1987-2000 (Kain et al., 2002).

Rio-Navarro et al. using data from the Mexican National Health Survey 2000 showed that overweight prevalence varied by age from 10.8 to 16.1% among 10-17 yrs boys and 14.3 to 19.1% among girls within the same age range; obesity prevalence were between 9.2 to 14.7% in boys and 6.8 to 10.6% in girls [Rio-Navarro et al., 2004].

Childhood obesity is also a fast emerging problem in Asia [Hara, 1988]. The prevalence of obesity in Chinese children increased from 2.1 to 5 % during 1986-98 [Pařízková & Hills, 2001]. The prevalence of childhood obesity in China reached 7.1 and 8.3% in Beijing and Shanghai, respectively, in year 2000 [WHO, 2000]. A population study on 6-12 year old children of Bangkok (Thailand) showed a fast increase of obesity from 12.2% in 1991 to 15.6% in 1993 [Pařízková & Hills, 2001]. In Malaysia, obesity has increased from 1% in 1990 to 6% in 1997 among 13-17 year-olds [Ismail & Vicknewar, 1999].

Among west Asian countries, Arab states have also encountered the problem of childhood obesity during recent past 2 decades. For example, El-Hazmi and Warsy showed that the prevalence of overweight among 1-18 yr olds Saudi children was 10.7 and 12.7% among boys and girls, respectively; obesity was found in 6 and 6.7% of boys and girls, respectively [EL-Hazmi & Warsy, 2002]. The maximum prevalence of obesity was seen among 2-3 yrs old children in both genders. Similar evidence has been provided from other Arab countries such as Bahrain, Kuwait, United Arab Emirates, and Lebanon (Table 2).

Although Africa is the continent with the highest prevalence of under-nutrition, it seems that even in this region the problem of overweight and obesity is increasing. For example, in a Yaoundé population, 18.2 % of girls and 1.7 % of boys aged 12-19 years were obese [Oppert & Rolland-Cachera, 1998]. Coexistence of wasting with an emergent obesity among 3 to 6 year old children in Cape Town population has been shown [Bourne et al, 1994].

Table 2. Prevalence of overweight and obesity among children in some countries in the Middle East

Country/City	Sex	Age	Sample Size	Prevalence (%)		Index/ Reference	Reference
				Overweight	Obesity		
Lebanon/ Beirut	M F	6-8 6-8	131 103	26 25	7 6	BMI/ IOTF	*Jabre et al. 2005*
Turkey/ Central Edirne	M F	12-17 12-17	538 526	11.3 10.6	1.6 2.1	BMI/ IOTF	*Oner et al. 2004*
Kuwait	M F	10-14 10-14	7205 7454	30 31.8	14.7 13.1	BMI/ NCHS	*Al-Isa 2004*
United Arab Emirates	F	11-18	898	14	9	BMI/ NHANES	*Al-Hourani et al. 2003*
Bahrain	M F	12-17 12-17	249 257		21 35	BMI/ WHO	*Al-Sendi et al. 2003*
Saudi Arabia/ Riyadh	M	12-20	894	13.8	20.5	BMI	*Al-Rukban 2003*
Kuwait	M F	0-5 0-5	3749 3670		7.5 9.0	Weight for Height/ NCHS/CDC	*Al-Isa & Moussa 1998*

Ansa et al. reported the prevalence of obesity among 6-12, 13-15 and 16-18 yr Nigerian children as 2.3, 4 and 3 %, respectively [Ansa et al. 2001]. Salzar-Martinez et al. has recently reported the prevalence of overweight and obesity as 12.1 and 6.2%, respectively among children and adolescents in Egypt [Salazar-Martinez et al. 2006].

1.3 Iran

Overweight and obesity among Iranian children and adolescents have been recently considered as a public health issue [Mohammadpour-Ahranjani et al., 2004; Mirmiran et al., 2003]. During last decades, investigators mainly focused on thinness, underweight and stunting. In spite of evidence which suggest that energy-protein undernutrition, and micronutrients deficiencies still exist among Iranian children [Mohammadpour-Ahranjani et al., 2004; MOH/NNFTRI, 2001; NNFTRI, 2002], epidemiologic and nutrition transition phenomena [Ghassemi et al., 2002] have persuaded researchers to carry out over-nutrition-related studies [Mohammadpour-Ahranjani et al., 2004; Dorosty et al., 2002; Kelishadi et al., 2003].

In this section, studies have been divided to 2 categories based on their coverage (i.e. national and sub-national). We reviewed those studies which have been published in 2000 onwards using age-specific BMI to define overweight and obesity. In 2 national studies on under-5 and 6 yr children, described below, underweight and overweight were defined as weight-for-age <2SD and >2SD of NCHS reference values, respectively. In all other studies overweight, pre-obesity, and obesity were defined as BMI $\geq 85^{th}$, 85th-95th, and $\geq 95^{th}$ percentile of age and sex-specific BMI values, respectively.

Table 3. Prevalence of pre-obesity and obesity among 5-19 yr Iranian children

Weight Status Age group (yr)	Boys				Girls			
	Pre-obese N (%)		Obese N (%)		Pre-obese N (%)		Obese N (%)	
	Urban	Rural	Urban	Rural	Urban	Rural	Urban	Rural
5-10	82(6.9)	46(4.8)	68(5.8)	18(1.9)	68(6.1)	35(3.8)	36(3.2)	19(2.1)
11-14	100(8.9)	26(3.5)	42(3.7)	18(2.4)	107(9.1)	54(6.6)	43(3.6)	21(2.6)
15-19	99(6.9)	31(4.2)	65(4.6)	12(1.6)	175(10.8)	87(9.1)	66(4.1)	30(3.2)

Ref. NNFTRI, 2001-03.

Table 4. Prevalence of pre-obesity and obesity among 14-20 yr Iranian adolescents

Code	Region	Boys		Girls	
		Pre-obesity	Obesity	Pre-obesity	Obesity
1	Tehran Province	10.1	4.7	9.1	2.1
2	Gilan and Mazandaran	8	4	15.5	5.8
3	East and West Azarbayejan and Ardebil	4.6	2.3	8.8	3
4	Charmahal-and-Bakhtiari, Isfahan, Yazd and north of Kerman	3	0.8	7	2.3
5	Zanjan, Qazvin, Qom, and Markazi	4.2	2.5	8.7	1.7
6	Hormozgan, Boushehr and south of Khouzestan	4.7	2	9.5	4.3
7	South of Khorasan, Sistan-and-Balouchestan and south of Kerman	2.5	2.5	6	3.8
8	Golestan and north of Khorasan	5.3	1.5	7.8	2.8
9	Semnan and centre of Khorasan	5.3	2	8	2
10	Kordestan, Hamedan, Lorestan, Kermanshah, Ilam and north of Khouzestan	2.8	1.5	8.7	2.5
11	Fars, Kohkilouyeh and Boyerahmad, and centre of Kerman	4	0.8	5.8	2.8
-	Total	5.3	2.4	8.7	2.8

Ref. MOH/NNFTRI, 2005

1.3.1 National Studies

In the "National Comprehensive Study on Household Food Consumption Pattern and Nutritional Status in Iran (2001-2003)", height and weight were measured in all household members in a nationally representative sample [NNFTRI[1], 2001-03]. The results are shown in graph 1 and Table 4 (figures of underweight are also included to emphasise that this type of malnutrition is still of great importance among under-5 Iranian children, especially in rural areas).

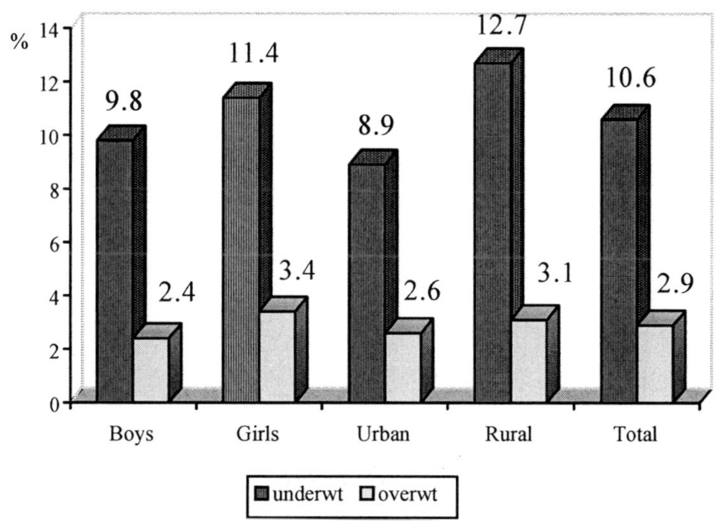

Ref. NNFTRI, 2001-03

Figure 1. Prevalence of under- and overweight among under-5 children in Iran

Another recent national survey was "National Assessment of Iron, Zinc, Vitamin A and Vitamin D in Different Age Groups, 2001" in which data on the prevalence of overweight among 6 yr as well as 14-20 yr children were collected [MOH[2]/NNFTRI, 2005]. In this study, 28 provinces of Iran were classified to 11 regions based on their health and nutritional profiles. Relevant findings are presented in figures 2 and 3 and Table 4. Significant inter-regional and gender differences are seen in the prevalence of overweight.

1.3.2 Sub-national Studies

Studies in Tehran. Tehran, as the biggest and most populated district in Iran, has its special characteristics which make it different from all other districts. Adoption of modern life style, higher food availability, easier access to facilities, air pollution (which significantly decrease the level of physical activity), and environmental design, result in a considerable distinct pattern of behaviours and diseases compared to other geographical locations in the country.

[1] National Nutrition and Food Technology Research Institute
[2] Ministry of Health

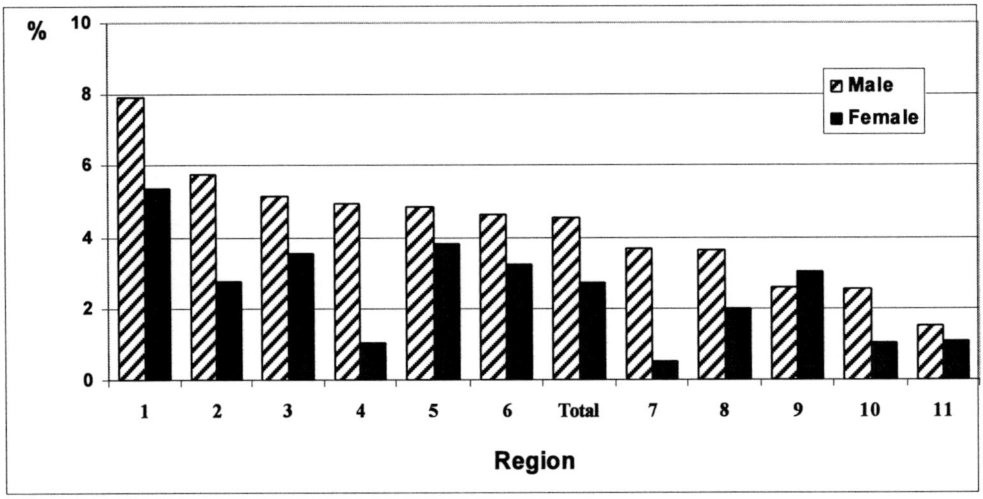

Definition of region numbers (codes) is given in Table 4. Ref. MOH/NNFTRI, 2005

Figure 2. Prevalence of overweight among 6 yr Iranian children by region and gender

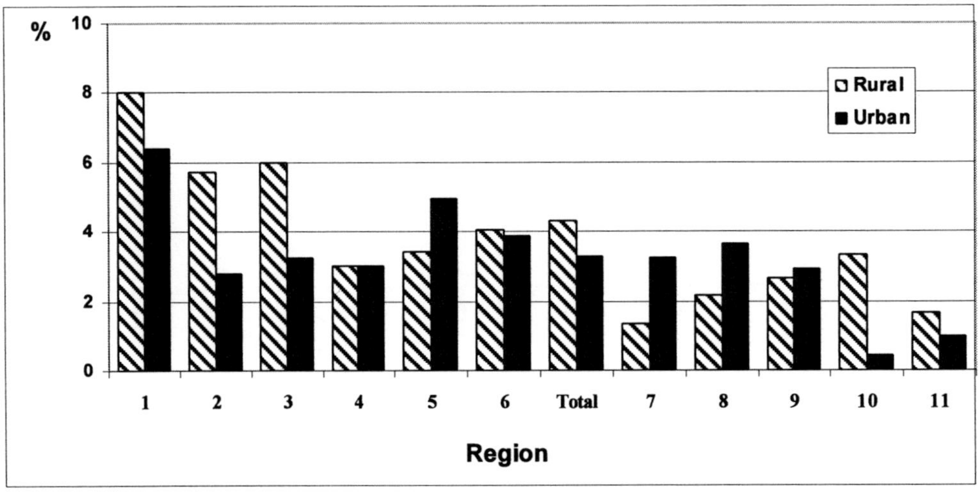

Definition of region numbers (codes) is given in Table 4. Ref. MOH/NNFTRI, 2005

Figure 3. Prevalence of overweight among Iranian 6-yr children by region and place of residence.

In table 5, prevalence of pre-obesity and obesity among Tehrani children and adolescents by gender are presented (based on data collected in the "National Comprehensive Study on Household Food Consumption Pattern and Nutritional Status in Iran (2001-2003)") [NNFTRI, 2001-03]

Table 5. Prevalence of pre-obesity and obesity among Tehrani children and adolescents by gender

Total		Girls		Boys		Age group
Obesity	**Pre-obesity**	**Obesity**	**Pre-obesity**	**Obesity**	**Pre-obesity**	
6.5	9.8	4.9	7.6	7.9	11.7	**5-10**
5.8	11.7	5.4	12.3	6.3	11.1	**11-14**
4.4	9.4	3.5	11.1	5.5	7.3	**15-19**

Ref. NNFTRI, 2001-03

Another recent study in Tehran city (2000-01) showed that 21.1 and 7.8% of adolescent students (11-16 yrs) were overweight and obesity, respectively. Prevalence of overweight in girls (23.1%) was significantly ($p<0.001$) higher than boys (18.8%) [Mohammadpour-Ahranjani et al., 2004].

Dadkhah et al. in 2003 reported that prevalence of overweight among 15-17 yr female students in one of the representative educational zones in Tehran city was 20.5% [Dadkhah et al., 2004].

Results of an analysis in a selected population (n=421) of a cohort study which has been performed in one of the municipal zone in Tehran city, showed that prevalence of overweight in 10-19 yr boys and girls were 10.7 and 18.4%, respectively. Prevalence of obesity was reported as 5.1 and 2.8%, respectively [Azizi et al., 2001].

In another recent study, prevalence of overweight and obesity among 6-14 yr male students (n=3782) was in the range of 5-12 and 3-5%, respectively [Ashrafi et al., 2001].

Studies in other cities/provinces. Ghavamzadeh conducted an overweight prevalence study in a representative sample of 7-18 yr primary, secondary and high school students in 2002 in *Urmia* city (north-west Iran) [Ghavamzadeh, 2004]. The study methodology was the same as Mohamadpour-Ahranjani's study in Tehran city (see above) which made the between-city comparisons possible. Prevalence of overweight among 7-10, 11-14, and 15-18 yr boys were found to be 13.3, 13.6, and 12.9%, respectively. Corresponding figures among girls were 15.4, 14.4 and 15.7%, respectively.

In another study among 1518 girl students aged 14-20 in *Tabriz* city (north-west Iran), prevalence of overweight was found to be 14.6% (with 11.1% pre-obesity) [Gargari et al., 2004].

Prevalence of overweight and obesity in 14-17 yr girl students (n=400) in *Lahijan* city (north Iran), was 14.8 and 5.3%, respectively [Bajan, 2002].

In a survey conducted among 4315 2-5 yr children using IOTF reference to define overweight and obesity in two provinces of Iran with totally different socio-economic status, i.e. *Sistan-and-Baloochestan* (as a poor province; south-west Iran) and *Gilan* (as an affluent province; north Iran), prevalence of overweight and obesity among 2-3 yr children were 23.5 and 10.9%, respectively. In 4-5 yr children, prevalence reported as 18.3 and 7.5%. Differences in overweight and obesity prevalence were not significant between provinces [Dorosty et al., 2002].

Results of a study performed in 3953 children and adolescents between the ages of 6 and 17 years in *Ahwaz* city (south-west Iran), showed that 18 and 17% of boys and girls were overweight, respectively. Prevalence of obesity in boys and girls were 9.2 and 5.7%, respectively [Veisi & karandish, 2002].

The prevalence of overweight was reported as 7.4 and 10.7% in male and female adolescents aged 11-18 yr in *Arak* and *Isfahan* cities (central Iran), respectively.The prevalence of obesity was 1.9 and 2.9% among girls and boys, respectively [Kelishadi et al., 2003].

Map of overweight in 5-19 yr Iranian children produced based on data collected in the "National Comprehensive Study on Household Food Consumption Pattern and Nutritional Status in Iran (2001-2003)" is shown in figure 4.

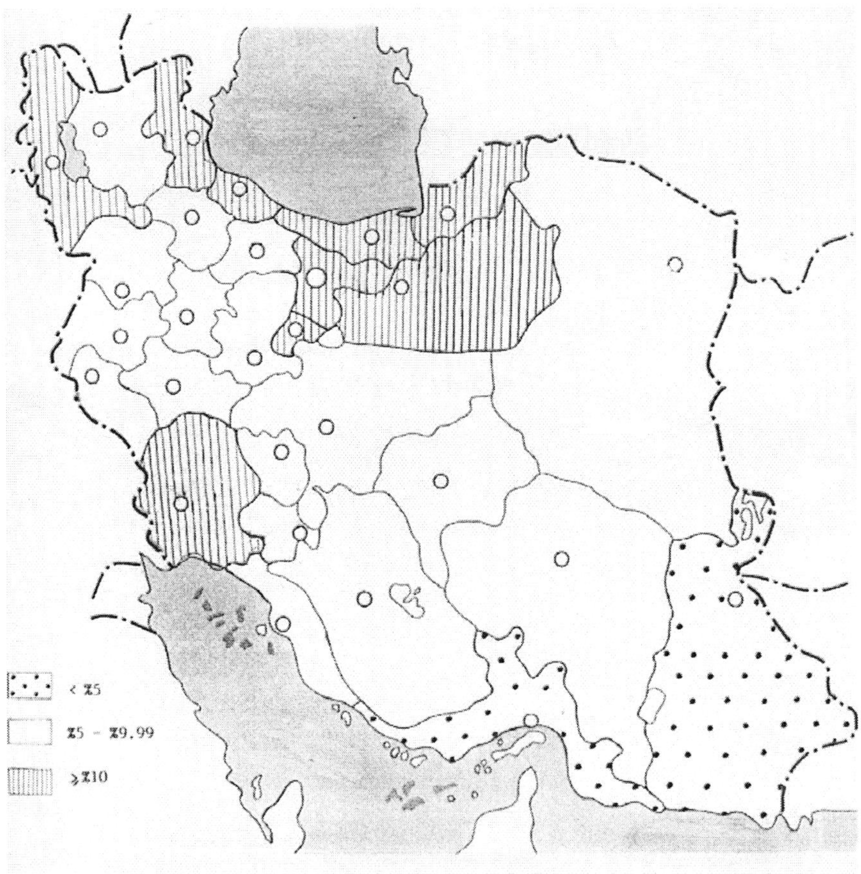

Ref. NNFTRI, 2001-03

Figure 4. Distribution of overweight among 5-19 yr children and adolescents in Iran

2 Determinants and Risk-Factors for Overweight and Obesity

2.1 Food and Nutrition Transition: Popkin's Hypothesis

Using food and nutrition data from developed countries, Barry Popkin in 1993 coined the term "Food and Nutrition Transition (FNT)" to explain the dramatic changes happened in food and nutrition situation among populations over time [Popkin, 1993]. The phenomenon has simultaneously occurred with other well-known transitions, i.e. "epidemiologic" and "demographic" transitions as well as the "technologic revolution". The concept of epidemiologic transition, proposed by Abdel Omran [Omran, 1971], describes the shift from a pattern of high prevalence of infectious diseases and nutritional deficiencies, resulting from pestilence, famine, and poor environmental sanitation, to a pattern of high prevalence of chronic and degenerative diseases strongly associated with lifestyle. Demographic transition describes the shift from a pattern of high fertility and high mortality to one of low fertility and low mortality, typical of modern industrial nations [Popkin et al., 2001]. Migration from rural to urban areas is also part of the latter transition. Finally, technologic progress has not only decreased the amount of energy needed for typical rural activities, but also changed the activity pattern into a much more sedentary one (e.g. by introducing cars and motorbikes, TV and computers, lifts, etc.)

In the first paper on FNT, Popkin explained the changes in diet and other lifestyle characteristics in five patterns of collection of food, famine, receding famine, degenerative diseases, and behavioural change [Popkin, 1993]. The "earlier" patterns are not restricted to the periods in which they first arose, but continue to characterise certain geographic and socioeconomic subpopulations [Popkin, 2001]. From the available evidence it could be seen that changes similar to those have occurred in developed countries are rapidly happening in most developing countries.

The FNT itself is marked by a shift from relatively monotonous diets based on indigenous staple grains or starchy roots, locally grown legumes, other vegetables and fruits, and (except for prosperous subpopulations) limited foods of animal origins, toward more varied diets that include more pre-processed food, more foods of animal origins, more sugar and fat, especially in processed drinks and foods, and often more alcohol. The most immediate result of the combination of such relatively energy-dense diets with physically inactive lives is a rapid increase in overweight and obesity. This is a usual, though not inevitable, consequence of urbanisation [Popkin et al., 2001].

Many researchers seeking to explain the worldwide increases in childhood obesity emphasise similar basic dietary changes within the developing world as a result of rapid globalisation and urbanisation [Brody, 2002]. With replacing industrialised agro-food systems for local subsistence farming, massive population move to urban areas has taken place [Cleves, 1993]. Demographic trend studies show that the number of Asian mega-cities (>8 million population) will increase from 2 in 1970 to 19 by 2015 [Popkin, 2001]. Other accompanying changes related to physical activity levels are inexpensive public transportation as well as communication systems [Schneider, 2000; Sobal, 2001], lack of safe play-grounds for children [Schneider, 2000], and dependence on mechanised transportation from suburbs to cities [Brody, 2002]. These factors can increase the risk of overweight and obesity in all population groups, including children.

Detailed reviews on FNT at global level [Popkin & Caballero, 2002; Popkin et al., 2002; Popkin, 2004] are recommended for interested readers.

2.2 Genetic and Biological Determinants of Overweight/Obesity

2.2.1 Genetic Factors

Evidence supports genetic predisposition to obesity. Children of obese parents have a higher risk of becoming obese. Many researchers showed that adopted children as adults had greater similarity in BMI and other features with their biological than their adopting parents [Maffeis et al., 1994]. Genes can contribute to obesity in a variety of ways: variations in metabolism, fat cell number, and how excess fat is distributed in the body (fat location). Resting metabolic rate (RMR) is also under genetic control. RMR is associated with the amount of energy expended during inactivity. It accounts for approximately 70% of daily energy expenditure in sedentary individuals [Ravussin & Bogardus, 1992] and can vary greatly between individuals (by as much as 1,000 Calories per day) [Foster et al., 1988]. Although the main determinant of RMR is the amount of fat-free mass, the RMR of individuals with the same fat-free mass and of the same age and gender can differ greatly [Brownell & Wadden, 1992]. Astrup et al. conducted a meta-analysis to investigate this relationship further. These authors found that formerly obese individuals had a 3-5% lower RMR than a never-obese control group of individuals [Astrup et al., 1999]. It is however difficult to determine if those previously obese individual had a lower RMR because of their weight loss (i.e. adaptive response) or because of their biological make-up. Several other physiological characteristics that may be genetically determined can mediate the regulation of body weight; some of these include neurotransmitters, the endocrine system, the gastrointestinal tract, adipose tissue, thermogenesis, and appetite and satiety [Beamer, 2003; Clark & Goldstein, 1995]. A genetic predisposition towards anxiety or depression can also contribute to obesity in some individuals. The genetics of obesity and the various studies of twins, families, adoption and populations have been well documented [Bouchard & Perusse, 1993].

It seems that the genetic effects account for at least 25-30% of obesity in the overall population [Bouchard & Perusse, 1993]. More recently estimates however run as high as 50-70% [Beamer, 2003]. Several single-gene mutations have been shown to cause obesity in animal models, however, the situation in humans is considerably more complex [Comuzzie & Allison, 1998]. As yet, no specific genes have been found that are associated with obesity in all cases. Beamer asserted that it is unlikely that all people who are obese have a single gene mutation that has a major effect on their body weight [Beamer, 2003].

It should be however noted that while genetic factors may help explain some inter-individual differences in BMI from a population perspective, genetic mutation is unlikely to explain the recent epidemic of overweight and obesity in children [Bray, 2003].

The theory that emphasises the role of biological processes in regulating an individual's weight is set-point theory. According to this, there is a specific weight range, called set-point, at which the body tends to remain. An individual with a weight above or below his/her set-point range will experience physiological and psychological pressure to return to the set-point range. The set-point can be compared to other relatively constant physiological mechanisms such as body temperature, blood pressure, or blood glucose level. The body will defend against a change in weight by making compensations in the mechanisms that govern the set-point. For example, one study revealed that overfed rats increased their metabolic rates, whereas the metabolic rate of underfed rats decreased [Keesey, 1986]. On the other hand, opponents to the set point theory simply point to the increase in obesity rates in the last three decades. Obviously, factors other than biological ones must play a role when it comes to weight regulation since a sharp increase in the rates of obesity has occurred [Wadden et al., 2002]. It may be logical to accept the fact that while set point theory may applicable to many individuals, there might be other factors such as exercise, diet, binge eating, and eating to deal with negative states which can cause a person's weight to move outside of this range [Garrow, 1978].

There are several genetic disorders where obesity is nearly always present. These include Prader-Willi syndrome, Laurence-Moon-Biedl-Bardet syndrome and Albright's hereditary osteodystrophy. Rare syndromes with genetic abnormalities of leptin or the leptin receptor have also been found recently. Usually, in these disorders obesity is expressed almost regardless of the environment. Indeed, these disorders probably have little to do with the current epidemic, although the study of individuals with these disorders can help us to understand the complex pathways that result in obesity [Anjali, 2004].

Differences in the prevalence of overweight and obesity between different races may also confirm the important role of genetics in determination of response to dietary energy intake, energy expenditure and regulation of body weight [Kimm & Obarzanek, 2002].

2.2.2 Early Programming of Later Overweight and Obesity: Barker's Hypothesis

Early nutrition and growth, reflected in birth weight, can determine later occurrence of many health outcomes, especially those related to the development of common non-communicable diseases. David Barker has coined the concept of "foetal origin of adult diseases" or "developmental origins of health and disease (DOH&D)" for the first time in mid-1980s to explain the whole process of maternal under-nutrition leading to obesity and its main non-communicable complications such as glucose intolerance and type 2 diabetes, coronary heart disease, stroke, hypertension, dyslipidemias, and some types of cancer in offspring. Since these conditions mostly show and impose themselves during adulthood, we just briefly touch the issue in this section.

Low birth weight (LBW) is still a serious public health problem in less-developed and developing world [UNICEF, 2005]. Intra-uterine growth retardation, mainly due to maternal under-nutrition, is the major cause of LBW in developing countries [Pojda & Kelly, 2000]. Evidence show that key body organs (e.g. hypothalamus) of full-term neonates who were LBW, are structurally and metabolically programmed to support life in a scarce environment in terms of dietary energy and nutrients. In fact, adaptations associated with foetal malnutrition become detrimental to health of the offspring, if they experience a period of adequate or plentiful nutrition leading to postnatal obesity [Stocker et al., 2005]. This phenomenon is increasingly happening in developing world due to coincidence of high prevalence of LBW and FNT in these countries.

It is important to mention that the relationship between birth weight and adulthood obesity is U-shape. It means that not only with low, but also with high birth weight, the risk of obesity will increase later in life [McMillen et al., 2004].

2.3 Non-Biological Factors

Although many authors have emphasised on the importance of genetic susceptibility to obesity, it seems that such a factor will not act unless a suitable environment is provided. Non biologic determinants of overweight and obesity are the main part of such an environment.

It has been shown that several environmental factors including television watching, low physical activity, lower socioeconomic status in white adolescents, consumption of sugar-containing beverages, skipping breakfast and unstructured meals are associated with obesity among U.S. children [Stettler et al., 2004].

2.3.1 Socioeconomic Factors

It seems that the social class difference in the prevalence of obesity were negligible during childhood, but were quite marked in early adulthood, with a greater percentage of overweight and obesity in lower social classes [Pařízková & Hills, 2001].

Gerald et al. pointed out that lower social class position, lower level of social support, and unmarried primary care-giver were all associated with high food intake and higher weight-for-height among children [Gerald et al., 1994]. Strauss & Knight showed those children from obese mothers, low-income families, and who had exposed to less cognitive stimulation, had an increased risk of obesity, independent of other demographic factors [Strauss & Knight, 1999].

Social beliefs and preferences is a major determinant of nutritional practices among mothers which can ultimately determine childhood overweight and obesity.

While before 1990s it was the general opinion that obesity is essentially a disease of socioeconomic elite in developing countries, more recent reviews have shown that obesity can no longer be considered solely a disease of groups with higher socioeconomic status. In fact the burden of obesity in each developing country tends to shift towards the groups with lower socioeconomic status as the country's GNP increases. A very important finding is that the shift of obesity towards women with low socioeconomic status apparently occurs at an earlier stage of economic development than it does for men [Monteiro et al., 2004].

A clear inverse U curve has been observed in the relation between household income as well as education and the prevalence of obesity in Brazil [Monteiro et al., 2001]. In fact, obesity among poor household with lowest education can be justified by the fact that there is an inverse relation between energy density and energy cost. Poverty and food insecurity are associated with lower food expenditures, low fruit and vegetable consumption, and lower-quality diets. A reduction in diet costs in linear programming models leads to high-fat, energy-dense diets that are similar in composition to those consumed by low-income groups. Such diets are more affordable than are prudent diets while having high palatability because of more sugar and fat. [Drewnowski & Specter, 2004]

2.3.2 Sudden Changes in Lifestyle

In some cases, the starting of obesity in childhood life may accompanied by sudden changes like recovery from illness or accident, when parents or care-givers allow increased food intake (particularly delicious high fat and sugar items), while the child has still limited physical activity.

Some investigators reported that obesity might appear in children, who had adapted to a high level of energy expenditure, but due to whatever reason, decrease their energy expenditure, for example young athletes, who stop their sport training [Gutin, 1998].

2.3.3 Physical Activity

In spite of the recent trend towards decreased dietary fat consumption, the increased prevalence of obesity might reasonably be considered to have increased due to the lack of health and dietary instructions, including inadequate physical activity and exercise [Hills, 1995; Hills & Byrne, 1998].

3 Potential Determinants and Risk Factors of Overweight and Obesity in Iran

Available evidence show that a rapid nutrition transition is happening in Iran. Ghassemi et al have recently documented this transition by systematic analysis of available information on socioeconomic, demographic and nutritional variables in the country [Ghassemi et al., 2002]. Significant socioeconomic and demographic changes (e.g. increased number of towns from 186 to 615 in the period of 1955-95) as well as nutritional changes (e.g. high proportion of households with "over-consumption" of dietary energy, double burden of malnutrition, etc) can be observed. Mohammadpour-Ahranjani et al have also recently reported significant increase in the prevalence of adolescent overweight in Tehran city during 1990s [Mohammadpour-Ahranjani et al., 2004].

According to the recent National Food Consumption Survey (2001-03), 35.6% of Iranian households consume more than 120% of their energy requirement, and fat provides 25% of total energy intake [NNFTRI, 2001-03]. Considering inter-provincial differences, it might be concluded that in some provinces and population segments, the intake have been much higher than these average figures. While the relationship between dietary fat and obesity is less consistent within populations [Willett, 1998], experimental studies have shown a mechanism through which fat may be associated with an increased risk of obesity [Poppitt & Prentice,1996]. Moreover, ecological analyses demonstrated a positive association between the proportion of energy from fat and the prevalence of overweight and obesity [Bray & Popkin,1998].

Over consumption of simple sugars is a potential risk factor for overweight [Jebb, 2005]. Therefore, current intake at the level of 9% of total energy among Iranian households [Houshyar-Rad et al., 2005] which is at the upper limit of the current recommendation (i.e. 10%) [WHO/FAO, 2003], may be added to dietary risks of overweight in Iranian population.

Average intake of dietary energy in urban areas has increased as about 65 Kcal/d from 1990-95 to 2001-03 [MOA[3]/NNFTRI 2003; NNFTRI, 2001-03]. This extra energy intake with constant physical activity level can lead to about 3 kg weight gain per year. It seems that with access to modern technology, the level of physical activity has also decreased during past decade. If so, both key components of lifestyle, i.e. diet and physical activity, have simultaneously acted in favour of weight gain at population level.

In a study among 10-19 yr adolescents in Tehran, Azizi et al showed that overweight/obese boys had an apparently higher energy intake than their normal weight counterparts [Azizi et al., 2001]. The composition of diet was however not different between overweight/obese and normal weight subjects. This observation is not consistent over all studies. For example findings of a study among adolescents in Isfahan and Arak cities (central Iran) found no difference in mean total energy intake between overweight or obese and normal-weight individuals. However, percentage of energy derived from carbohydrates was significantly higher in overweight or obese group ($P<0.05$). Among the same group of adolescents, investigators found a direct linear association between BMI and the frequency of rice (6.8 *vs* 11.6 times), and bread/pasta and an inverse relationship for fruit (6.2 *vs* 4.2 times)

[3] Ministry of Agriculture

and vegetable consumption [Kelishadi et al., 2003]. Increased satiety and decreased risk of obesity with diets high in vegetables and fruits have been shown elsewhere [Jebb, 2005].

Fast food/Ready-to-eat. In a study which was carried out among Tehrani high school students, the investigators found that adolescents from high socio-economic class consumed significantly more fast/ready-to-eat foods compared to those who were belonged to medium or low classes [Omidvar, 2002]. High-energy high-fat foods as well as soft drinks usually offered in fast food shops are an important feature of an obesity-promoting environment especially for the young.

Availability is another important factor which should be taken into consideration. Fast food establishments have become more ubiquitous in large cities, especially in capital city, Tehran. About 5 years ago, there was no fast food chain restaurant in Tehran, but nowadays these establishments may be seen less than every 2 kilometres and one may find websites which advertise fast food chains in Iran or even assess consumers preferences for different fast food establishments through voting systems.

In Iran, there are numerous types of traditional mixed dishes which are nutrient-dense, tasty, and diverse. Many years ago, all mothers/housewives used to cook mixed dishes for lunch and dinner spending couple of hours to prepare each meal. These kind of foods were usually made from fresh materials. Over the past two decades, home environment has been changed tremendously. Nowadays, there are more families having working mothers and time limitation has become an important issue. Beside this, industrial production of ready-to-eat/cooked foods, expansion of fast food restaurants, heavy marketing on junk foods, as well as heavy traffic jam and long rush hours in large cities makes women to spend fewer hours in the kitchen. As a result, housewives may preclude preparation of healthy meals and family members tend to eat less traditional dishes or eat the same dishes which are not as fresh and nutrient-dense as were in the past.

Socio-economic factors. In a study among Iranian households, investigators revealed that in higher quintiles of socio-economic status, consumption of bread and cereals, sugar and sweets significantly decreased and meats, vegetable and fruits increased [Abdollahi et al., 2005]. While this dietary pattern is regarded as beneficial to optimum body weight, intra-household food allocation can not be analysed by the methodology used to collect the data.

On the other hand, we showed that more years of formal education among mothers may lead to overweight in 14-17 yr Tehrani boy students [Mohammadpour-Ahranjani et al., 2004]. However, we did not find such a difference in girls [Mohammadpour-Ahranjani et al., 2001]. A similar association was found for fathers' educational level in boys. We demonstrated that obesity among boys whose fathers had academic degrees was 3.2-fold of those who had illiterate father (25 *vs* 7.7%). In the same study, overweight was more prevalent among boys who had working mothers. These findings may suggest that earning more money by mothers enables them to purchase more high-calorie foods; on the other hand, time limitation is an obstacle for working mothers in caring their children. It is possible that adolescent girls are more independent in terms of preparing and eating homemade meals, so less supervision by mothers may have a greater impact on boys.

At the same time, Kelishadi et al. showed that a BMI>85th percentile among Isfahani adolescents (centre Iran) was more prevalent in families with an average income than in high-income families ($P<0.05$) and in those with less-educated mothers [Kelishadi et al., 2003].

As mentioned earlier, social preferences can act as determinants of childhood overweight and obesity. In a study in centre of Iran, it was shown that mothers of overweight or obese adolescents preferred an overweight child and adolescent and agreed with the belief that these children would outgrow their obesity or overweight more often than mothers of adolescents with normal weight [Kelishadi et al., 2003].

Findings of a study carried out among high school girl students in *Tabriz* city (north-west Iran), revealed an inverse significant correlation between family size ($r=-0.12$, $p<0.05$), parity ($r=-0.13$, $p<0.01$), and birth order ($r=-0.12$, $p<0.05$), and BMI [Eizadifar et al., 2004].

Role of advertisements as a powerful marketing strategy should not be ignored when analysing the risk factors for overweight and obesity among adolescents. A number of experimental studies support the notion that young children's preference for a food increases as exposure to the food increases [Birch et al., 1982; Birch et al., 1987; Amini, 2002]. In a study among Tehrani school-aged students aimed at evaluation of the food advertisements on children's TV programmes and their recalled, demanded, and consumption, Amini et al. showed that the most frequent advertised brand was reminded more than others and the students' demand for the mentioned brand was ranked second. On the other hand, they revealed that the students, who reminded a brand name, consumed it about twelve times compared to those who did not remember the same brand [Amini, 2002]. Considering the increasing share of snack food advertisements on Iranian broadcast (currently the 3rd rank with 10% share of all advertisements) [Dibaji & Aghakiant, 1996], this factor has to be dealt with in future preventive strategies. Pournorouz in a content analysis study on the children targeted advertisements demonstrated that the most frequent advertisement was snacks/junk foods (42%). They also found that 12% of the advertisements were misleading [Pournorooz & Naghibossadat, 1996]. Through a content analysis study of Iranian newspapers, 17% of messages identified as ambiguous [Mohammadpour-Ahranjani et al., 2003]. However, it should be taken into consideration that 45% of Tehrani school students believed that only few of the food advertisements transferred true facts and 22% thought that all of the messages were false [Amini, 2002]. Amini did find that 37% of the food advertisements relied on nutrition related issues and half of these messages were incorrect or confusing [Amini et al., 2005].

Physical activity. Having adequate physical activity, as a main component of healthy lifestyle, needs its own pre-requisites. Designing our big cities, especially the capital city Tehran, has focused on facilitating automobile transportation. Most of our streets, especially in downtown, do not have wide sidewalks, and pedestrians do not feel safe while walking. Moreover air pollution is known as a major threat to health and a barrier to physical activity in the capital city and other big cities. While green areas is a limitation especially in the capital city, in most other big provinces vast green areas are accessible which may suggest that we can benefit green areas in physical activity programmes.

As we suggested elsewhere, type of climate/geographical characteristic of our country, i.e. long warm season in some parts of Iran may be considered as an important limiting determinant for physical activity [Rashidi et al., 2005]. The absolute maximum temperature may reaches than 50 degree centigrade in August in some cities in Iran [Iran Statistics Centre, 2001].

Nowadays, because of factors such as striking number of car accidents and air pollution, parents prefer to find home-based entertainments for their children. Road traffic accidents are considered to be the second highest cause of mortality in Iran [Montazeri, 2004]. Since streets are tremendously crowded and motorways have been extended largely, students have to go to school by car. Nearly all young families who have school students live in small flats and there is no room for children to spend their energy. As a result, children have to use their extra time by replacing energy consuming activities with sedentary manner. For example, in a study among Tehrani adolescent students, we found that 11-16 yr students reported watching television for 2.8±1.6 hours/day while they exercised for about half an hour daily [Mohammadpour-Ahranjani et al., 2001]. Moreover, we demonstrated that overweight boys and girls spent more hours on computer than their non-overweight counterparts (P=0.002 and 0.06, respectively). In a study carried out on 7-18 yr school students in *Urmia* (north-west Iran), students reported to watch television for 2.2 hours/day and to exercise for less than one hour per day. It may be interesting to mention that exercise duration among girls was about half of the boys [Ghavamzadeh, 2002]. In another study among 15-17 yr female students in *Rasht* city (north Iran), investigators found that about 15% of students walked more than 45 minutes/day, while about 27% of them reported to watch television for 3-5 hours/day [Maddah, 2005]. In some other big cities, however, a more traditional pattern of lifestyle might be seen. For instance, findings of a study carried out among school children in *Ahwaz* city (south-west Iran) revealed that 36.7 and 61.3% of 6-17 yr school children go to school by car and on foot, respectively [Veisi & Karandish, 2001]. Moreover, about 47% of the children reported that they performed physical activity regularly. Not surprisingly, only 23.8% of the children had PC (personal computer) at their home [Veisi & Karandish, 2001]. In a study among adolescents in *Isfahan* and *Arak* cities, it was reported that regular extracurricular physical activity during the school year and participation on sport teams was lower in girls than boys and also inversely associated with BMI [Kelishadi et al., 2003]. They also reported that time spent watching television was significantly greater for subjects with BMI>85th percentile.

4 Preventive Strategies for Childhood Obesity

Undoubtedly, the best strategy to prevent childhood overweight and obesity is promotion of a healthy lifestyle which involves eating healthy and being more physically active [Ebbeling et al., 2002]. We may classify strategies according to 1) Setting, i.e. home, school, home and school-based programmes to which we may add even community/local, national and global campaigns; 2) Coverage, i.e. universal and selected; and 3) Level of intervention including community (overall reduction of BMI), at-risk children (those who have obese parents), and secondary prevention (treatment of childhood obesity).

Since our knowledge on prevention of childhood overweight and obesity comes from other societies, there is an urgent need to develop specific causal webs for overweight and obesity among Iranian children, preferably by each province.

According to Müller et al., risk factors for childhood overweight may defer from obesity [Müller et al., 2005]. However, it should be stated that many strategies, programmes or guidelines which have been adopted or developed so far by others, can be of use in Iranian society. For example, all 11 tips for parents towards prevention of obesity in Malaysian children [Sidik & Ahmad, 2004] seems to be fitted to our society; and from all 16 approaches suggested for prevention and treatment of childhood obesity, 14 approaches seems appropriate for our country [Ebbeling et al., 2002].

It has been argued that conventional weight loss programmes developed for adults is not sustainable, and after 5 years nearly all weight looser reach their initial weight [Anonymous,

1993]. Since children and adolescents are more susceptible to environmental factors/pressure and being less mature, most efforts to reduce obesity in children have used either family-based or school-based programmes rather than individual treatments [Ebbeling et al., 2002].

It has been suggested that health promotion within a school setting, as a measure of universal prevention, is necessary, but not enough. Regarding "selected" prevention, interventions aimed at children within higher limits of normal weight as well as overweight children from obese parents and low socio-economic level seem to be promising [Müller et al., 2005].

Dietary strategies. There is sufficient evidence to develop clear dietary guidelines for preventing weight gain. Such a guideline is strongly consistent with cardio vascular disease and cancer prevention guidelines. If these guidelines are to be translated into sustainable changes in eating habits, coordinated actions across multiple stakeholders are also required [Jebb, 2005].

Findings of the latest two consumption surveys in Iran show that energy intake as Cal/capita has slightly decreased during the past decade [MOA/NNFTRI, 2003; NNFTRI, 2001-03]. We may deduce that recent dramatic increase in the prevalence of overweight and obesity in Iranian population might not be attributable to excess dietary energy intake. The share of energy comes from dietary fat is however gradually increasing.

Physical activity. Physical activity oriented approaches need a broad range of changes from transport expenses to environmental design to being well established in a community. Therefore, for adopting such strategies we have to consider all relevant factors/links. However, Wareham et al. in a review of physical activity and obesity prevention evidence suggested that it is not amenable to determine effective approaches according to current evidence on physical activity and obesity. They noted that if trials are based on an explicit causal model with a clear theoretical foundation, it would be possible to analyse different aspects of an intervention and assess the effectiveness of each part separately [Wareham et al., 2005]. Yet they concluded that current suggestion of 45-60 minutes activity with moderate intensity should be advised for obesity prevention on a daily basis.

Past experiences. "Planet health" is a famous and successful school-based programme in this field. It was carried out among the 6th-8th grades American students for 2 years aiming at evaluating the impact of a health behaviour intervention "an interdisciplinary, integrated health education curriculum" on obesity. Regarding obesity relevant outcomes, results indicated a decrease in obesity and a greater remission of obesity among female subjects [Gortmaker et al., 1999].

There are however many less to moderately efficient programmes in developed countries. The NSFS (National School Fruit Scheme) in England showed a short-term positive effect on fruit consumption among 4-6 yr children, but the difference disappeared after 3 years [Wells & Nelson, 2005]. Other programmes such as CATCH (Child and Adolescent Trial for Cardiovascular Health) [Luepker et al., 1996] and APPLES (Active Programme Promoting Lifestyle Education in Schools) [Sahota et al., 2001] were not successful in BMI reduction. It has to be mentioned however that these programmes were not specifically designed for overweight and obesity.

It was shown that 11-14 yr Tehrani students spent the greatest amount of their pocket money for buying snacks and they reported school buffets as the main supplier (52.7%) [Amini, 2002]. An implication of these findings would be to educate students and increase healthy choices through school buffets. However, such an alteration may lead students to provide their desirable junks outside schools. This may confirm the idea that it would be better to use a holistic approach which covers school and home simultaneously [Müller et al., 2005].

Actually, despite genetic predisposition to obesity, parents are able to build a healthy environment in which their children get used to appropriate eating behaviours and physical activity. It seems that the close relation between school educational curriculum and family support lead to designing school and family-based interventions. KOPS (Kiel Obesity Prevention Study) is an 8-year example of such a combination in Germany. The aim of the project was to improve health-related behaviours among 5-7 yr school children. The researchers found a significant age-dependent increase in median triceps skinfold of the whole group and percentage of fat mass in overweight children [Müller et al., 2001].

In the mean time, it should be taken into consideration that intervention setting is a key determinant of success for a given strategy. For example, it has been documented that increasing physical activity levels through physical education sessions and behavioural change are most likely to be achieved by implementation of comprehensive school-based programmes [Wareham et al., 2005].

Conclusion

Currently, while overweight and obesity is going to be a major public health problem among Iranian children and adolescents, we lack required analytical data to adopt evidence-based childhood overweight and obesity prevention strategies in the country. Immediate, underlying, and basic risk factors of childhood overweight and obesity in different age- and sex-groups of Iranian children and adolescents as well as information about relevant characteristics of all stake-holders' knowledge and attitudes towards childhood overweight and obesity as a public health problem shall be explored and addressed. Communication and advocacy for the issue seems to be a very important strategy to prevent childhood overweight and obesity.

Since efforts have to be focused mainly on primary prevention of overweight and obesity, community nutritionists and other health professionals are expected to obtain adequate knowledge on both biological and social aspects of obesity and understand the existing biosocial link through their educational curriculum. This will need a strong and efficient capacity-building programme within the country.

To strengthen positive aspects of the traditional behaviours and technologies is an option when designing community-based programmes. For example, we do not have any vending machines in schools. As another instance, we may refer to our usual consumption of raw green leafy vegetables like watercress, mint, and parsley with main dishes. Mean daily intake of these kinds of vegetables in Iranian households is presently about 42 grams [NNFTRI, 2001-03].

Improving nutritional knowledge of mothers has been highlighted as an important component of nutrition security achievement in Iran [Ghassemi, 1998]. Since we have encountered under-nutrition for many years, parents' views are mostly in favour with their children's weight gain. This traditional belief should be modified based on stages of nutrition transition in different parts of the country. It will be very important to devise educational programmes at family level when dealing with childhood overweight and obesity. According to available evidence, it seems that specific educational programmes should target parents and caregivers especially grandparents who play an important role in taking care of children in Iran.

At the same time, it should be noted that in a country like Iran where the double burden of under- and over-nutrition exist, much emphasis on prevention of overweight and obesity might result in aggravation of under-nutrition among vulnerable subgroups such as adolescent girls because of fearness of fatness [WHO/FAO, 2003]. Therefore, potential undesirable effects should also be taken into account when adopting any preventive strategy for overweight and obesity problem.

References

Abdollahi, M; Mohammadi, F; Houshiar-Rad, A; Ghaffarpour, M; Ghodsi, D; Kalantari, N. Socio-economic differences in dietary patterns and nutrient intakes: the comprehensive study of household food consumption patterns and nutritional status of I.R. Iran, 2001-2003. Annals of Nutrition and Metabolism, *18th International Congress of Nutrition*, 19-23 September 2005, Durban, South Africa, p.72.

AIHW/NHFA. The relationship between overweight, obesity and cardiovascular disease. A literature review prepared for the National Heart Foundation of Australia (NHFA). Canberra: *Australian Institute of Health and Welfare* (AIHW), November 2004.

Al-Hourani, HM; Henry, CJ; Lightowler, HJ. Prevalence of overweight among adolescent females in the United Arab Emirates. *Am J Hum Biol*, 2003 15(6),758-64.

Al-Isa, AN; Moussa, MA. Obesity among Kuwaiti pre-school children aged 0-5 years: prevalence and comparison with the NCHS/CDC reference population. *Nutr Health*, 1998 12(4),235-46.

Al-Isa, AN. Body mass index, overweight and obesity among Kuwaiti intermediate school adolescents aged 10-14 years. *Eur J Clin Nutr,* 2004 58(9),1273-7.

Al-Rukban, MO. Obesity among Saudi male adolescents in Riyadh, Saudi Arabia. *Saudi Med J,* 2003 24(1),27-33.

Al-Sendi, AM; Shetty, P; Musaiger, AO. Prevalence of overweight and obesity among Bahraini adolescents: a comparison between three different sets of criteria. *Eur J Clin Nutr*, 2003 57(3),471-4.

Amini, M. Evaluation of food advertisements on children's TV programmes and determination of relationship between TV food advertisements recalled and foods demanded and consumed by students of junior high school, district 6, Tehran 2000-01. Thesis submitted for partial fulfilments of MSc in nutrition, Faculty of Nutrition Sciences and Food Technology, Shaheed Beheshti University of Medical Sciences, Tehran, 2002 [in Farsi].

Amini, M; Mohsenian-Rad, M; Kimiagar, M; Omidvar, N; Mehrabi, Y. Food advertising on Iranian children's television: a content analysis and an experimental study with junior high school students. *Ecology of Food and Nutrition*, 2005 44, 123-133.

Anderson, PM; Butcher, KF; Levine, PB. Economic perspectives on childhood obesity. Federal Reserve Bank of Chicago: *Economic Perspect*, 2003 3Q, 30-48.

Andreyeva, T; Sturm, R; Ringel, JS. Moderate and severe obesity have large differences in health care costs. *Obes Res*, 2004 12(12), 1936-43.

Anjali J. What works for obesity? *A summary of the research behind obesity interventions*. BMJ Publishing Group Limited, London, 2004.

Anonymous. Methods for voluntary weight loss and control: NIH technology assessment conference panel. *Ann Intern Med*, 1993 119,764-70.

Anonymous. Reports on tasks for scientific cooperation, Collection of data on products intended for use in very-low-calorie-diets. *Report of experts participating in Task 7.3*, September 2002.

Ansa, VO; Odigwe, CO; Anah, MU. Profile of body mass index and obesity in Nigerian children and adolescents. *Niger J Med*, 2001 10,78-80.

Ashrafi, MR; Abdollahi, M; Houshiar-rad, A. The prevalence of obesity among Tehrani 6–14 year male students using BMI, 2000– 01. *Presented in the 6th Iranian Nutrition congress, 12–15 February 2001, Ahwaz, Iran [in Farsi].*

Azizi, F; Allahverdian, S; Mirmiran, P; Rahmani, M; Mohammadi, F. Dietary factors and body mass index in a group of Iranian adolescents: Tehran Lipid and Glucose Study-2. *Int J Vitam Nutr Res*, 2001 71, 123-127.

Bajan, M. Prevalence of obesity, fat distribution and its relationship with food consumption pattern in secondary school girls in Lahijan. Thesis submitted for partial fulfilment of MSc in Nutrition, Faculty of Nutrition Sciences and Food Technology, Shaheed Beheshti University of Medical Sciences, June 2002 [in Farsi].

Beamer, BA. Genetic influences on obesity. In: Anderson RE (Ed.) Obesity: Aetiology, assessment, treatment and prevention. *Champaign: Human Kinetics*, 2003; 43-58.

Beccaria, L; Galli, L; Tonini, G; Calori, G; Gallus, G; Chiumello, G; Balsamo, A; et al. Multicentric study on the frequency of obesity in school-age children in Italy. *Riv Ital Pediatr*, 2000, 26: 115-120.

Birch, LL; Birch, D; Marlin, D; Kramer, I. Effect of instrumental eating on children's food preferences. *Appetite*. 1982 3, 125-34.

Birch, LL; Martin DW. I don't like it; I never tried it: effects of exposure on two-year-old children's food preferences. *Appetite*, 1982 3, 353-60.

Birch, LL; Mcphee, L; Shoba, C; Piroc, E; Steinburg, L. What kind of exposure reduced children's food neophobia? *Appetite*, 1987 9, 171-8.

Biró, G. First Hungarian Representative Nutrition Survey. Albaswiss Press, Budapest, 1993.

Booth, ML; Chey, T; Wake, M; Norton, K; Hesketh, K; Dollman, J. et al. Change in the prevalence of overweight and obesity among young Australians, 1969–1997. *Am J Clin Nutr*, 2003 77,29–36.

Bouchard, C; Perusse, L. Genetic aspects of obesity. *Ann N Y Acad Sci*, 1993 29(699), 26-35.

Bourne, LT; Langenhoven, ML; Steyn, K; Jooste, PL; Laubscher, JA; Bourne, DE. Nutritional status of 3-6 year-old African children in the Cape Peninsula. *East Afr Med J*, 1994 71(11),695-702.

Brody, J. The global epidemic of childhood obesity: poverty, urbanisation and the nutrition transition. *Nutrition Bytes*, 2002 8(2), Article 1. through [http://repositories.cdlib.org/uclabiolchem/nutritionbytes/vol8/iss2/art1]. downloaded on 20th Oct., 2005.

Brownell, KD; Wadden, TA. Aetiology and treatment of obesity: Understanding a serious, prevalent, and refractory disorder. *J Consult Clin Psychol*, 1992 60(4), 505-517.

Bray GA, Popkin BA. Dietary fat intake does affect obesity! *Am J Clin Nutr*, 1998 68, 1157-1173.

Bray, GA. Contemporary diagnosis and management of obesity, 2nd Edition. Newton: *Handbooks in Healthcare*, 2003.

Bundred, P; Kitchiner, D; Buchan, I. Prevalence of overweight and obese children between 1989 and 1998 population based series of cross sectional studies. *BMJ* 2001 322(7282), 326-8.

Caterson, ID; Van Hubbard; Bray, GA; Grunstein, R; Hansen, BC; Hong, Y; et al. Obesity, a worldwide epidemic related to heart disease and stroke. AHA Conference Proceedings, Prevention Conference VII, Group III: Worldwide Comorbidities of Obesity. *Circulation*, 2004 110, e476-e483.

Chinn, S; Rona, RJ. Trends in weight for height and triceps skinfold thickness for English and Scottish children, 1972±1982 and 1982±1990. *Paediatr Perinat Epidemiol*, 1994 8: 90-106.

Chopra, M; Galbraith, S; Darnton-Hill, I. A global response to a global problem: the epidermic of over nutrition. *Bull World Health Organisation*, 2002 80,952-58.

Clark, MM; Goldstein, MG. Obesity: A health psychology perspective. In Goreczny, AJ (Ed.), Handbook of health and rehabilitation psychology. New York: *Plenum*, 1995; 157- 173.

Cleves, MJ. Half the World, Half the Chance: *An Introduction to Gender and Development*. Oxford: Oxfam; 1993.

Comuzzie, AG; Allison, DB. The search for human obesity genes. *Science*, 1998 29 (280-5368), 1374-77.

Dadkhah-Piraghag, M; Omidvar, N; Mehrabi, Y. Assessment and comparison of weight status of female high school adolescents and their parents in Tehran, district 6, 2002. *Proceedings of 2nd Congress of Non-communicable Diseases Prevention*, 8-10 March 2004, Tehran, P.203.

De Onis, M; Blössner, M. Prevalence and trends of overweight among preschool children in developing countries. *Am J Clin Nutr*, 2000 72, 1032-9.

De Spiegelaere, M; Dramaix, M; Hennart, P. The influence of socioeconomic status on the incidence and evolution of obesity during early adolescence. *Int J Obes Relat Metab Disord*, 1998, 22: 268-274.

Dibaji, F; Aghakiant, H. Determination of the time proportion of TV advertisements on I.R.I.B. in one week. Final Report of research project, Centre for Studies and Evaluation of I.R.I.B. Programmes, 1996, No.76/54 [in Farsi].

Dietz, WH. Health consequences of obesity in youth: childhood predictors of adult disease. *Paediatrics*, 1998 101, 518-25.

Dorosty, AR; Siassi, F; Reilly, JJ; Rona, RJ; Chinn, S. (2002). Obesity in Iranian children. *Arch Dis Child* [10.1136/adc.87.5.388], 87 (5).

Drewnowski, A; Specter, SE. Poverty and obesity: the role of energy density and energy costs. *Am J Clin Nutr*, 2004 79, 6-16.

Ebbeling, CB; Pawlak, DB; Ludwig, DS. Childhood obesity: public-health crisis, common sense cure. *The Lancet*, 2002 360,473-82.

Eisenstein, EL; Shaw, LK; Nelson, CL; Anstrom, KJ; Hakim, Z; Mark, DB. Obesity and long-term clinical and economic outcomes in coronary artery disease patients. *Obes Res*, 2002 10, 83–91.

EL-Hazmi, MAF; Warsy, AS. The prevalence of Obesity and overweight in 1-18 year old Saudi Children. *Ann Saudi Med*, 2002 22(5-6): 303-7.

Elmadfa, I; Godina-Zarfl, B; König, J; Dichtl, M; Faist, V. Prevalence of overweight and plasma lipids in 7-18 year old Austrian children and adolescents. *Int J Obes Relat Metab Disord,* 1993, 17 (Suppl. 2): 35.

Eizadifar, Sh; Eghtesadi, Sh; Omidvar, N; Ghodsi, D; Koushavar, H. Prevalence of overweight and obesity in adolescent girls in Tabriz and its associated factors. *Proceedings of 2nd Congress of Non-communicable Diseases Prevention*, 8-10 March 2004, Tehran, P.265.

Foster, GD; Wadden, TA; Mullen, JL; Stunkard, AJ; Wang, J; Feurer, I D; et al. Resting energy expenditure, body composition, and excess weight in the obese. *Metabolism*, 1988 37(5), 467-472.

Friedrich, MJ. Epidemic of obesity expends its spread of developing countries. *JAMA*, 2002 287, 1382-6.

Gargari, BP; Behzad, MH; Ghassabpour, S; Ayat, A. Prevalence of overweight and obesity among high-school girls in Tabriz, Iran, in 2001. *Food Nutr Bull*, 2004 25,288-291.

Garrow, JS. Energy balance and obesity in man. Amsterdam: Elsevier/North Holland *Biomedical*, 1978.

Garrow, J; Summerbell, C. Obesity. *Health Care Needs Assessment third series.* Radcliffe Medical Press, 2002. http://ncna.radcliffe-online.com/obesity.html

Gerald, LB; Anderson, A; Johnson, GD; Hoff, C; Trimm, RF. Social class, social support and obesity risk in children. *Child Care Health Dev*, 1994 20,145-163.

Ghassemi H. Food and nutrition security in Iran: studies of planning and implementation models. Final report of research project, *NNFTRI*, Tehran, 1998 [in Farsi].

Ghassemi, H; Harrison, G; Mohammad, K. An accelerated nutrition transition in Iran. *Public Health Nutr,* 2002 5(1A), 149–155.

Ghavamzadeh, S. Prevalence of overweight and obesity among school aged students in Urmia, Iran, 2001. Final report of research project. Urmia University of Medical Sciences and Health Services, 2004 [in Farsi].

Goran, MI; Ball, GDC; Cruz, ML. Obesity and risk of type 2 diabetes and cardiovascular disease in children and adolescents. *J Clin Endocrin Metab*, 2003 88(4), 1417–1427.

Gortmaker, SL; Peterson, K; Wiecha, J; Sobol, AM; Dixit, S; Fox, MK; et al. Reducing obesity via a school-based interdisciplinary intervention among youth: Planet Health. *Arch Pediatr Adolesc Med*, 1999 153,409-18.

Gutin, B. Exercise, body composition, and health in children. In: Lamb, D; Murray, R. (Eds.) Perspectives in exercise science and sports medicine. Vol. 11, Exercise, *Nutrition and Weight Control.* Cooper, Carmel, 1998.

Hara, M. Trends in obesity. *Nippon Rinsho*, 1988; 46,2361-4.

Hills, AP. Physical activity and movement in children: its consequences for growth and development. *Asia Pacific J Clin Nutr*, 1995 4, 43-45

Hills, AP; Byrne, NM. Exercise prescription for weight management. *Proceedings of the Nutrition Society*, 1998 57(1), 93-103.

Hope, AA; Kumanyika, SK; Whitt, MC; Shults, J. Obesity related comorbidities in obese African Americans in an outpatient weight loss programme. *Obes Res*, 2005 13, 772–779.

Houshyar-Rad, A; Abdollahi, M; Hajirasouli, A; Esmaeili, M; Kalantari, N. Dietary risk factors of CVD in food consumption pattern of Iranian Households (2001-2002). Annals of Nutrition and Metabolism, *18th International Congress of Nutrition*, 19-23 September 2005, Durban, South Africa, p.165.

IOTF. *Childhood Obesity Report*, May 2004. www.iotf.org/childhood.

Iranian Statistics Centre. Annual Statistical Report. Tehran: Iranian Statistics Centre, 2001.

Ismail, MN; Vicknewary, EN. Prevalence of obesity in Malaysia: Data from three ethnic groups. *Country report at the Asian BMI/Obesity Workshop*, Milan, Italy, 1999.

Jabre, P; Sikias, P; Khater-Menassa, B; Baddoura, R; Awada, H. Overweight children in Beirut: prevalence estimates and characteristics. *Child Care Health Dev*, 2005 31(2), 159-65.

Jebb, SA. Dietary strategies for the prevention of obesity. *Proceedings of the Nutrition Society*, 2005 64,217-227.

Kafatos, AG; Panagiotakopoulos, G; Bastakis, N; Trakas, D; Stoikidou, M; Pantelakis, S. Cardiovascular risk factors of Greek adolescents in Athens. *Prev Med*, 1981, 10: 173- 186.

Kain, J; Burrows, R; Uauy, R. Obesity trends in children and adolescents: *basic determinants. In: Chen, C; Dietz, WH. [Ed.] Obesity in childhood and adolescents. Nestlé Nutrition Workshop Series*, Paediatric Programme, Vol. 49, Lippincott Willians & Wilkins, 2002; 54-67.

Keesey, R. E. A set-point theory of obesity. In Brownell, KD; Foreyt, JP (Eds.), Handbook of eating disorders: *Physiology, psychology, and treatment of obesity, anorexia, and bulimia.* New York: Basic Books, 1986; 63-87.

Kelishadi, R; Hashemipour, M; Sarrafzadegan, N; Sadry, G; Ansari, R; Alikhassy, H; et al. Obesity and associated modifiable environmental factors in Iranian adolescents: Isfahan Healthy Heart Program- Heart Health Promotion from Childhood. *Paediatr Int*, 2003 45, 435-442.

Kimm, SYS; Obarzanek, E. Childhood Obesity: A New Pandemic of the New Millennium. *Paediatrics*, 2002 110(5), 1003-7.

Luepker, RV; Perry, CL; McKinlay, SM; Nader, PR; Parcel, GS; Stone, EJ, et al. Outcomes of a field trial to improve children's dietary patterns and physical activity: the Child and Adolescent Trial for Cardiovascular Health (CATCH). *JAMA*, 1996 275,768-76.

Lobstein, T; Frelut, ML. Prevalence of overweight among children in Europe. *Obe Rev*, 2003 4,195–200.

Maddah, M. Personal communication, 15 August, 2005.

Maffeis, C; Talamini, G; Tato, L. Influence of diet, physical activity and parents' obesity on children's adiposity: a four-year longitudinal study. *Int J Obes Relat Metab Disord*, 1998 22(8), 758-64.

Martorell, R; Khan, LK; Hughes, ML; Grummer-Strawn, LM. Obesity in Latin American women and children. *J Nutr*, 1998 128,1464-73.

McMillen, IC; Muhlhausler, BS; Duffield, JA; Yuen, BSJ. Prenatal programming of postnatal obesity: fetal nutrition and the regulation of leptin synthesis and secretion before birth. *Proceedings of the Nutrition Society*, 2004 63, 405-12.

Mirmiran, P; Mirblouki, M; Mohammadi, F; Azizi, F. Prevalence of underweight, overweight and obesity among Tehrani adolescent students during 1998-2001. *IJEM* (Iranian Journal of Endocrinology and Metabolism), 2003 5, 369-377 [in Farsi].

MOA/NNFTRI. National Household Food Consumption Survey, I.R.Iran, 1990-95. *Final report of national survey,* Second edition, Tehran, *NNFTRI*, 2003.

MOH/NNFTRI. National assessment of iron, zinc, vitamin A and vitamin D in different age groups, 2001. *Final report of national survey*, Tehran, Iranian MOH, 2005 [in Farsi].

Mohammadpour-Ahranjani, B; Kalantari, N; Rashidi, A; Karandish, M; Eshraghian, MR; Kalantari N. Prevalence of overweight and obesity among secondary and high school students in Tehran-2000. *Data bank of research project*, Tehran, NNFTRI, 2001.

Mohammadpour-Ahranjani, B; Abdollahi, M; Pakravan, M. Content analysis of nutritional messages in Iranian newspapers, 1999-2000. *Proceedings of the 9th European Nutrition Conference*, Italy, 2003, p.583.

Mohammadpour-Ahranjani, B; Rashidi, A; Karandish, M; et al. Prevalence of overweight and obesity in adolescent Tehrani students, 2000-2001: an epidemic health problem. *Public Health Nutr,* 2004 7, 645-8.

Mohammadpour-Ahranjani, B; Zellipour, L; Rashidi, A; Kalantari, N; Karandish, M; Eshraghian, MR. Mothers' educational level is positively associated with overweight among Tehrani adolescent boy students. Obesity: taking theory into practice, *Proceedings of the Nutrition Society,* volume 63 OCB 2004, Dublin, Republic of Ireland, 5-8 July 2004.

Montazeri, A. Road-traffic-related mortality in Iran: a descriptive study. *Public Health*, 2004 118(2),110-3.

Monteiro, CA; Conde, WL; Popkin, BM. Independent effects of income and education on the risk of obesity in the Brazilian adult population. *J Nutr*, 2001 131, 881S-886S

Monteiro, CA; Moura, EC; Conde, WL; Popkin, BM. Socioeconomic status and obesity in adult populations of developing countries: a review. *Bull WHO*, 2004 82, 940-46.

Müller, MJ; Asbeck, I; Mast, M; Langnase, K; Grund, A. Prevention of obesity-more than an intention. Concept and first results of the Kiel Obesity Prevention Study (KOPS). *Int J Obes Relat Metab Disord*, 2001 25 (suppl 1), S66-74.

Müller, MJ; Danielzik, S; Pust, S. School- and family-based interventions to prevent overweight in children. *Proceedings of the Nutrition Society*, 2005 64,249-54.

NNFTRI. National Comprehensive Study on Household Food Consumption Pattern and Nutritional Status in Iran (2001-2003). Data bank of research project, Tehran, NNFTRI, 2005.

Ogden, CL; Flegal, KM; Carroll, MD; Johnson, CL. Prevalence and trends in overweight among US children and adolescents, 1999-2000. *JAMA* 2002 288:1728-32.

Olshansky, SJ; Passaro, DJ; Hershow, RC; Layden, J; Carnes, BA; Brody, J; et al. A potential decline in life expectancy in the United States in the 21st century. *N Engl J Med*, 2005 352(11), 1138-45.

Omidvar, N. Psychological determinants of food choice and nutritional status in high school adolescents in the city of Tehran. Dissertation submitted for partial fulfillments of PhD in nutrition, Faculty of Nutrition and Health, Tabriz University of Medical Sciences and Health Services, Tabriz, 2002 [in Farsi].

Omran, AR. The epidemiologic transition: A theory of epidemiology of population change. *Midbank Mem Fund Q*, 1971 49: 509-538.

Oner, N; Vatansever, U; Sari, A; Ekuklu, E; Guzel, A; Karasalihoglu, S; Boris, NW. Prevalence of underweight, overweight and obesity in Turkish adolescents. *Swiss Med Wkly*, 2004 134(35-36),529-33.

Oppert, JM; Rolland-Cachera, MF. Prévalence, évolution dans le temps et conséquences économiques de l'obésité. *Med Sci,* 1998 14,939-943.

Pařízková, J; Hills, A. [Ed.] *Childhood Obesity: Prevention and Treatment*. CRC Press, Florida, 2001; 21-29.

Pojda J; Kelly L (Eds.) Low Birth Weight. A report based on the international low birth weight symposium and workshop held on 14-17 June 1999 at the international centre for diarrhoeal disease research, Dhaka, Bangladesh; *Nutrition Policy paper* No **18**, Geneva: The UN ACC/SCN, 2000.

Popkin, BM. Nutritional patterns and transitions. *Popul Dev Rev*, 1993 19: 138-157.

Popkin, BM. The nutrition transition and its relationship to demographic change. In: Semba, RD; Bloem MW (Eds.) *Nutrition and Health in Developing Countries*. New Jersy: Humana Press, 2001: 427-445.

Popkin, B; Horton, S; Kim, S. The nutrition transition and prevention of diet-related chronic diseases in Asia and the Pacific. Asian Development Bank *Nutrition and Development Series* No **6**, Manila: Asian Development Bank, 2001.

Pokin, BM; Caballero, B. The nutrition transition: diet and disease in the developing world. Washington: Academic Press, 2002.

Popkin, B; Lu, B; Zhai, F. Understanding the nutrition transition: measuring rapid dietary changes in transitional countries. *Public Health Nutrition*, 2002 5 (6A): 947-953.

Popkin, BM. The nutrition transition: an overview of world patterns of change. *Nutr Rev*, 2004 62 (7 Pt 2): S140-S143.

Poppitt, S; Prentice, AM. Energy density and its role in the control of food intake: Evidence from metabolic and community studies. *Appetite*, 1996 26, 153-174.

Pournorooz, M; Naghibossadat, R. Content analysis of advertisements aimed at children, broadcast from Iran TV during the first half of year. *Final report of research project, Centre for Studies and Evaluation of I.R.I.B. Programmes*, 1996, No.77/54 [in Farsi].

Power, C; Lake, JK; Cole, TJ. Body mass index and height from childhood to adulthood in the 1958 British birth cohort. *Am J Clin Nutr*, 1997, 66, 1094-1101.

Puhl, R; Brownell, KD. Bias, Discrimination, and Obesity. Obes Res, 2001 9, 788–805.

Raebel, MA; Malone, DC; Conner, DA; Xu, S; Porter, JA; Lanty, FA. Health services use and health care costs of obese and nonobese individuals. *Arch Intern Med*, 2004 164, 2135-2140.

Rashidi, A; Mohammadpour-Ahranjani, B; Vafa, MR; Karandish, M. *Prevalence of obesity in Iran. Obes Rev*, 2005; 6, 191-2

Ravussin, E; Bogardus, C. A brief overview of human energy metabolism and its relationship to essential obesity. *Am J Clin Nutr*, 1999 55, 242S-245S.

Rio-Navarro, BE; Velázquez-Monroy, O; Sánchez-Castillo, CP. The high prevalence of overweight and obesity in Mexican children. *Obes Res*, 2004 12,215-23.

Sahota, P; Rudolf, MCJ; Dixey, R; Hill, AJ; Barth, JH; Cade, J. Randomised controlled trial of primary school based intervention to reduce risk factors for obesity. *BMJ*, 2001 323,1029-32.

Salazar-Martinez, E; Allen, B; Fernandez-Ortega, C; Torres-Mejia, G; Galal, O; Lazcano-Ponce, E. Overweight and obesity status among adolescents from Mexico and Egypt. *Arch Med Res*, 2006 37,535-42.

Schneider, D. International trends in adolescent nutrition. *Soc Sci Med*, 2000 15: 955-967.

Sidik, SM; Ahmad, R. Childhood obesity: contributing factors, consequences and intervention. *Mal J Nutr*, 2004 10,13-22.

Sjöberg, RL; Nilsson, KW; Leppert, J. Obesity, shame, and depression in school-aged children: A population-based study. *Paediatrics*, 2005 116, 389-92.

Stettler, N; Signer, TM; Suter, PM. Electronic games and environmental factors associated with childhood obesity in Switzerland. *Obes Res*, 2004 12,896-903.

Strauss, RS; Knight, J. Influence of the home environment on the development of obesity in children. *Paediatrics*, 1999 103,E851.

Sobal, J. Commentary: Globalisation and the epidemiology of obesity. *Intl J Epidemiol*, 2001 30: 1136-1137.

Sorof, J; Daniels S. Obesity hypertension in children*: A problem of epidemic proportions. Hypertension*, 2002 40, 441-447.

Stocker, CJ; Arch, JRS; Cawthorn, MA. Foetal origins of insulin resistance and obesity. *Proceedings of the Nutrition Society*, 2005 64, 143-151.

UNICEF. The State of the World's Children 2005. New York: UNICEF, 2005.

Veisi, M; Karandish, M. Determination of body mass index percentiles of 6-16 years old students in Ahwaz city, Iran, 2001. Final report of research project. Ahwaz Jondi-Shapour University of Medical Sciences and Health Services, 2004 [in Farsi].

Wadden, TA; Brownell, KD; Foster, GD. Obesity: Responding to the global epidemic. *J Consult Clin Psych,* 2002 70(3), 510-525.

Wang G; Dietz WH. Economic burden of obesity in youths aged 6 to 17 Years: 1979–1999. *Paediatrics*, 2002 109(5), 81-86.

Wareham, NJ; van Sluijs, EM; Ekelund, UIF. Physical activity and obesity prevention: a review of the current evidence. *Proceeding of the Nutrition Society*, 2005 64,229-47.

Wee, CC; Phillips, RS; Legedza, ATR; Davis, RB; Soukup, JR; Colditz, GA; et al. Health care expenditures associated with overweight and obesity among US adults: importance of age and race. *Am J Public Health*, 2005 95, 159–65.

Wells, L; Nelson, M. The National School Fruit Scheme produces short-term but no longer-term increased in fruit consumption in primary school children. *BJN*, 2005 93,537-42.

Willett, WC. Is dietary fat a major determinant of body fat? *Am J Clin Nutr*, 1998 67 (suppl),556S-562S.

Whitaker, RC; Wright, JA; Pepe, MS; Seidel, KD; Dietz, WH. Predicting obesity in young adulthood from childhood and parental obesity. *N Engl J Med,* 1997 337(13), 869-73.

WHO. Non communicable diseases, including mental health: childhood obesity in China. Geneva: *WHO*, 2000.

WHO/FAO. Diet, nutrition and the prevention of chronic diseases. *WHO Technical Report Series,* No.916, Geneva: WHO, 2003.

Young, SYN; Gunzenhauser, JD; Malone, KE; McTiernan, A. Body mass index and asthma in the military population of the north western United States. *Arch Intern Med*, 2001 161, 1605-11.

In: Global Dimensions of Childhood Obesity
Editor: Richard K. Flamenbaum, pp. 127-138
ISBN: 1-60021-037-6

Chapter 6

THE ENDOGENOUS OBESITY WE STILL DON'T RECOGNIZE

Geni Balaban*[*] *and Gisélia Alves Pontes da Silva
Nutrition Department and Mother & Child Health Department,
Federal University of Pernambuco, Brazil

Abstract

Introduction: Obesity etiology is multifactorial, including genetic and environmental factors. Traditionally, obesity is classified as endogenous (due to genetic syndromes and endocrine diseases) and exogenous (due to excessive intake in relation to energy expenditure). It has been related that endogenous obesity is responsible only for a small percentage of the total of obesity cases. We defend the idea that this approach is too much simplistic and reflects a gap between clinical and research settings. We believe that this small endogenous obesity percentage is actually due to our still limited knowledge about the energy balance regulation and the several obesity causes. Objective: to review the literature concerning energy balance regulation, genetic and neuroendocrine factors involved in obesity etiology and future perspectives for obesity treatment. Sources of data: articles published in indexed scientific journals, books, dissertations and thesis. Most articles were obtained from Medline and Scielo databases using the keywords "obesity", "energy balance", "genetic", "hormone", "treatment", for the period between 1985 and 2005. Results: here we discuss the following topics: energy balance regulation, obesity genetics and gene – environment interactions, metabolic imprinting and future perspectives for obesity treatment. Conclusion: The recent advances in our understanding of neuroendocrine energy balance regulation, obesity genetics and gene – environment interactions demand a paradigm shift in obesity classification and therapeutic approach. In the future, patients previously classified in the same group, as having exogenous obesity, may have their obesity cause identified and individualized at the endogenous level. An individualized approach of the different obesity causes may lead us to safer and more effective treatments.

[*] E-mail address: genibalaban@hotmail.com, R. Sgto. José M. Brasileiro, 530, Lagoa Seca Juazeiro do Norte-CE Brasil, Cep: 63040-170

Introduction

Obesity etiology is multifactorial, including genetic and environmental factors. Traditionally, obesity is classified as endogenous (due to genetic syndromes and endocrine diseases) and exogenous (due to excessive intake in relation to energy expenditure). It has been related that endogenous obesity is responsible only for a small percentage of the total of obesity cases.

We defend the idea that this approach is too much simplistic and reflects a gap between clinical and research settings. We believe that this small endogenous obesity percentage is actually due to our still limited knowledge about the energy balance regulation and the several obesity causes.

The energy balance is regulated by a complex neuroendocrine system, only partly understood. The leptin discovery, in 1994, marked a revolution in our energy balance understanding. White adipose tissue is now recognized as an important endocrine and secretory organ, releasing a wide range of protein factors termed adipokines. Other important discoveries came, like the gut hormones ghrelin and peptide YY_{3-36}.

In addition, it has been shown that genetics can modulate the response to environmental alterations, like dietary changes and physical activity programs. On the other hand, it has been related that early nutritional experiences can alter gene expression. We agree with other authors that obesity is a phenotype of different diseases, some of them still don't identified.

In this article, our objective is to review the literature concerning energy balance regulation, genetic and neuroendocrine factors involved in obesity etiology and future perspectives for obesity treatment. Our sources of data included articles published in indexed scientific journals, books, dissertations and thesis. Most articles were obtained from Medline and Scielo databases using the keywords "obesity", "energy balance", "genetic", "hormone", "treatment", for the period between 1985 and 2005.

Energy Balance Regulation

The energy balance of the human body is under the regulation of a complex and still poorly understood neuroendocrine system. This network is composed by an afferent system, a processing unit located in the ventromedial hypothalamus in the central nervous system, and an efferent system [1].

The afferent system brings information about the hunger and satiety balance, as well as on the body energy reserves. The afferent signals may be of short or long term duration, and of peripheral or central origin [1].

Peripheral factors signaling hunger include low glucose plasma levels, cortisol and ghrelin, a recently described hormone produced in the stomach [1-3]. Ghrelin was first identified in 1999, initially as a stimulatory agent for the growth hormone secretion and, later on, as a regulator of the energy balance. Fasting results in increased secretion of ghrelin, whereas feeding decreases its secretion [1-3]. The hormone has also been identified in umbilical cord blood, although its role on the feeding behaviour of the newborn is still not clearly established [4].

Peripheral signs for satiety include gastrointestinal distension, the activity of nutrients and several hormones, such as insulin, cholecystokinin and the peptide YY_{3-36} (PYY_{3-36}) [1], [5]. The intestinal hormone PYY_{3-36} is secreted postprandially and in amounts proportional to the caloric value of the meal. Infusion of normal postprandial concentrations of the hormone decreases appetite significantly and reduces food ingestion in around 33% during 24 h [5].

Leptin, first described in 1994, is a long-term peripheral afferent factor which inhibits the appetite and anabolic pathways, stimulating catabolic pathways [6], [7]. It is mainly produced by adipocytes, and informs the hypothalamus on the availability of stored energy represented by the adipose tissue [1], [6], [7]. Other sources of leptin have been identified, such as the liver, stomach and placenta [7]. Vatten et al [8] observed a positive association between leptin levels in umbilical cord blood and weight and length at birth. A review by Sandoval & Davis [9] describes the integrated regulation of leptin and insulin, suggesting that alterations in leptin levels could be involved in the physiopathology of diabetes.

Besides these peripheral signals, the ventromedial hypothalamus receives information from other portions of the brain concerning the energy balance regulation. Dopamine, gamma-amino butyric acid, neurotensin and corticotropin-releasing hormone provide information related to stress, alert state and pain, which exert an inhibitory effect on appetite. Serotonin and norepinephrine have also been suggested to have an important role in inducing satiety. The activity of serotonin over satiety seems to have a central as well as a peripheral component, with intestinal secretion of serotonin [1], [10]. Metenkephalin, orexin-A and -B, the melanin-concentrating hormone and galanin, on the other hand, stimulate food intake and energy storage [1].

Peripheral and central afferent signals reach the neurons on the ventromedial hypothalamus, where they are integrated by a "central processing unit" designed for the stimulation or inhibition of food intake and energy expenditure. This central processing unit has an anorexigenic branch which includes neurons expressing the POMC (proopiomelanocortin) peptide, with its clivage product alpha-MSH (alphamelanocyte-stimulating hormone) and the CART (cocaine-anphetamin-regulated transcript) peptide. The orexigenic branch, on the other hand, contains neurons expressing the NPY (neuropeptide Y) and AgRP (agouti gene-related protein) peptides. These two branches compete for melanocortin receptors [1].

The synthesis of POMC e alpha-MSH is stimulated by overfeeding and leptin infusion. Alfa-MSH binds to the melanocortin receptor and induces anorexia. The synthesis of CART is also induced by leptin, and reduced by fasting [1].

NPY is the main orexygenic peptide, and has specific receptors. Its expression is stimulated by fasting and weight loss and inhibited by leptin. The AgRP peptide is a competitive antagonist of the melanocortin receptors, blocking the binding of alpha-MSH to the receptor and thus preventing the induction of satiety [1].

According to Kalra et al [11], rhythm and synchronism in the secretion of leptin, ghrelin and NPY are important for the daily feeding pattern. The authors suggest that subtle and progressive disturbances of this mechanism result in a positive energy balance, leading to excessive weight gain and obesity.

The efferent system relates to appetite and energy storage versus energy expenditure. The sympathetic nervous system induces energy expenditure, whereas the parasympathetic system stimulates storage [1]. The total energy expenditure has three components: resting energy expenditure (representing in general 50 to 65% of total expenditure), thermogenesis (around 10% of total expenditure) and voluntary energy expenditure (which ranges between 5 to 50% of total expenditure) [1]. Bachman et al [12] showed that rats submitted to ablation of the three known kinds of adrenergic receptors become obese due to a deficiency in the food-induced thermogenesis mechanism.

Obesity Genetics and Gene – Environment Interactions

Obesity etiology is multifactorial, with genetic and environmental factors involved [13-22] (Figure 1- Obesity Causal Model). Persons with obese parents have increased risk for developing obesity, evidencing a familial trait in the disease [16]. The relative role of genetics and environment, however, is difficult to establish since, besides genetic factors, feeding habits and physical activity are also shared among parents and children [16], [18], [19]. Furthermore, that is evidence that genetic factors can modulate body response to environmental changes such as those involving diet and physical activity [22].

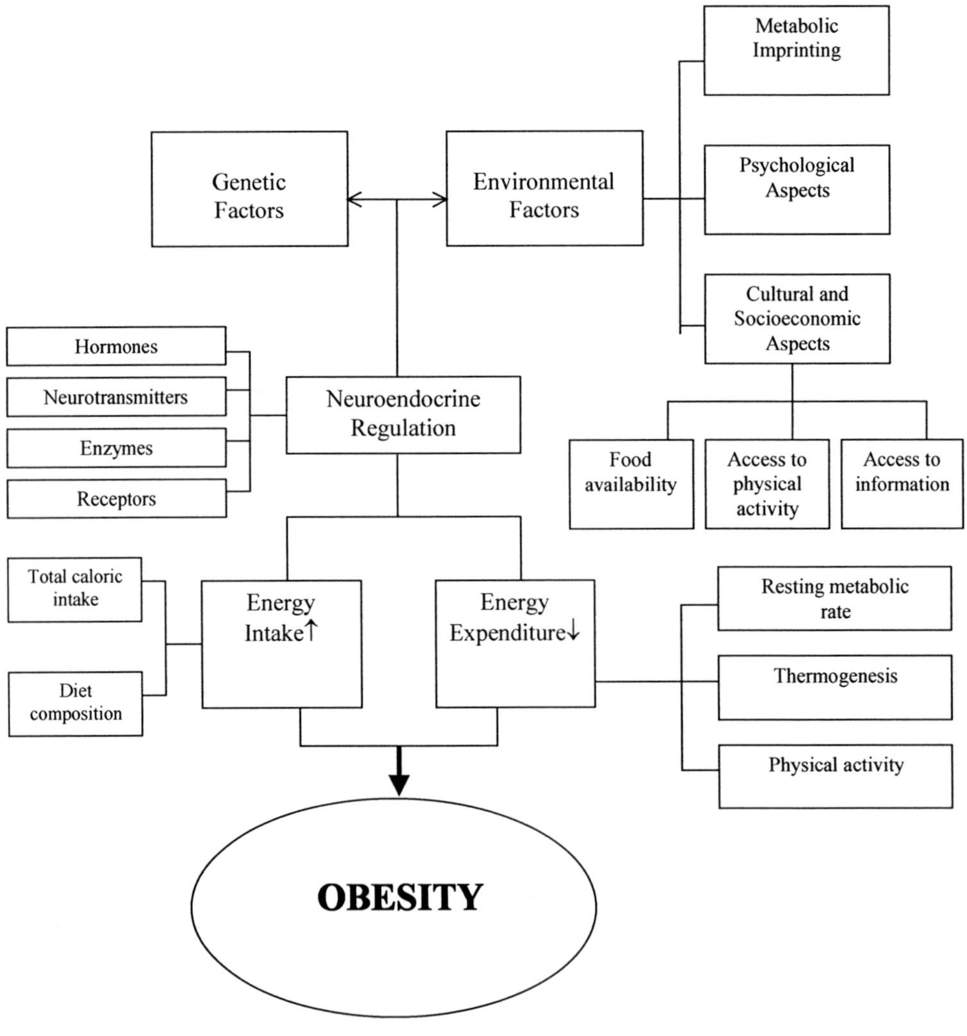

Figure 1 – Obesity Causal Model.

A significant individual variation in lipid plasma concentration in response to modifications in the amount of ingested fat and cholesterol, for instance, has already been reported. Some individuals are less sensitive to diet modifications, whereas others respond more easily to these interventions [22].

Studies with monozygotic twins have also indicated a role for genetic components in the response to environmental changes [22]. An investigation involving 12 pairs of monozygotic twins submitted to a hypercaloric diet showed considerable variation in weight gain, increase in body fat and in visceral fat among the individuals, with larger between-pair than within-pair differences. In a study with monozygotic twins submitted to a negative energy balance, reached through a program of physical exercise, greater within-pair concordance was observed for weight variation, and body, subcutaneous and visceral fat.

While a genetic modulation of the response to environmental changes is apparent, on the other hand, some evidences suggest that environmental conditions can, during critical developmental periods, induce modifications on the pattern of expression of specific genes, as discussed below (see *metabolic imprinting*) [23],[24]. It is believed that the initial nutritional experiences of an individual may influence his/her susceptibility for particular chronic diseases in adulthood, including obesity [23-33].

Hoffman et al [33], for instance, reported results showing that children with a history of malnutrition and classified as stunted (with a deficit in the height/age index) present deficient processes of lipid oxidation, and are thus more susceptible to obesity. It was suggested that this mechanism could explain the increased prevalence of obesity in developing countries.

Increased energy intake and decreased energy expenditure have been pointed as the main causes of obesity [13], [34], [35]. Some studies, however, have not detected differences in the energy intake patterns of obese and nonobese individuals. It is possible that the information provided by the person about his/her energy intake is not a valid measure [13], [36]. The interaction between genetic and environmental factors described above can also explain these results [22].

Obesity has been classified as endogenous (secondary to genetic syndromes and endocrinopathies, such as the Prader-Willi or Down syndromes, hypothyroidism, etc...) or exogenous (resulting from excessive food intake in relation to energy expenditure). Currently, endogenous obesity is considered to account for only around 1% of the cases [37].

Recent advances in the understanding of the neuroendocrine regulation of the energy balance, the genetic factors responsible for obesity and the interaction between genetics and environment, however, suggest that this classification should be reviewed in the future, and that the frequencies observed today will be significantly altered. It is probable that the small frequency of cases diagnosed as endogenous obesity is actually due to our incomplete understanding of these phenomena. As new hormones, neurotransmitters, receptors and genes are identified, the etiology of obesity acquires new dimensions. Patients now assigned to a single group, such as the so-called exogenous obesity, may have the cause of the disease particularized and identified at the endogenous level.

Lustig [1] described childhood obesity as a phenotype of several diseases, most of them not yet identified. According to Warden & Warden [38], around 15 chromosome loci related to weight, body fat and other characters associated to obesity have been identified in humans, and over 90 of them in animal models. Seven of these genes were already identified as responsible for obesity in humans, and in most cases obesity results from the interaction of multiple genes and not from one gene alone [38].

Cases of childhood obesity due to leptin deficiency have been reported, but human obesity is more frequently associated to resistance to the activity of this hormone than to its deficiency [38].

Mutations of the gene coding the melanocortin receptor MC4R have been suggested as the most frequent known genetic cause of obesity in humans [38]. Children presenting a syndrome characterized by obesity, adrenal insufficiency and red hair, assigned to mutations on the gene coding proopiomelanocortin resulting in inhibition of alpha-MSH production, have been reported. Alpha-MSH affects hair colour by binding to the MC1R receptor in the skin, and food intake and energy expenditure by binding to the MC3R and MC4R receptors in the hypothalamus. Adrenal insufficiency in these children can be explained by the fact that alpha-MSH is composed by the first 13 aminoacids of the adrenocorticotrophic hormone [38].

An association between mutations in the MC4R receptor and some mental disorders characterized by behaviour disturbances and obesity has been suggested [39].

Obesity caused by mutation of the gene coding the prohormone convertase 1, an enzyme involved in the conversion of POMC into active components, including alpha-MSH, has also been identified [38].

Metabolic Imprinting

Epidemiologic studies as well as experiments with animal models have suggested that the first nutritional experiences of an individual may affect his/her susceptibility for chronic diseases of adulthood, such as obesity, hypertension, cardiovascular disease and type 2 diabetes [23-33], [40-42]. The term metabolic imprinting or metabolic programming describes the phenomena that an early nutritional experience, occurring during a critical developmental stage (opportunity window), results in a permanent effect predisposing to specific diseases throughout the life [23].

The investigation reported by Ravelli et al [27] with 19-year old Dutch youngsters, who had been prenatally exposed to hunger and deprivation between 1944 and 1945, is classical among epidemiologic studies. Individuals whose mothers had been deprived during the first two trimesters of pregnancy presented an overweight prevalence 80% higher than those who had not been exposed to these conditions. The phenomena can be explained, according to the authors, by the fact that these individuals were submitted to nutritional deprivation during a critical period of hypothalamic differentiation, affecting the development of the centres regulating appetite. On the other hand, for youngsters exposed to deprivation during the last trimester of pregnancy, or during the first five months of postnatal life, the overweight prevalence was 40% lower than among nonexposed individuals. The phenomena was, in this case, attributed to nutritional deprivation during a critical period for adipocyte proliferation.

Waterland & Garza [23] suggested some mechanisms for the metabolic imprinting. They include induction of modifications in the structure of some organs (affecting vascularization, innervation or the distribution of the different types of cells), or in the number of cells and metabolic differentiation (alterations in the expression of particular genes, resulting in variations in the production of enzymes, hormones, hormone receptors, transmembrane transporters, etc…).

Breastfeeding represents one of the earliest nutritional experiences for the newborn, in continuity to the nutrition process began during intrauterine life. The nutrients present in breastmilk are qualitative and quantitatively different from those contained in formulas. Furthermore, many bioactive factors present in the human milk, such as hormones and growth factors, have a role in growth, differentiation and functional maturation of specific organs, influencing different aspects of development [43-45].

Wagner [43] points out that the amniotic fluid and breastmilk share some characteristics, such as bioactivity, emphasizing the concept of a continuity between the intrauterine and extrauterine growth processes. Hirai et al [44] showed the importance of some growth factors present in the amniotic fluid as well as in breastmilk for the process of perinatal gastrointestinal adaptation.

The unique composition of breastmilk could thus be involved in the establishment of metabolic imprinting, affecting for instance the number and/or size of adipocytes or inducing metabolic differentiation. A great number of potential mechanisms could be suggested by the complexity of the neuroendocrine network regulating the energy balance, with its multiple components and the great number of bioactive factors present in breastmilk. Many studies have investigated the possibility of a protective role of breastmilk against obesity, with controversial results [46-65].

Insulin, adrenal steroids, T3 and T4 are among the hormones present in breastmilk [45]. Casabiell et al [66] identified leptin in human milk, with a possible regulatory effect in the newborn due to its role in inhibiting appetite and anabolic pathways and in stimulating catabolic pathways [8].

Lucas et al [67] described different endocrine responses, concerning the secretion of pancreatic and intestinal hormones, among breastfed and formula-fed newborns.

Some groups have reported a greater consumption of protein by newborns fed with baby formula than by those who are breastfed, a possible mechanism to explain increased risk for obesity. The increased ingestion of protein would result in increased secretion of IGF-1 (insulin-like growth factor type 1), which would stimulate adipocyte proliferation. This hypotheses, however, has not been confirmed and demands more detailed investigation [31].

Future Perspectives for Obesity Treatment

The successfully use of recombinant leptin to treat leptin deficiency related obesity was already described in humans [68] . Vickers et al [69] reported that neonatal leptin treatment reverses developmental programming in rats. According to these authors, adult offspring of rats subjected to undernutrition during pregnancy develop obesity, hyperinsulinemia, hyperleptinemia, reduced locomotor activity, hyperphagia and increased fat mass, especially in the presence of a high fat diet. The authors found that leptin neonatal treatment (day three to thirteen) resulted in a transient slowing of neonatal weight gain and normalized caloric intake, locomotor activity, body weight, fat mass and fasting plasma glucose, insulin and leptin concentrations in contrast to saline treated offspring. Klebanov et al [70] reported that adipose tissue transplantation protects leptin deficient mice from obesity and normalizes insulin sensitivity. Boghossian et al [71] reported that a stable increase in leptin availability in the hypothalamus with the aid of leptin gene therapy suppresses fat accretion for nearly the lifetime of laboratory rodents.

Gurwitz [72] suggests that nicotinic agonists may play a role as anti-obesity drugs.

It has been reported that after bypass surgery used to treat obesity, ghrelin levels are lower and there is elevation in PYY_{3-36}, suggesting that the success of bypass surgery may be as much hormonal as mechanical, as induced malabsorption is usually only temporary whereas the loss of appetite is permanent [2], [73-76].

Future therapeutic targets against obesity include cholecystokinin, PYY_{3-36} or their analogues and ghrelin antagonists [1], [11], [76], [77].

Yanovski [78] enphazaises that as obesity is a chronic condition that requires continuous treatment, both the immediate and long-term risks and benefits of pharmacotherapy must be carefully weighed.

Conclusion

The recent advances in our understanding of neuroendocrine energy balance regulation, obesity genetics and gene – environment interactions demand a paradigm shift in obesity classification and therapeutic approach. As new hormones, neurotransmitters, enzymes, receptors and genes are identified, obesity etiology takes another dimension.

In the future, patients previously classified in the same group, as having exogenous obesity, may have their obesity cause identified and individualized at the endogenous level. An individualized approach of the different obesity causes may lead us to safer and more effective treatments.

References

[1] Lustig RH. The neuroendocrinology of childhood obesity. *Pediatr Clin North Am* 2001; 48: 1-14.

[2] Flier JS, Maratos-Flier E. The stomach speaks – ghrelin and weight regulation. N *Engl J Med* 2002; 346: 1662-3.

[3] Horvath TL, Diano S, Sotonyi P, Heiman M, Tschüp M. Minireview: ghrelin and the regulation of energy balance – a hypotalamic perspective. *Endocrinology* 2001; 142: 4163-9.

[4] Chanoine JP, Yeung LPK, Wong ACK, Birmingham CL. Immunoreactive ghrelin in human cord blood: relation to anthropometry, leptin and growth hormone. *JPGN* 2002; 35: 282-6.

[5] Batterham RL, Cowley MA, Small CJ, Herzog H, Cohen MA, Dakin CL et al. Gut hormone PYY_{3-36} physiologically inhibits food intake. *Nature* 2002; 418: 650-4.

[6] Friedman JM. Genetics of obesity. (1999; October; 19) Available from: http://www.hhmi.org/science/genetics/friedman.htm.

[7] Hoppin AG, Kaplan LM. The leptin era: new insight into the mechanisms of body weight homeostasis. *J Pediatr Gastroenterol Nutr* 1999; 29: 250-64.

[8] Vatten LJ, Nilsen ST, Odergard RA, Romundstad PR, Austgulen R. Insulin-like growth factor I and leptin in umbilical cord plasma and infant birth size at term. *Pediatrics* 2002; 109: 1131-5.

[9] Sandoval DA, Davis SN. Leptin: metabolic control and regulation. *J Diabetes Complications* 2003; 17: 108-13.

[10] Silva SRF. *Pharmachological stimulus to serotonine reuptake: effects on neonatal growth and development in rats.* [Master degree dissertation]. Recife (PE), Brazil: Federal University of Pernambuco, Nutrition Department; 2002.
[11] Kalra SP, Bagnasco M, Otukonyong EE, Dubc MG, Kalra PS. Rhythmic, reciprocal ghrelin and leptin signaling: new insight in the development of obesity. *Regul Pept* 2003; 111: 1-11.
[12] Bachman ES, Dhillon H, Zhang CY, Cinti S, Bianco AC, Kobilka BK et al. Adrenergic receptor signaling required for diet-induced thermogenesis and obesity resistance. *Science* 2002; 297: 843-5
[13] Schonfeld-Warden N, Warden CH. Childhood obesity: etiology and treatment. *Clin Pediatr Am Norte* 1997; 2: 343-66.
[14] Parra-Cabrera S, Hernández B, Durán-Arenas L, López-Arellano O. Alternative models to obesity epidemiologic analysis as a public health problem. *Rev Saúde Pública* 1999; 33: 314-25.
[15] Monteiro CA. Conde WL, Popkin BM. Independent effects of income and education on the risk of obesity in the brazilian adult population. *J Nutr* 2001; 131: 881S-6S.
[16] Zlochevsky ERM. Obesity in childhood and adolescence. *Rev Paul Ped* 1996; 14: 124-33.
[17] Fonseca VM, Sichieri R, Veiga GV. Factors related to obesity in adolescents. *Rev Saúde Pública* 1998; 32: 541-9.
[18] Nguyen VT, Larson DE, Johnson RK, Goran MI. Fat intake and adiposity in children of lean and obese parents. *Am J Clin Nutr* 1996; 63: 507-13.
[19] Oliveria AS, Ellison RC, Moore LL, Gillman MW, Garrahie EJ, Singer MR. Parent-child relationship in nutrient intake: the Framingham Children's Study. *Am J Clin Nutr* 1992; 56: 593-8.
[20] Golan M. Environmental factors influence in childhood obesity development and treatment. *Anais Nestlé* 2002; 62: 31-42.
[21] Ukkola O, Bouchard C. Genetic factors and chilhood obesity. *Anais Nestlé* 2002; 62: 12-21.
[22] Pérusse L, Bouchard C. Gene diet interections in obesity. *Am J Clin Nutr* 2000; 72: 1285S-90S.
[23] Waterland RA, Garza C. Potential mechanisms of metabolic imprinting that lead to chronic disease. *Am J Clin Nutr* 1999; 69: 179-97.
[24] Waterland RA, Garza C. Potential for metabolic imprinting by nutritional pertubation of epigenetic gene regulation. *Public Health Issues Infant Child Nutr* 2002; 48: 317-33.
[25] Baker SS, Motil KJ, Heyman MB. Research agenda for pediatric gastroenterology, hepatology and nutrition: Nutrition and obesity: Report of the North American Society for Pediatric Gastroenterology, Hepatology and Nutrition for the Children's Digestive Health and Nutrition Foundation. *JPGN* 2002; 35: S281-5.
[26] McClellan R, Novak D. Fetal nutrition: how we become what we are? *J Pediatr Gastroenterol Nutr* 2001; 33: 233-44.
[27] Ravelli GP, Stein ZA, Susser MW. Obesity in young men after famine exposure in utero and early infancy. *N Engl J Med* 1976; 295: 349-53.
[28] Singhal A, Farooqi S, Rahilly SO, Cole TJ, Fewtrell M, Lucas A. Early nutrition and leptin concentrations in later life. *Am J Clin Nutr* 2002; 75: 993-9.

[29] Martorell R, Stein AD, Schroeder DG. Early nutrition and later adiposity. *J Nutr* 2001; 131: 874S-80S.
[30] Morley R, Dwyer T. Early exposures and later health and development. *Public Health Issues Infant Child Nutr* 2002; 48: 257-78.
[31] Michaelsen KF, Hoppe C, Schack-Nielsen L, Molgaard C. Does an excessive protein intake early in life cause health problems such as obesity later in life? *Public Health Issues Infant Child Nutr* 2002; 48: 279-93.
[32] Davis MK. Breastfeeding and chronic disease in childhood and adolescence. *Pediatr Clin North Am* 2001; 48: 1-10.
[33] Hoffman DJ, Sawaya AL, Verreschi I, Tucker KL, Roberts SB. Why are nutritionally stunted children at increased risk of obesity? Studies of metabolic rate and fat oxidation in shantytown children from São Paulo, Brazil. *Am J Clin Nutr* 2000; 72: 702-7.
[34] Troiano RP, Briefel RR, Carrol MD, Bialostosky K. Energy and fat intakes of children and adolescents in the United States: data from the National Health and Nutrition Examination Surveys. *Am J Clin Nutr* 2000; 72: 1343S-53S.
[35] Atkin LM, Davies PSW. Diet composition and body composition in preschool children. *Am J Clin Nutr* 2000; 72: 15-21.
[36] Bandini LG, Schoeller DA, Cyr HN, Dietz WH. Validity of reported energy intake in obese and nonobese adolescents. *Am J Clin Nutr* 1990; 52: 421-5.
[37] 96-Damiani D, Carvalho DP, Oliveira RG. Childhood obesity – a great challenge. *Ped Mod* 2000; 36: 489-528.
[38] Warden NAS, Warden CH. Biological influences on obesity. *Pediatr Clin North Am* 2001; 48: 1-8.
[39] List JF, Habener JF. Defective melanocortin 4 receptors in hiperphagia and morbid obesity. *N Engl J Med* 2003: 1160-3.
[40] Klein S, Wadden T, Sugerman HJ. AGA technical review on obesity. *Gastroenterology* 2002; 123: 882-932.
[41] Koletzko B, Girardet JP, Klish W, Tabacco, O. Obesity in children and adolescents worldwide: current views and future directions-Working group report of the First World Congress of Pediatric Gastroenterology, Hepatology and Nutrition. *J Pediatr Gastroenterol Nutr* 2002; 35: S205-S212.
[42] Goran MI. Metabolic precursors and effects of obesity in children: a decade of progress, 1990-1999. Am J Clin Nutr 2001; 73:158-71.
[43] Wagner CL. Amniotic fluid and human milk: a continuum of effect? *JPGN* 2002; 34: 513-4.
[44] Hirai C, Ichiba H, Saito M, Shintaku H, Yamano T, Kusuda S. Trophic effect of multiple growth factors in amniotic fluid or human milk on cultured human fetal small intestinal cells. *JPGN* 2002; 34: 524-8.
[45] Hamosh M. Bioactive factors in human milk. *Pediatr Clin North Am* 2001; 48: 1-19.
[46] Kramer MS. Do breast-feeding and delayed introduction of solid foods protect against subsequent obesity? *J Pediatr* 1981; 98: 883-7.
[47] Kramer MS, Barr RG, Leduc DG, Boisjoly C, McVey-White L, Pless B. Determinants of weight and adiposity in the first year of life. *J Pediatr* 1985; 106: 10-4.
[48] Kramer MS, Barr RG, Leduc DG, Boisjoly C, Pless B. Infant determinants of childhood weight and adiposity. *J Pediatr* 1985; 107: 104-7.

[49] Fomon SJ, Rogers RR, Ziegler EE, Nelson SE, Thomas LN. Indices of fatness and serum cholesterol at age eight years in relation to feeding and growth during early infancy. *Pediatr Res* 1984; 18: 1233-8.
[50] Agras WS, Kraemer HC, Berkovitz RI, Hammer LD. Influence of early feeding style on adiposity at 6 years of age. *J Pediatr* 1990; 116: 805-9.
[51] Zive MM, McKay H, Frank-Spohrer GC, Broyles SL, Nelson JA, Nader PR. Infant-feeding practices and adiposity in 4-y-old anglo- and mexican-americans. *Am J Clin Nutr* 1992; 55: 1104-8.
[52] O' Callaghan MJ, Williams GM, Andersen MJ, Bor W, Najman JM. Prediction of obesity in children at 5 years: a cohort study. *J Pediatr Child Health* 1997; 33: 311-6.
[53] Wadsworth M, Marshall S, Hardy R, Paul A. Breastfeeding and obesity: relation may be accounted for by social factors. *BMJ* 1999; 319: 1576.
[54] Tulldahl J, Pettersson K, Andersson SW, Hulthen L. Mode of infant feeding and achieved growth in adolescence: early feeding patterns in relation to growth and body composition in adolescence. *Obes Res* 1999; 7: 431-7.
[55] Von Kries R, Koletzko B, Sauerwald T, Von Mutius E, Barnert D, Grunert V et al. Breast feeding and obesity: cross sectional study. *BMJ* 1999; 319: 147-50.
[56] Liese AD, Hirsh T, von Mutius E, Keil U, Leupold W, Weiland SK. Inverse association of overweight and breast feeding in 9 to 10-y-old children in Germany. *Int J Obes Relat Metab Disord* 2001; 25: 1644-50.
[57] Gillman MW, Rifas-Shiman SL, Camargo CA, Berkey CS, Frazier L, Rockett HRH et al. Risk of overweight among adolescents who were breastfed as infants. *JAMA* 2001; 285: 2461-7.
[58] Hediger ML, Overpeck MD, Kuczmarski RJ, Ruan J. Association between infant breastfeeding and overweight in young children. *JAMA* 2001; 285: 2453-60.
[59] Armstrong J, Reilly JJ, Team CHI. Breastfeeding and lowering the risk of childhood obesity. *Lancet* 2002; 359: 2003-4.
[60] Toschke AM, Vignerova J, Lhotska L, Osancova K, Koletzko B, von Kries R. Overweight and obesity in 6-to-14-year-old czech children in 1991: protective effect of breast-feeding. *J Pediatr* 2002; 141: 764-9.
[61] Butte NF. The role of breastfeeding in obesity. Pediatr Clin North Am 2001; 48: 1-7.
[62] Koletzko B, von Kries R. Is early interruption of breastfeeding associated to posterior risk of obesity? *Anais Nestlé* 2002; 62: 22-30.
[63] Dewey KG. Is breastfeeding protective against child obesity? *J Hum Lact* 2003; 19: 9-18.
[64] Balaban G, Silva GAP, Motta MEFA, Carneiro CQ, Silva CRA, Nunes GJB, Vieira MPG, Rodrigues VO. *Early interruption of breastfeeding and other potential risk factors for overweight in preschool children.* (submited for publication)
[65] Balaban G, Silva GAP, Dias MLCM, Dias MCM, Fortaleza GTM, Morotó FMM, Rocha ECV. Does breastfeeding prevent childhood overweight? *Rev Bras Saúde Matern Infant* 2004; 4(3): 263-8.
[66] Casabiel X, Pineiro V, Tome MA, Peino R, Dieguez C, Casanueva FF. Presence of leptin in colostrum and/or breast milk from lactating mothers: a potential role in the regulation of neonatal food intake. *J Clin Endocrinol Metabol* 1997; 82: 4270-3.

[67] Lucas A, Blackburn AM, Aynsley-Green A, Sarson DL, Adrian TE, Bloom SR. Breast vs bottle: endocrine responses are different with formula feeding. *Lancet* 1980; 14: 1267-9.

[68] Farooqi IS, Jebb AS, Langmack G, et al: Effects of recombinant leptin therapy in a child with congenital leptin deficiency. *N Engl J Med* 1999; 341: 913-5.

[69] Vickers MH, Gluckman PD, Coveny AH, Hofman PL, Cutfield WS, Gertler A, Breier BH, Harris M. Neonatal leptin treatment reverses developmental programming. *Endocrinology* 2005; 146 (10): 4211-6.

[70] Klebanov S, Astle CM, DeSimone O, Alblamunits V, Harrison DE. Adipose tissue transplantation protects ob/ob mice from obesity, normalizes insulin sensitivity and restors fertility. *J Endocrinol* 2005; 186(1): 203-11.

[71] Boghossian S, Lecklin A, Torto R, Kalra PS, and Kalra SP. Suppression of fat deposition for the life time with gene therapy. *Peptides* 2005; 26(8): 1512-19.

[72] Gurwitz D. The therapeutic potential of nicotine and nicotinic agonists for weight control. *Expert Opin Investig Drugs* 1999; 8(6): 747-60.

[73] Cummings DE, Weigle DS, Frayo RS, et al. Plasma ghrelin levels after diet - induced weight loss or gastric bypass surgery. *N Engl J Med* 2002; 346:1623-30.

[74] Naslund E, Gryback P, Hellstrom PM, et al. Gastrointestinal hormones and gastric emptying 20 years after jejunoileal bypass for massive obesily. *Int J Obes Relate Metab Disord* 1997; 21: 387-92.

[75] Le Roux CW, Shuurey S, Ghatei MA, et al. PYY and decreased appetite following jejunum intestinal bypass in rats. British Endocrine Society. Glaasgow, 2003: endocrine abstracts.

[76] Neary NM, Small CJ, Bloom SR. Gut and mind. *Gut* 2003; 52:918-21.

[77] Asakawa A, InuiA, Kaga T, et al. Antagonism of ghrelin receptor reduces food intake and body weight gain in mice. *Gut* 2003; 52: 947-52.

[78] Yanovski JA. Aggressive therapy for childhood and adolescent obesity. In: Chen C, Dietz WH. *Obesity in Childhood and Adolescence*. Philadelphia: Lippincott Williams & Wilkins; 2002; 223-44.

In: Global Dimensions of Childhood Obesity
Editor: Richard K. Flamenbaum, pp. 139-153

ISBN: 1-60021-037-6

Chapter 7

CHILDHOOD OBESITY. THE VIEW FROM THE FAMILY

Anders Lindelof *

Social Anthropology, Denmark

Abstract

The current article is based on a qualitative study exploring overweight and obese children and their families' perceptions and understandings of the child's obesity. The study involved 60 obese children and 40 parents. Three analytical areas of interests are elaborated. 1) Which factors do the child and his or her family believe initially to have caused the child's obesity? 2) How does the child's obesity influence the daily life of the obese child and its parents? 3) How does the family try to help and support the child towards weight loss?

The results showed that many families either partly or not at all believed that factors related to diet and exercise had caused the child's obesity. However, these families were aware of the medical explanation of obesity but believed that their child was an exception from this. As these families did not associate the obesity with diet or exercise they believed that external and non-adjustable factors had caused the obesity. Compared with families associating the child's obesity with diet and exercise these families were less affected by the child's obesity and were thus less willing to achieve weight loss by changing their way of living.

I relate the empirical findings to the currents Danish ways of treating childhood obesity. I show that these weight reducing strategies are characterized by a goal of changing the child's eating and exercising habits regardless of the perception of the family. I propose that this imbalance between the families' perception of the obesity and the strategies focus on diet and exercise might explain the depressing results weight reducing strategies are generating.

This leads to my final supposition that future intervention programs aiming at reducing the child's weight must deal with the perceptions of the family simultaneously or even prior to traditional focus on diet and exercise.

---

* E-mail address: A_lindelof@hotmail.com, Ny Munkegade 12,3, 8000 Århus C, Denmark

Introduction

It is almost commonplace to begin an article on childhood obesity with mentioning the increasing prevalence of overweight Childhood Obesity: New Research and obesity among children, youth and adults nearly all over the world [1]. However, the situation is now so alarming that a recent report estimated that for the first time in a century future generations are likely to die before their parents due to obesity in the United Kingdom [2] and it is only a matter of years before obesity has exceeded smoking of tobacco as the leading cause of death [3]. We are, as the WHO [4] has pointed out, facing one of the most serious threats to public health in modern time and it is of great importance that we fight the obesity problem by preventing people from becoming overweight and obese, and reduce the number of already overweight and obese individuals[1].

There is a general acceptance that two of the major factors contributing to the so-called obesity epidemic are increased levels of sedentary activities and a diet with increased levels of fat and sugar [5]. In explaining these phenomena it has been suggested that we live in an obesogenic environment [6], [7], which encourages a minimum level of physical activity, and which provides a host of cheap and unhealthy foods and drinks heavily marketed by the respective industries.

However, this still leaves us with two important questions that this article will try to address: First, why do some children become obese while others do not? Second, why can some obese children lose weight while others cannot? There are no easy answers to these questions and although growing research has focused on childhood obesity much still needs to be investigated. Especially qualitative research is lacking and it is widely accepted that insights into knowledge, perceptions and behaviour surrounding the traditional fields of nutrition and exercise [8], [9] are much needed if we are to understand the obese and thereby be able to create effective ways of preventing and treating childhood obesity.

In 2003 I conducted an anthropological and qualitative study of obese children and their families exploring their shared and individual perceptions of the child's obesity.

My research showed that many families did not associate their child's obesity with causes directly related to food or exercise. However, they were very well aware of the medical or physiological explanation of obesity but believed that their child was an exception from this, and that his or her obesity was caused by non-adjustable factors, which made them believe that the child's weight could not be reduced. Because the family believed that the child's obesity was permanent the child did not receive any home based support towards weight reduction and hence, the child did not lose weight.

One might argue that a scientific understanding of these perceptions is of little importance since the treatment of obesity is the same regardless of what the child and family believe. However, my argument is that knowledge exploring these perceptions is essential when establishing effective intervention strategies aiming at reducing childhood obesity. It is, I propose, of great importance when treating childhood obesity that the child's and the family's perceptions of the child's obesity are dealt with simultaneously or even prior to the attempt to change the child's eating and exercising behaviour.

---

[1] In the rest of this article there will be no further distinction between overweight and obesity and the latter term "obesity" will be used synonymously with overweight.

To support this argument I first focus on the current ways of treating childhood obesity, primarily focusing on Danish weight-loss programs for children and youth. Secondly, I present my own research findings. These lead me to a critique of the way childhood obesity is mostly dealt with regarding lifestyle intervention. I argue that the strategies used are focusing on a too narrow goal of changing the children's eating and exercising habits regardless of the attitudes and perceptions of the child and its family. I then propose that future intervention strategies must pay attention to these perceptions if a greater rate of success is achieved.

Current Ways of Preventing and Treating Childhood Obesity

Due to the dramatic increase in the prevalence of overweight and obese children and youth, a growing focus on preventing and treating childhood obesity has appeared. It is of course preferable to prevent children and other age groups from growing obese compared to treating the already obese. The reason for this is both associated with the personal consequences (physiological, psychological and sociological) that obese people suffer from either as child, adolescent [10], or adult [11] and on the societal economical perspectives. It has been estimated that in direct health care cost (preventing, diagnosis, treatment) obesity counts for 5 – 7 % of the total annual medical expenditures in the United States [[12]]. Due to the still increasing number of obese individuals this number will rise. Finally, early prevention is important due to the life long persistency of obesity and the relation between late childhood/adolescent obesity and adult obesity [13].

However, if preventing people and especially children from becoming obese at all, a societal change encouraging healthy eating habits and physical activity is necessary. This cannot be carried out solely by the health professionals, and it is of great importance that many different institutions and departments working with children participate in creating favourable surroundings. Lissau and colleagues [14] have argued that besides health professionals this includes families, schools, governments as well as the relevant industries and one could add the media. Although some changes in this direction are beginning to occur, for example healthier food in schools or safer bicycle tracks, there is still a long way to go if we are to write off the obsogenic society. Therefore, effective strategies aiming at reducing the already obese need to be established.

In the remaining part of this chapter focus will be on the treatment of childhood obesity, as it is practised today[2]. However, to limit my focus I will only discuss lifestyle modification as practiced in Denmark in 2005.

In order to understand one of the most common intervention strategies of treating childhood obesity, it is useful to consider the aetiology of obesity. Simply stated obesity is the result of a positive energy balance caused by an excess of calories in the diet compared to energy expended on physical activity. Logically the way to lose weight is to reverse the equation and create a negative energy balance, where the body uses the stored fat as energy and thereby reduces body fat. Therefore, to introduce a healthier diet and reduce sedentary activities are key elements in current ways of treating childhood obesity.

[2] The following are only addressing intervention strategies aiming at reducing childhood obesity and not national campaigns or other strategies targeting the whole population.

In Denmark (2005) 94 projects aiming at reducing childhood and youth obesity are listed on an online published database by Learning Lab Denmark [15]. The following analysis is based on a thorough reading on the standardized online information of these projects.

Although different in scope all the intervention programs have a common denominator, namely diet and exercise. All projects have some sort of nutritious focus. Either as one-way information about healthy meals and foods or more participatory based activities like food shopping excursions, cooking or other food-related activities. The projects also focus on physical exercise either by encouraging participation in non-formalized exercise like walking or biking to school or more formalized activities like joining a sports club or special sports events for obese children only. In all projects, these two areas are considered the focal points of the intervention programs.

Depending on the scope and intentions of the project there may be secondary focus areas guided by a specialist. Eighteen (19 %) of the projects did involve a psychologist and 1 project (1 %) did involve an anthropologist. The rest of the projects did not involve other subject boundaries than those concerning knowledge about nutrition (e.g. dietician, scientist of food technology, nutritionist) or physical activity (e.g. physiotherapist, instructor of gymnastics or fitness).

Although children are the primary targets of the programs it is widely accepted that the family must be involved at some level and the majority of the programs do in fact involve the child's family (81 projects, 86 %). Unfortunately no further specialisation is given in what these projects do to involve the families.

The duration of the different intervention projects varies. The vast majority (58 projects, 61 %) is under one year. Eleven (11 %) projects are planned for one year and six (6 %) projects for more than one year. Eighteen (19 %) projects did not inform about the duration or their program.

All projects had as their primary aim to promote a healthier lifestyle by reducing the child's weight or stop further weight gain. As a secondary aim the projects worked to create a positive environment for the child and thereby increase the level of self-perception, self-esteem and other psycho-social areas. Regarding the promotion of a healthier lifestyle and a permanent weight loss the effect is not fully known. This is partly because the majority of the projects are still running and the long term effects have not been obtained and partly because those projects that have been running for a longer time has not been evaluated in a sufficient and satisfactory manner.

The lack of sufficient evaluation is not only a Danish issue but reflects an overall problem of the various intervention strategies used when aiming at reducing childhood obesity [16]. However, even though the exact quantitative effect of many intervention strategies is unknown, the global history of treating childhood obesity is depressing [17], [18] and effective strategies generating and securing a long term weight loss are much needed.

Although a host of different strategies of intervention has been established to promote and secure a healthier lifestyle, a far too common pattern is that the obese lose weight when beginning to participate in the program but when finishing the involvement the obese regains the lost pounds [19]. Therefore, the different task is not to help the children lose weight per se, but to make sure they stay slim in the future.

But how is this ensured? The following will argue that if a higher rate of success, measured as long term and permanent weight loss, is to be achieved the strategy used must involve a high degree of patient involvement [20] where the obese child is empowered in respect to his or her own treatment. This means, that the strategy of intervention must target the family's resources (both financial and non-physical), perception and knowledge of the child's obesity. Similar thoughts have been proposed by Funnel and colleagues [21] in relation to postoperative care after obesity surgery.

Based on empirical data, the following will give an insight into these areas. Later I will return to the current ways of treating obesity and point out some of the problems we are facing.

Investigation

The academic field involving childhood obesity is dominated by results of quantitative research rather than qualitative.

However, recently qualitative studies exploring different topics like, for example, teenagers' perceptions of their own and others' bodies [22], children and parents' perception of the barriers towards a healthy diet and physical activity [23] and parents' views about their children's television viewing behaviours [24] have been published.

This growing interest in qualitative data reflects the need for new strategies in treating childhood obesity with an increased focus on other areas than the traditional fields of nutrition and exercise. In other words it is not enough to know how many hours obese children watch TV per day or how many calories he or she consumes. The important issues are why the children watch so much TV, or why he or she consumes so many calories.

The present study was qualitative. The thesis and main question were broadly defined; how does an obese child and his or her parents understand and perceive the child's obesity?

I did not operate with pre-decided minor research questions since this could have limited the information to topic areas already decided upon by the researcher. In addition, by operating with a narrow thesis or too many minor research questions it is assumed that the informants have an opinion about these matters, and that their opinion reflects their view on the problem under investigation. For example He et al. [25] focused on parents' views on their children's TV behaviour and Hesketh et al. [26] explored children and their parents' view on physical activity. Despite the relevance and importance of these studies the narrow research questions of these two researchers assumed that the informants associate the child's obesity with behaviour related to either watching television or physical exercise. Hence, the informant is not encouraged to elaborate on other aspects of obesity that they might find more or equally important.

My study involved 60 children equally divided between boys and girls. The average age was 11 ranging between six and 18 years of age. The children's weight and other measurements were not recorded. Thirty-seven parents of the children were also involved. Twenty six parents were divorced and in all except three cases I had contact with the child's mother only.

The children and their parents were located from 3 settings within Denmark:

1) Fifteen children and parents were recruited from a locally based weight loss program for children and youth. The informants were contacted by letter by the program, which besides information from the program included my project description and a stamped addressed envelope for those who wanted to participate. Forty two % answered.

2) Ten children and parents were recruited from schools in Århus. These informants were contacted by the school nurse who asked, if they wanted to participate in the study. All asked agreed to participate.

3) Thirty five children and 12 parents from a "Julemærkehjem"[3]. In Denmark there are four "Julemærkehjem", which function as free boarding schools for socially troubled and mostly obese children for 10 weeks. At the "Julemærkehjem" the children are given regular school education, but are also exposed to a wide range of physical activity and a healthy diet which result in weight losses for nearly everybody.

My data were gathered primarily through qualitative interviews [27]. The children from the Julemærkehjem" were interviewed on the school grounds whereas the rest were interviewed at the children's homes. Separate interview guides for children and parents were created focusing on topics like social surrounding, school relations, the child's diet and exercising habits and so on.

At the "Julemærkehjem" the children were interviewed first individually and later in smaller groups allowing the children to inspire and exchange ideas with each other. The interviews conducted at the children's homes were primarily done separately for both the child and the parents without the other(s) being present. If this could not be achieved the parents were asked to remain quiet while the child was being interviewed.

Apart from the interviews I conducted a two-week fieldwork [28] at the "Julemærkehjem" interacting with the children in their daily life.

The interviews were recorded and later transcribed. In average they lasted 73 minutes. The data from the fieldwork were written down later and added to the transcript.

After finishing the empirical research all data were analyzed according to the principles initially developed by James Spradley [29]. First different themes that carried common meanings were identified and categorized. These themes were then compared and related to each other trying to establish a pattern related to the child's obesity. Finally areas of specific interest were pointed out for detailed discussion.

Three areas will now be summarized and elaborated upon.

1. Which factors do the obese child and his or her family believe to have caused the child's obesity initially?
2. How does the child's obesity influence the daily life of the obese child and its parents?
3. How does the family try to help and support the child towards weight loss?

1, Which factors do the obese child and his or her family believe to have caused the child's obesity initially

To start with, all children and parents were aware of the physiological understanding of obesity. All families knew that in general obesity is the result of an imbalance between diet and exercise. This has been demonstrated elsewhere [30] and Murphy and colleagues [31] even showed that children

down to the level of kindergarten have a thorough understanding of healthy vs. non-healthy food.

[3] The free translation goes "an institution financed by selling Christmas stamps".

However, when analyzing data from the empirical research, a pattern related to the belief of how the family[4] believed the obese child initially became obese emerges. Although the following analysis suggests a clear distinction between two groups the complexity should not be ignored as the families obviously cannot be divided into two homogenous groups. Therefore, these two groups represent either end in a continuum.

One group of families believed that their child's obesity was caused by factors related to an imbalance between nutrition and physical exercise. These families thought that either the child or the whole family had had an unhealthy diet and/or a sedentary lifestyle.

The other group of families had a different view. They believed that the child and the family had lived a relatively active life and had enjoyed a healthy diet. This made them believe that the primary cause of the child's obesity could not be associated with factors related to food and exercise. These families then believed unique and individual factors to have caused the child's obesity. Although different explanations were revealed many were related to earlier events in the child's life or congenital characteristics. For example some families believed that the child had had an illness as infant or had lived a rough early childhood which somehow had caused the obesity. Other families believed that the child was born "big-boned" or with "low metabolism" or "weak nerves" which had caused the obesity. Explanations varied from being very specific like the family who believed it was the abnormally high amount of carrots the child ate, which caused the obesity to more non-specific explanations like "this is the way we look in our family".

However, as I will show later my point is not what the family believes, but that they believe something which is not directly related to factors associated with an unhealthy diet and a sedentary lifestyle.

There was a social stratification which divided these two groups. Although I did not collect data about the families' financial positions and the educational level of the parents, I visited the homes of the families and asked the children at the "Julemærkehjem" to describe their home. The following is therefore based on a subjective account.

The families who believed the child was obese due to an imbalance between food and exercise were generally from a higher societal level. In comparison to the other group they held more prestigious jobs, and their housing situation was better with the majority living in a house with a closed garden. Furthermore and in comparison to the other group, it was in the most cases only the obese child, who was obese in the family. Finally, the children in this group had more friends and liked school better than the children of the other group.

The group of families who held an explanation not directly related to food and exercise generally came from a lower societal level. The parents were often unemployed and they lived in large apartment complexes with no closed garden the child could use for play. In comparison to the other group there was a tendency towards the whole family being obese. Also, in comparison with the other group there were far more divorced parents in this group, and it was the rule rather than the exception that the child's biological parents did not get along very well. The children often expressed that they were bullied at school and the majority of them disliked going to school at all. The children in this group had only a few if any friends and often spent their free time alone.

[4] In the following "family" is synonymous with both child and parent since views and perceptions between child and parent were alike.

To summarize: one group of families believed their child's obesity was related to factors associated with nutrition and exercise and one group of families believed that factors not related to nutrition and exercise had caused the child's obesity. However these families were aware of the medical explanation of obesity but believed that their child had had healthy eating and exercising habits and hence, believed something out of their reach had caused the obesity.

As the following will show the difference in perception of what causes the problem of obesity generates a difference in the way obesity could be handled as well.

2, How does the child's obesity influence the daily life of the obese child and its parents?

When interviewing the families I tried to get an understanding of how their child's obesity affected their daily lives. A clear connection emerged between the two groups described.

The group of families, who believed that factors related to food and exercise had caused the child's obesity, were generally much more concerned about the obesity. The parents often felt directly responsible for the child's weight and believed that they in some way had failed in raising the child. The parents therefore tried their best to make up for past mistakes and help the child achieve a weight reduction. In general these families considered their child's obesity a major problem and they spent many resources thinking about how to support the child.

The group of families who believed the child's obesity was caused by factors not associated to food and exercise were in comparison to the other group far less affected by the child's obesity. These families did not feel a personal responsibility for the child's weight and did not feel they had failed in raising the child. Naturally they were sorry for the child and wished that the child did not have weight problems. However, they did not consider the child's obesity a major problem and they did not in any substantial way support the child in reducing weight.

I was very interested in exploring the reason for this difference between the two groups of families and especially why the latter group did not seem to be affected in any major negative way by the child's obesity. It seems that because this group of families did not associate the child's obesity with factors related to food and exercise but rather with non-adjustable factors, they also believed that the child's obesity was inevitable and chronic. As these families believed that their child's obesity was inevitable, they did not trouble themselves by being affected by the child's weight in their daily lives.

To summarize, the group of families who believed factors related to food and exercise had caused the child's obesity were also feeling a personal responsibility for the child's weight problem and supported the child in losing weight. In all, this group of families were very concerned about the child's weight. In contrast to this, the group of families who believed that factors not related to food and exercise had caused the child's obesity did not feel a personal responsibility and did not in any major way try to support the child in losing weight. These families were sad about the obesity and the related consequences the obesity caused but believed that the obesity was an inevitable condition the child had to get used to and live with.

Below I will show that there is a close relation between the families' levels of concern with the child's obesity and the practical support the child receives in order to lose weight in the family.

3, How does the family try to help and support the child towards weight reduction?

There was a difference in the way the two groups of families tried to help reduce the child's weight.

The group of families who believed that factors related to food and exercise had caused the child's' obesity, and at the same time were affected by the complications of the child's obesity, did more to make the child lose weight than the other group did. This is no surprise. Since these families knew what to do to reduce the weight by introducing a healthier diet and/or increase the level of physical exercise, and were highly motivated to reduce their child's obesity, they were also willing to create a favourable environment for the child in order for him or her to lose weight.

All families in this category had changed the child's or the whole family's diet primarily by reducing the levels of fat and sugar or reduce the amount of food the child ate. The majority of the families had also made restriction on how much candy, junk food and other non-healthy "extra" meals the child was allowed to buy for him/herself. In other words, these families did well concerning the diet.

All the families in this group had also tried to reduce the child's sedentary activities by increasing the amount of physical exercise. But in comparison to the success in changing the diet only a few families succeeded in increasing the level of physical activity over a longer period of time. The pattern was very often that the child had started to increase the level of physical exercise like riding the bike to school or joining a sports club. However, for the majority of the children this was only maintained for a short period of time just to be resumed the next time the child experienced negative attention due to his or her obesity and wanted to lose weight.

The other group of families who did not believe the child was obese due to causes directly related to food and exercise and who were not in their daily life influenced by the child's obesity did not in any major way try to encourage the child to lose weight. This is not surprising either. First of all they believed the child had healthy eating and exercising habits. This made them believe that the obesity were inevitable and related to non-adjustable and external factors. Thus, the families did not feel responsible for the obesity and did not believe that weight could be reduced and hence were not motivated to support the child in reducing his or her weight. Therefore the majority of the families in this category did not put any serious effort into making the child lose weight.

However, many families in this group had tried and tried occasionally to change the family diet. To explain these initiatives I suggest that the reasons are grounded in the heavy attention childhood obesity attracts. Both child and parents were often told by others what to eat and what not to eat. Doctors, school nurses, teachers, and even unknown people at the supermarket often tried to correct the family in buying and eating the right food. And of course the family tried their best to live up to these expectations, but since they did not believe the diet to be seriously responsible for the obesity the initiatives reflected this attitude and were of no significance. As an example, a mother told me that the only diet related problem she could think of was her child using too much sugar in his tea, which she had tried to reduce.

This last section has described the way the two groups handled the child's obesity practically. One group of families did try to help the child lose weight by primarily reducing fats and sugars in the child's diets. Being successful at this the majority of the families failed in supporting the child in increasing the level of physical exercise over time. The other group did not do any serious attempt to reduce the child's weight. Although this last group's lack of intervention is problematic, it is understandable due to their belief in how the child initially became obese. As they did not feel responsible for the weight, they were therefore not motivated to make changes in the child's eating and exercising habits.

Comments

Before I go into detail with the practical implications of the results of the study a brief discussion of some of the above findings is suitable to anticipate some common objections. This is primarily related to the group of families who did not associate their child's obesity with nutrition and physical activity since this group is the most difficult group to help and support by intervention strategies, as one can easily imagine.

It is a common objective put forward by both health professionals and lay people that even though some of the families mentioned in the above believe that their child's obesity is caused by factors not related to diet and exercise, this is not to be taken seriously but is rather a poor excuse in the attempt to disclaim responsibility for the child's weight problem. The families themselves were certainly well aware of this way of understanding their explanations and they often felt dismissed when explaining their point of view to others. For example many families expressed in the interviews, that when visiting their medical practitioner they were seldom taken seriously and listened to. Regardless of what they believed had caused the obesity they were always informed about healthy nutrition and the importance of exercise.

Although this critical attitude towards the families' understanding of the child's obesity is understandable I am cautious in reducing the families' understandings to poor excuses only, and it is my conviction that we have to take their understandings seriously no matter how odd they seem. The reason is, I believe, that whether a poor excuse or not, these understandings and perceptions have shaped and still shape the families' handling of the child's obesity. As shown, this means that since the families believed that the child's weight problem was a chronic condition, they also believed that the success of changing eating and exercising habits would be limited leaving the families with no motivation in trying to introduce a healthier diet and reduce sedentary activities.

From this perspective the lack of motivation and action in supporting the child to lose weight is rational. By reducing these beliefs to poor excuses we fail to understand the families' logical association between motives and action and instead tend to dismiss the families as lazy and ignorant; a view common among doctors and students of medicine, as has been shown elsewhere [32], [33]. Therefore, if a positive relation to the families is to be established it is of primary concern when dealing with obese children and their families that their perspectives are taken seriously.

This brings me back to the beginning of this article and the intervention strategies used when trying to reduce childhood obesity.

Implications

As shown in the above a common way of treating childhood obesity reflects the aetiology of obesity and focus is on nutrition and exercise. This, of course, is supported by science and cannot be denied. You will without doubt lose weight if you consume a non-fattening diet and exercise regularly. Therefore, as the brief description of the Danish intervention strategies showed in the beginning of this article, current intervention strategies try to make the obese lose weight by introducing a healthier diet and increase the level of physical exercise. The implicit philosophy behind this strategy seems to be, first; that the obese is obese because of unhealthy habits regarding diet and exercise and, second; that these habits can be changed by increasing the knowledge of healthy nutrition and the importance of exercise.

But as shown in this material and supported by other studies obese individuals are not obese due to a lack of knowledge about healthy dieting or because he or she does not know that exercise is important. Hence, the result of educating about these factors is limited as it is not a higher level of knowledge the obese are in need of, but, put simply, tools to implement the already realized knowledge into action. In other words, the effect of using an intervention strategy defining actions into right (us) or wrong (them) and perceive "them" as somehow irrational and non-compliant just waiting to be transformed is not high. Unfortunately this is a common way of doing health promotion and has been criticised elsewhere [34], [35].

The point is, that far too much obesity intervention is based on the assumption that an increased knowledge of diet and exercise will lead to a change in behaviour and a weight reduction. It is as if a change of lifestyle is paralleled with a traditional disease and its biomedical treatment. Like a hormone irregularity treated with pills. But instead of pills weekly doses of exercise and information on healthy nutrition is given and, after a while, it is expected that the child and family can monitor their own treatment.

Although the above description may seem exaggerated my proposal is that the treatment of childhood obesity needs to abandon its scientific and biomedical background. Instead, I suggest, focus needs to be placed on a practical or phenomenological notion of obesity where the complexity of everyday practice and reasoning is understood and integrated in the intervention programs.

This means, that consideration has to be taken towards the families own perception of the problem. As shown in the above many families believed that the child's obesity was caused by other factors than those directly associated with food and exercise and hence, these families did not make any serious effort to reduce fat in the child's diet or increase the level of physical activity. Although this attitude is problematic, it is logical seen from the families' perspective and a major barrier to achieve weight reduction since it cannot be expected that the family act in a non-logical way. Therefore, it is of central concern that intervention programs address and alters these perceptions prior or simultaneously to the focus on nutrition and physical activity. In other words, the family has to be ready to change their behaviour before an actual change can occur, as described by Rhee et. al.[36]. Based on the above empirical investigation this means, first, that the family has to understand that food and exercise are connected with the child's obesity and second, that the family needs to change their current ways of living in order to make the child loose weight.

The French sociologist Pierre Bourdieu's (1930 – 2002) notion of habitus might be helpful in conceptualizing this[37].

Although habitus is a complex concept, the relevance in this context lies in the fact that habitus is the product of earlier experiences and refers to the social and material world a subject has been and is exposed to. The point is that these earlier experiences functions as a profound structuring principle that direct the choices people make in respect to the overall life situation. In other words, habitus is the link between experience and practice. By introducing a concept as habitus two important issues appears, first, that behaviour and action does not exist in a vacuum but is formed by a more profound structure of cognition. And second, that a permanent change of behaviour cannot be achieved without changing this structure of cognition.

In the present context, it is of course well known that behaviour can be altered by information. This is probably why the majority of obese children actually lose weight when beginning a formalized program targeting childhood obesity. But it is also well known that it is dubious whether this initial weight loss will lead to a permanent weight reduction. Related to the concept of habitus this lack of permanent weight loss is understandable since habitus has not changed and still influence the child's daily choices. Because habitus is a profound, but not a static structure, it will not change by weekly information on diet and exercise. For this to happen far more intensive and thorough intervention must be established. Compared to the above mentioned strategies used by Danish intervention programs this means, that instead of a weekly session the intervention must integrate as many aspects of the child's and its family's life as possible. It also means that the duration of the intervention must last for a number of years, however, not necessarily with the same intensity. But perhaps must importantly it means that the basis of the intervention must be related to the resources and understandings of the child and family and not perforce to diet and exercise.

Only by a long lasting, intensive, and interdisciplinary effort will it be possible to change the underlying structure, what Bourdieu termed habitus, and only when this is done, can it be expected, that the family engage in a permanent weight reduction.

Conclusion

This article has attempted to demonstrate complexity of childhood obesity as it is experienced by those who are obese as well as their families. Contrary to the majority of scientific research in this field I have not per se focused on the traditional areas related to diet and exercise. Rather, I have focused on the views expressed by the family concerning the child's obesity regardless of their opinion on diet and physical activity. I demonstrated that in a continuum with the medically correct view (explanations involving diet and exercise) at one end and more alternative views (explanations not involving diet and exercise) at the other end the families could be placed at different spots on this continuum. Some families were very aware that the child's obesity was caused by either an unhealthy diet and/or too many sedentary activities and some families believed that the obesity was caused by other factors. These factors could either be non-reachable, e.g. an early childhood disease causing a permanent low metabolism, or they could be partly non-reachable, e.g. social or psychological problems which caused the child to eat too much. However, it is important to note that regardless of the families' beliefs they knew the correct general medical explanations to the origin of obesity.

Based on data from the families' home, the parents' educational background and a personal view on the families I demonstrated that these views or believes had a social aspect. The families believing that unhealthy diet and/or lack of sufficient physical activity had caused the obesity were generally from the upper social levels of society. Whereas the families who believed that these factors either did not or only partly involved exercise generally came from a lower societal layers.

I then went on to show, that these believes shaped both the mental and practical handling of the obesity. Families explaining the child's obesity with factors related to food and exercise were very concerned and motivated to support the child towards weight reduction. Hence, they carried out initiatives governing the child's weight. In opposition to this, the families who did not believe the obesity to have been caused by unhealthy diet and/or insufficient physical activity were not motivated for weight reduction and did not support the child towards weight reduction. I argued that since these families believed that the origin of the child's obesity was out of their reach they also assumed that no change in diet or exercise would reduce the weight. Hence, they did not carry out any initiatives of importance that would benefit the child.

The implications above are important. If a permanent change of behaviour is to be achieved it is of great importance that a family comprehend that a change in the child's eating and exercising behaviour has influence on the child's health and weight. I have argued that serious effort to do this has to be made prior to or simultaneously with traditional intervention strategies. This led me to a critique of the current Danish intervention strategies targeting obese children. These intervention programs need to be far more intense than is the case today. If a permanent change of lifestyle is to be initiated a weekly session involving healthy diet and exercise is not going to work. It has to be realized that a change of behaviour is a far more complex procedure or project, than, say, a more traditional disease which can be cured with medicine.

Therefore, future intervention programs targeting obese children must integrate as many institutions as possible (e.g. schools, medical practitioners, infra structure, media, and so on) initiating a change in the daily life of the child and not just on the weekly meeting day. They also need to involve different levels of professional expertise (e.g. psychologists, anthropologists, behavioural experts and the like) and not just a dietician and a physical therapist working with diet and physical activity. Another important factor is time. A permanent change of behaviour is not changed in a few months but takes many years. However, perhaps most important, all these initiatives must be made according to the child and families' own perceptions of the problem problem. A change of lifestyle cannot be forced but needs to be generated and maintained by the people in question.

Seen in this light it is not merely the goal as the actual weight loss that is important but rather the journey to reach the goal, as Cheryl Mattingly has shown [38] in her excellent analysis of occupational therapists trying to support newly and severely injured patients. As previously mentioned, the task is not to reduce the weight but rather to teach the child and its family how to live a healthy life. The goal of permanent weight loss among obese children will not and cannot be achieved until the journey to a healthy life has been realized.

References

[1] International Obesity Task Force. Task force about obesity. www.iotf.org. Accessed 21-10-05

[2] House of Commons. Health Committee. Obesity. Third Report of Session 2003–04. Volume I. www.publications.parliament.uk/pa/cm200304/cmselect/cmhealth/23/23.pdf. Accessed 21-10-05

[3] Mokdad AH, Marks JS, Stroup DF, Gerberding JL. Actual Causes of Death in the United States, 2000. *JAMA*, 2004;291:1238-1245

[4] World Health Organization. (1998). Obesity: Preventing and managing the global epidemic, *Report of WHO Consultation on Obesity*, Geneva, 3-5 June, 1997,*WHO*, 1998

[5] Crossly N. Fat is a Sociological Issue: Obesity Rates in Late Modern, 'Body-Conscious' Societies, *Social Theory & Health*, 2004;2:222-253

[6] Booth KM, Pinkston MM, Carlos Poston WS. Obesity and the Built Environment. *J Am Diet Assoc*. 2005;105:S110-S117

[7] James WPT. The Future. In: Burniat W, Cole TJ, Lissau I, Poskitt EME (EDS). Child and Adolescent Obesity. Causes and Consequences, Preventing and Management. Cambridge: Cambridge University Press; 2002:389-402

[8] Gordon-Larsen P. Obesity-related Knowledge, Attitudes, and Behaviors in Obese and non-obese Urban Philadelphia Female Adolescent. *Obesity Research* 2001;9,2:112-8

[9] Allison DB. Dietary Supplements for Weight Loss: Challenges in Evaluation. *Obesity Reviews,* 2005;6:89–92

[10] Hill AJ, Lissau I. Psychosocial Factors. In: Burniat W, Cole TJ, Lissau I, Poskitt EME (EDS). Child and Adolescent Obesity. Causes and Consequences, *Preventing and Management.* Cambridge: Cambridge University Press; 2002:109-127

[11] Puhl R, Brownell KD. Bias, Discrimination, and Obesity. *Obesity Research*, 2001;9, 12: 788-805

[12] Finkelstein EA, Ruhm CJ, Kosa KM. Economic Causes and Consequences of Obesity. *Annu. Rev. Public Health* 2005;26:239–57

[13] Whitaker RC, Wright JA, Pepe MS, Seidel KD, Dietz WH. Predicting Obesity in Young Adulthood from Childhood and Parental Obesity. *New England Journal of Medicine* 1997;337:869-73

[14] Lissau I, Burniat W, Poskitt EME, Cole T. Prevention. In: Burniat W, Cole TJ, Lissau I, Poskitt EME (EDS). Child and Adolescent Obesity. Causes and Consequences, Preventing and Management. Cambridge: Cambridge University Press;2002:243-269

[15] http://www.kropogvaegt.lld.dk. Accessed 18-10-05

[16] Summerbell CD, Ashton V, Campbell KJ, Edmunds L, Kelly S, Waters E. Interventions for Treating Obesity in Children. *The Cochrane Database of Systematic Reviews* 2003, Issue 3. Art. No.: CD001872. DOI: 10.1002/14651858.CD001872

[17] Summerbell CD, Ashton V, Campbell KJ, Edmunds L, Kelly S, Waters E. Interventions for Treating Obesity in Children. *The Cochrane Database of Systematic Reviews* 2003, Issue 3. Art. No.: CD001872. DOI: 10.1002/14651858.CD001872

[18] Summerbell CD, Waters E, Edmunds LD, Kelly S, Brown T, Campbell KJ. Interventions for Preventing Obesity in Children. *The Cochrane Database of Systematic Reviews* 2005, Issue 3. Art. No.: CD001871.pub2. DOI: 10.1002/14651858.CD001871.pub2

[19] Latner JD. Self-help in the Long-term Treatment of obesity. *Obesity Reviews*, 2001;2: 87-97

[20] Suarez-Balcazar Y, Harper GW (eds.*). Empowerment and Participatory Evaluation of Community Interventions: Multiple Benefits*. New York: Haworth Press, 2003

[21] Funnel MM, Anderson RM, Ahroni JH. Empowerment and Self-Manegament after Weight Loss Surgery. *Obesity Surgery*, 2005;15:417-422

[22] Wills W, Backett-Milburn K, Gregory S, Lawton J. Young Teenagers' Perceptions of Their Own and Others' Bodies: A Qualitative Study of Obese, Overweight and 'Normal' Weight Young People in Scotland. *Social Science & Medicine*, 2005;62:396-405
[23] Hesketh K, Waters E, Green J, Salmon L, Williams J. Healthy Eating, Activity and Obesity Preventing: a Qualitative Study of Parent and Child Perceptions in Australia. *Health Promotion International*, 2005;20; 1:19-26
[24] He M, Irwin JD, Sangster Bouck LM, Tucker P, Pollett G. Screen-Viewing Behaviours Among Preschoolers Parents' Perceptions. *An J Prev Med*, 2005;29, 2:120-125
[25] He M, Irwin JD, Sangster Bouck LM, Tucker P, Pollett G. Screen-Viewing Behaviours Among Preschoolers Parents' Perceptions. *An J Prev Med*, 2005;29, 2:120-125
[26] Hesketh K, Waters E, Green J, Salmon L, Williams J. Healthy Eating, Activity and Obesity Preventing: a Qualitative Study of Parent and Child Perceptions in Australia. *Health Promotion International*, 2005;20; 1:19-26
[27] Kvale S. InterViews: An Introduction to Qualitative Research Interviewing. London: Sage Publications, 1996
[28] Spradley JP. Participant Observation. New York: Holt, Rinehart and Winston, 1980
[29] Spradley JP. The ethnographic interview. New York: Holt, Rinehart and Winston, 1979
[30] Hesketh K, Waters E, Green J, Salmon L, Williams J. Healthy Eating, Activity and Obesity Preventing: a Qualitative Study of Parent and Child Perceptions in Australia. *Health Promotion International*, 2005;20; 1:19-26
[31] Murphy AS, Youatt JP, Hoerr SL, Sawyer CA, Andrews SL. Kindergarten Students' Food Preferences are not Consistent with their Knowledge of the Dietary Guidelines. *J Am Diet Assoc* 1995;95,2:219-23
[32] Foster GD, Wadden TA, Makris AP, Davidson D, Sanderson RS, Allison DB, Kessler A. Primary Care Physicians' Attitudes about Obesity and Its Treatment. *Obesity Research*, 2003; 11:1168-1177
[33] Wiese HJ, Wilson JF, Jones RA, Neises M. Obesity Stigma Reduction in Medical Students. *Int J Obes Relat Metab Disord*, 1992 Nov;16(11):859-68
[34] Balshem M. *Cancer in the Community*. Class and Medical Authority. London: Smithsonian Institution Press, 1993
[35] Buchanan D. An Ethic for Health Promotion. *Rethinking the Sources of Human Well-Being*. Oxford: Oxford University Press, 2000
[36] Rhee KE, DeLago CW, Arscott-Mills T, Mehta SD, Davis K. Factors Associated With Parental Readiness to make Changes for Overweight Children. *Pediatrics*, 2005;116;no1:e94 – e101
[37] Bourdieu P. *The Logic of Practice*. Oxford: Blackwell Publishers Ltd., 1990
[38] Mattingly C. Healing Dramas and Clinical Plots. The Narrative Structure of Experience. Cambridge: Cambridge University Press, 1998

In: Global Dimensions of Childhood Obesity
Editor: Richard K. Flamenbaum, pp. 155-168
ISBN: 1-60021-037-6

Chapter 8

Development of Child Food Preferences: The Role of Age, Experience, and Exposure

Meredith S. Dolan[1], Michael Henderson[1] and Myles S. Faith[1,2*]
1 The University of Pennsylvania School of Medicine, USA
2 The Children's Hospital of Philadelphia, USA

Abstract

The main objective of this chapter is to summarize the literature on early determinants and development of child food preferences. The chapter begins with a literature review of the earliest flavor preferences for sweet, salty, and bitter tastes during infancy and the effect of early exposure to infant formulas on the later taste preferences. The effects of exposure frequency, food experience, role modeling, parenting styles, and mass media are followed by behavioral techniques to modify children's food preferences. The final section of the chapter covers commonly used assessments of infant and child food preferences.

Introduction

Individuals' food preferences are shaped early in life, possibly beginning in utero [1, 2] or during early infancy [3]. Children's food preferences play a critical role in determining their eating patterns, eating habits, and overall diet quality, which may persist into adulthood. Therefore, understanding children's food preferences is important for developing child-based nutrition education and intervention programs to improve children's eating habits.

The main objective of this chapter is to summarize the literature on early determinants and development of child food preferences. The chapter begins with a literature review of the earliest flavor preferences for sweet, salty, and bitter tastes during infancy and the effect of early exposure to infant formulas on the later taste preferences. The effects of exposure frequency, food experience, role modeling, parenting styles, and mass media are followed by

* Correspondence: Myles S. Faith, Ph.D. Weight and Eating Disorders Program, University of Pennsylvania School of Medicine, 3535 Market Street – 3rd Fl., Philadelphia, PA 19104. Phone: 215-898-2953. Fax: 215-898-2878

behavioral techniques to modify children's food preferences. The final section of the chapter covers commonly used assessments of infant and child food preferences.

Innate Preferences for Taste

Sweet taste. A number of studies have demonstrated a large acceptability of sucrose solutions among newborn infants [4-6], which may have evolved from the need to obtain sufficient energy from plant sources [7]. Beauchamp et al. [8] investigated whether early dietary experiences could impact sweet taste preferences in 6-month-old human infants. In this study, 199 infants were tested for sucrose preference at birth and 140 of these infants were tested again at 6 months of age. According to seven-day diet histories, infants who were regularly fed sweetened water (sweetened with table sugar, Karo syrup, or honey) ingested a significantly larger volume of sucrose solution at age 6 months compared to infants who had no prior experience with sweetened water. In a subsequent study, Beauchamp et al. [9] showed that maintenance of sucrose acceptability at age 2 years was also dependent on post-natal exposure to sweetened water.

In contrast to these findings, another experiment by Beauchamp et al. [9] showed greater consumption of sucrose-sweetened Kool-Aid compared to unsweetened Kool-Aid, regardless of children's prior experience with sweetened water. The fact that prior experience with sugar water was not related to consumption of plain or sweetened Kool-Aid in this study could be explained by the relatively unpalatable taste of unsweetened Kool-Aid, or infants' prior experience with other sweetened beverages such as fruit juices.

Salt taste. While humans seem to have an innate preference for sweet tastes, their acceptance of salty tastes appears to follow a developmental shift with age. A study by Beauchamp et al. [10] investigated infants' responsiveness to sucrose and saline solutions between 2.5 and 6.7 months of age. Fifty-four infants were divided into groups based on age (Group 1 = 2.5 to 3.9 months, Group 2 = 4.0 to 5.3 months, Group 3 = 5.4 to 6.7 months), and were administered feedings with two different sucrose solutions (0.2 M vs. 0.4 M sucrose concentrations) and two different saline solutions (0.1 M vs. 0.2 M sodium chloride (NaCl). Infants' responses to each of the tastants was compared to their responsiveness following a control of 30 ml of sterile water. The youngest infants did not differentially consume sterile water and saline solutions. However, the two older infant groups ingested significantly more saline solution compared to sterile water. There was no significant age effect for sucrose intake. These results suggest an early developmental shift in salt taste preference, beginning at about 4 months of age, in human infants.

Beauchamp et al. [10] reported a second developmental shift in saline solution acceptance in older children, between ages 7-23 months and 31-60 months. Children were presented with NaCl solutions (0.17 M and 0.34 M) and deionized water, and were encouraged to drink ad lib during a 30-second time period. Infants 7 to 23 months of age consumed significantly more of the 0.17 M NaCl solution compared to water, whereas differential consumption between the 0.34 M NaCl solution and water was not significant. In contrast, children 31 to 60 months of age rejected both NaCl solutionx relative to water. There are no clear explanations for the increased preference for saline solutions in early infancy or for the shift toward rejection of saline solution in older children. Beauchamp et al. hypothesize that the early developmental shift may be secondary to the development of central and/or peripheral mechanisms for salt taste perception. Early experiences with salty foods in more familiar contexts also may be responsible for the rejection of saline solution in older children. Thus, context may have a critical role in determining taste preference.

Bitter taste. Compared to the literature on children's acceptance of sweet and salty taste, research for bitter taste is more limited. To investigate young children's acceptance of bitter taste, Kajiura et al. [11] compared the responses of infants to experimentally manipulated urea concentrations; infants were either 0-6 days old (newborns) or 14-180 days (older infants). Bitter taste responsiveness was measured by several outcomes including: intake of a diluent (0.07 M sucrose) vs. test solution (0.12, 0.18, and 0.24 M urea), infant sucking pressure, and hedonic responses based on infant facial expressions and body movements. Newborns tended to consume more of, and had a greater sucking response to, whichever solution was presented first. In contrast, older infants consumed more of the diluent than urea and responded with relatively more and stronger sucks for the diluent than urea, regardless of the order of presentation. Compared to newborns, a significantly greater number of older infants were classified as urea rejectors based on facial reactions and body movements. However, among those newborns who reacted differentially to diluent and urea, the majority rejected the bitter solution. This study suggests an early developmental shift in the acceptance of bitter taste.

The effect of early exposure on food preference

It has been suggested that there are sensitive periods during which infants are likely to develop flavor preferences and aversions [12]. Mennella et al. tested these potential critical periods for flavor learning involving early exposure to the differential sensory characteristics of commercially available infant formulas [13]. The three main classes of infant formulas include milk-based, soy-based, and protein hydrolysates. Milk-based formulas were slightly sweet and 'sour and cereal-type', while soy based formulas were slightly sweeter, more sour and bitter and with a 'hay/beany' odor [14]. Hydrolyzed protein-based formulas are characterized by unpalatable bitter and sour tastes and an unpleasant aftertaste [15]. Previous studies had shown that infants willingly accept feedings with protein hydrolysate formula if exposed to it before, but not after, 4 months of age [13].

Mennella et al. [16] tested whether early exposure to infant formula affects later acceptance of familiar and other formulas. Two groups of infants were exposed exclusively to either a protein hydrolysate or a milk-based formula, while the other two groups were assigned to both a protein hydrolysate and milk-based formula for specified periods of time during the intervention. When tested at the end of the 7-month exposure period, a dose-response acceptance of the protein hydrolysate formula was observed. Infants who were exposed exclusively to the protein hydrolysate formula were most accepting of this formula at 7.5 months of age, while infants who were exclusively fed the milk-based formula strongly rejected the protein hydrolysate at the end of the study period. Infants who were fed alternately with the protein hydrolysate and milk-based formulas were more accepting of the protein hydrolysate at 7.5 months compared to infants exclusively fed milk-based formula, but were less accepting compared to infants who were fed exclusively with the protein hydrolysate formula.

Mennella et al. [17] further explored the hypothesis that flavor learning during infancy affects flavor preference in childhood by evaluating the responses of 4-5 year-old children to various flavors and odors. Children who were fed hydrolysate formula as infants were more likely to prefer sour-flavored apple juice compared to those fed milk- or soy-based formula.

In contrast, children who were fed soy formula were more likely to prefer bitter-flavored apple juice compared to children who were fed milk-based formula. In addition, compared to children exposed to milk-based formula, children who were fed hydrolysate or soy formulas were more likely to rate the flavor of hydrolysate formula as pleasant. Children in the hydrolysate formula group were also more likely to rate the odor of hydrolysates as pleasant compared to those fed milk-based formulas. Interestingly, mothers whose children were fed hydrolysate or soy formula were more likely to rank broccoli as one of their children's favorite vegetables. Thus, early exposure to differential sensory characteristics may predict children's food preferences at 4-5 years of age.

Liem et al. [18] investigated the effects of early flavor experience on sweet and sour preferences in 4-5 year-old and 6-7 year-old children, reporting a significant interaction between age and formula group (milk vs. hydrolysate) in their preferences for sour tastes, but not sweetness. In this study, 4-5 year-old children who had been fed hydrolysate formula during infancy preferred higher levels of citric acid (added to increase its sourness) in their apple juice compared to older children who had been fed a similar formula. When presented with sweetened apple juice, there was no significant interaction between age or formula group in their preferences for juice with added sugar. Additionally, children whose mothers reported regularly adding sugar to their children's foods were significantly more likely to prefer juice with added sugar compared to those children whose mothers reported that they never added sugar to their children's foods. Thus, flavor learning during early infancy and childhood may influence taste preference in latter childhood and possibly beyond.

Effect of Frequent Exposure on Food Preference

Children's acceptance of novel foods can be enhanced by repeated exposure [19, 20]. Sullivan et al. [21] found that 8-15 exposures to an initially novel food item was necessary to achieve increased acceptance among 3-6 year-old children. However, it has been suggested that infants may require fewer exposures to an initially novel food before increasing their acceptance of that food, compared to older children [22]. Birch et al. [19] conducted one of the first studies documenting that child food preference is a function of exposure frequency. In Experiment 1, two year-old children received 2, 5, 10, 15, or 20 exposures to five initially novel cheeses; and in Experiment 2, children were exposed to five initially novel fruits 0, 5, 10, 15, or 20 times. The experimental foods were presented as "paired consumption trials" in which children were asked to taste and compare foods, rating which of the foods they would like to "eat more of." Child food preference was positively associated with exposure frequency in both experiments. These results are consistent with the exposure hypothesis [23] that repeated exposures to a stimulus enhances attitudes towards it.

Exposure may also explain the positive correlation between parent and child food preferences, as parents may only expose their children to parent-preferred foods. For example, Borah-Giddens and Falciglia [24] reported a strong concordance between a food that had never been offered to a child and maternal dislike for that particular food. In a study by Vereecken et al. [25], the reported food consumption frequency by mothers was significantly associated with that of their children, aged 2.5 - 7 years. Parental food preferences may influence child food preferences by providing home exposure to those items.

Food Experience

The previous section discussed the relationship between food exposure frequency and increased liking for those foods. However, the flavors with which the food is presented, or the "food experience," is also a determinant of children's food preferences. Sullivan et al. [21] recruited 39 preschool children, ages 3-6 years, to study the effect of repeated experience with an initially novel food (tofu) on food preferences. Children were assigned to one of three varieties of tofu: salty, sweet, or plain, for a total of 15 exposures over 9 weeks. On three occasions during the exposure period, children's food preferences were assessed for the three versions of tofu as well as a sweet, salty, and plain version of a similar novel food (i.e., ricotta cheese). As a post-assessment, children tasted and rated their preferences for the three versions of tofu and the same versions of a completely novel food, jicama. Results indicated that preference for the exposed version of tofu increased over time across the three groups, confirming the exposure effect [19, 20]. However, experience with one flavor of tofu did not result in a generalized liking of the other non-exposed flavors of tofu, nor did it translate to a greater preference for ricotta cheese. Similarly, experience with one version of tofu did not transfer to a generalized preference of the corresponding version of jicama. This suggests that the flavors with which a food are exposed, or the food experience, play an important role in shaping food preferences; although flavor preferences may not necessarily transfer to similar foods.

Birch and colleagues [22] conducted a similar study of the effect of infants' experience with a new food on their intake of similar foods. Infants were assigned to one of two target novel foods, either bananas or peas, which they consumed on 10 occasions. As a pre-assessment, infants were fed samples of their *target food*, the *same food* from a different brand, a *similar* food (peaches and pears instead of bananas, or carrots and corn instead of peas), and a *different* food (i.e., peas for infants receiving bananas as their target food, and bananas or beef for those infants receiving peas). Following 10 exposures to their target food, infants were given a post-assessment with those foods presented in the pre-assessment. As expected, exposure to the target food increased acceptance of that food. Acceptance for foods similar to the target foods also increased at post-exposure, while intake of the *different* foods remained constant from baseline to post-exposure. The results confirm that infants have an initial neophobic response to new foods, which can be overcome with increased exposure and that experience with certain flavors or foods can enhance acceptance for similar foods.

The Effect of Role Modeling on Children's Food Preferences

Children's social environment, including role modeling by parents, siblings, teachers, and peers, as well as parenting styles, can shape children's food preferences.

Family (parents/siblings). Borah-Giddens et al. [24] conducted a meta-analysis of seven child food preference studies, which specifically addressed the association between parent and child food preferences. They reported a significant correlation between the food preferences of parents and their children, aged 25 years or younger. Skinner et al. [26] also found a positive relationship between young children's food preferences and those of other family members including the mother, father, and older sibling.

Teachers, other role models. Teachers also play an important role in shaping child food preferences. Hendy and Raudenbush [27] performed a series of studies to investigate the impact of teacher role modeling on child food preferences in a classroom setting using questionnaires and quasi-experiments. Preschool teachers reported modeling as the most effective strategy in influencing child food preferences. "Teacher silent modeling," in which teachers took bites of target foods (i.e., fresh mango and dried cranberries) without saying anything, was ineffective at increasing food acceptance for both new foods and familiar foods in the classroom setting. However, "enthusiastic teacher modeling" in which the teacher tasted the foods and proclaimed "I love (novel food)!" or "These are delicious" increased child food acceptance across the five test meals.

Not only is teacher enthusiasm important in affecting child food preference, but the social-affective context of food presentation also has a large effect. In a study by Birch et al. [28], teachers presented a food perceived as "neutral" to 4 year-old children in one of four conditions: reward condition (i.e., children received food reward for good behavior), non-contingent attention condition (i.e., child presented with food and adult attention, but not contingent upon completing a task), nonsocial condition (i.e., child presented with food in their locker twice a day), or the snack-time familiarity condition (i.e., control group). Foods presented in reward conditions or non-contingently paired with adult attention were associated with increased child preference of those foods. However, no changes in preference were observed in the nonsocial or control conditions.

Peers. Children's peers are also very important in the development of food preferences. A series of experiments by Hendy and Raubenbush [27] found that teacher modeling was no longer an effective influence on preschool children's food preferences when used in competition with a peer model; peer influence was especially strong among females. In another experiment, Hendy [29] found that same age girl models were more effective than boy models in increasing food acceptance among both sexes of children, contrary to previous research suggesting that same sex models were more effective.

Effects of General Parenting Styles

Parents play a critical role in the development of their children's food preferences beginning with infant feeding practices and parental role modeling. However, general parenting styles and parental education levels have also been identified as predictors of child food preferences. Kremers et al. [30] explored the correlation between general parenting strategies and child eating habits (mean age = 16.5 years). Parents were defined as either "authoritative" (firm and supportive parenting), "authoritarian" (strict but less involved parenting), "indulgent" (involved but not strict parenting), and "neglectful" (low strictness and low involvement parenting) based on self-report questionnaires. Results indicated that an authoritative parenting style was associated with child fruit intake and healthy attitudes toward eating fruits and vegetables. The authoritarian parenting style was associated with low levels of fruit consumption, while the indulgent parenting style was associated with greater fruit intake compared to the authoritarian or neglectful styles.

Vereecken et al. [25] examined the link between maternal education level, parenting styles, and child food preferences. Highly educated mothers praised their children more, and increased verbal praise was a significant predictor of children's vegetable consumption. In contrast, lower maternal education levels were found to be more permissive, which was correlated with an increased consumption of refined sugars.

Mass Media Influences

A large percentage of commercials airing during children's programming are food advertisements. An analysis of commercials scheduled during weekend children's television showed that 37% of advertisements on American television and 49% of commercials on British television were food advertisements [31]. Most of these advertised products were snack foods, breakfast cereals, and fast food restaurants. Until recently, there were no studies that examined whether food advertisements directed at children had any effect on child eating preferences or behavior.

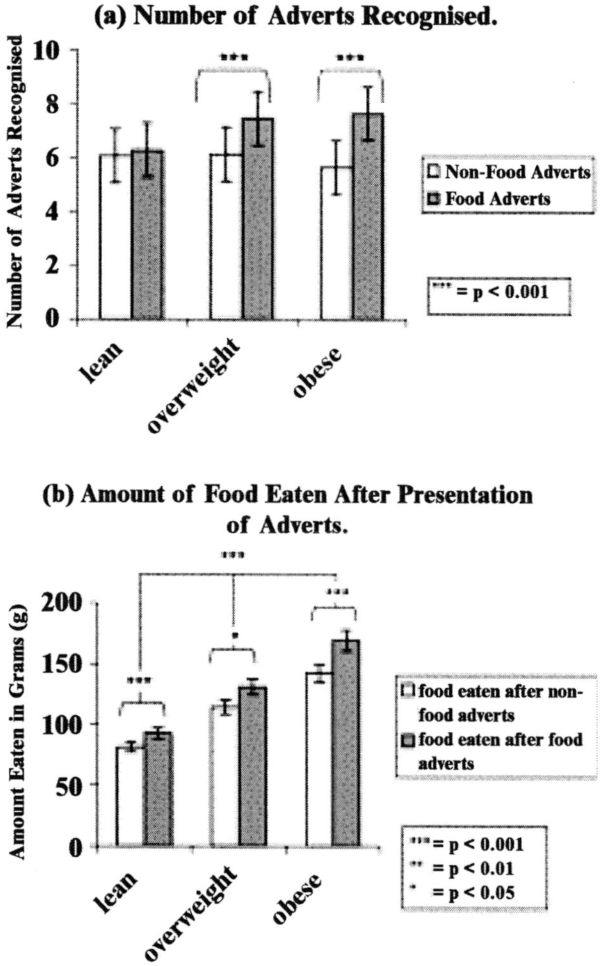

Fig. 1. The number of television advertisements recognized and the amount of food consumed after viewing the advertisements ***$p<0.001$, **$p<0.01$, *$p<0.05$.

Halford et al. [32] explored the differences between normal weight and overweight children in their ability to recognize television advertisements of food and non-food items as well as the total amount of food consumed after viewing TV ads. A total of 42 children, aged 9-11 years, participated in the study and were grouped according to their obesity status. On two separate occasions, the children watched a series of food-related advertisements or advertisements that did not pertain to food followed by a 10-minute cartoon video. Next, they were given permission to eat ad lib from an assortment of food items including a low-fat savory snack, a low-fat sweet snack, a high-fat sweet snack, and a high-fat savory snack.

When given a list of 16 food ads, from which 8 had been shown, overweight and obese children recognized significantly more food ads compared to normal weight children (Figure 1a). Across all groups, the number of recognized food-related TV advertisements was directly related to the amount of food consumed after watching those ads. In addition, participants ate more of the high-fat high-sugar snacks after viewing the food ads and more of the low-fat savory snack after viewing the non-food advertisements. These findings suggest that TV commercials can affect food preferences and eating behavior, and may especially encourage unhealthy food choices among overweight children.

Changing Children's Food Preferences

Behavior Modification. A number of studies have focused on strategies through which parents can influence and modify child food preferences. The results of a three year project by Hart et al. [33] on developing parent education programs suggest that behavioral techniques, rather than nutrition facts alone, have a greater impact on increasing healthy feeding behaviors in children. Similar results were found in a study by Wardle et al. [34] investigating the effects of parent-led exposure in influencing 2-6 year-old children's acceptance of a target vegetable rated marginally low on a pre-intervention test. Parents were randomized to the parent-led exposure group, the nutrition education group, or a control group which did not receive any instruction. Greater increases in liking and consumption of the target vegetable were found in the parent-led exposure group, and nutritional knowledge alone was not sufficient to influence target vegetable consumption. Wardle's results confirmed those from previous studies that repeated exposure is key to increasing child food acceptance.

Restriction. Whereas frequent exposure and role modeling have been identified as effective strategies to influence child food preferences, restrictive feeding practices may have drawbacks. Many parents believe that the most effective way to control their children's intake of high-fat high-sugar foods is to restrict access to those foods. However there is evidence to suggest that restricting children's food intake may be counterproductive. Liem et al. [35] conducted a study on kindergarten-aged children's food preferences in the Netherlands and reported that children whose intake of mono and disaccharides (MDS), or simple sugars, was highly restricted by parents consume fewer MDS beverages and foods during breakfast and lunch. However, 55% of these highly restricted children preferred an "orangeade" drink of highest sucrose concentration compared to 33% of children who were slightly restricted.

Fisher and Birch [36] examined the behavioral effects of restricting 3-5 year-old children's access to palatable foods for five weeks. Peach and apple-flavored fruit bar cookies were chosen as the experimental foods, as these were neither highly liked nor disliked by the children. Children were randomly assigned to receive one of the experimental foods as the control and the other was restricted. Prior to the experimental phase, there were no differences in children's responses to the restricted food and the control food. During the restriction period, however, the restricted food received more positive comments, more requests, and more attempts to obtain it compared to the control food.

In addition to restricting children's intake of certain foods, pressuring children to consume more food may also have unintended effects on child food preferences. Fisher et al. [37] assessed parental tendencies to pressure their 5 year-old daughters to eat more food. They found that parents who more frequently pressured their daughters to eat had children with lower fruit, vegetable, and micronutrient intakes. They also reported a negative correlation between parents' own fruit and vegetable intake and the use of pressure to eat, suggesting that role modeling may be more effective than pressuring children to eat or restricting children's intake of specific foods for changing child food preferences.

Opportune ages to change food preferences. Skinner et al. [38] tested longitudinal changes in children's food preferences from ages 2-8 years. Mothers completed a 196-item Food Preference Questionnaire at T1 (2-3 years), T2 (4 years), and T3 (8 years). Mothers reported that children liked ~60% of the listed foods at T1. The number of liked foods only increased by 3.7% at T3, whereas the number of disliked foods increased by 5.5%. Between T1 and T2, foods that were never tasted decreased from 55 to 37 foods. These results suggest that the majority of child food preferences are developed by the age of 2-3 years and that a critical period for increasing acceptance of novel foods may exist around age 4 years.

Barriers to Changing Food Preferences: Neophobia

Research has shown that omnivores are neophobic, or reluctant to try new foods, regardless of our need for a varied diet. This conflict has been termed the "generalist's dilemma" [39]. One possible mechanism responsible for the reluctance to try new foods is omnivores' self-protection against potentially poisonous substances. Individuals may learn to accept and increase their preference for initially novel food items through "learned safety," or after repeated exposure to a food item, and in the absence of accompanying gastrointestinal distress [40].

Cooke and Wardle [41] sent child eating behavior questionnaires to 564 mothers of 2-6 year-olds, and found no association between age, gender, or parental intake and neophobia among children. High levels of neophobia were associated with lower intake of vegetables, fruits, and meats, but did not affect consumption of high-fat, high-sugar snacks, starchy food items, or eggs. These results may provide evidence for the evolutionary avoidance of potentially toxic food items, as those foods associated with neophobia are the most potentially dangerous. Toxins are found in many plants, and protein-rich foods are most likely to cause food-borne illnesses.

Assessment of Children's Food Preferences

The most significant predictor of children's food intake is their liking of particular foods [42]. For this reason, it is important to develop reliable methods for the assessment of children's food preferences.

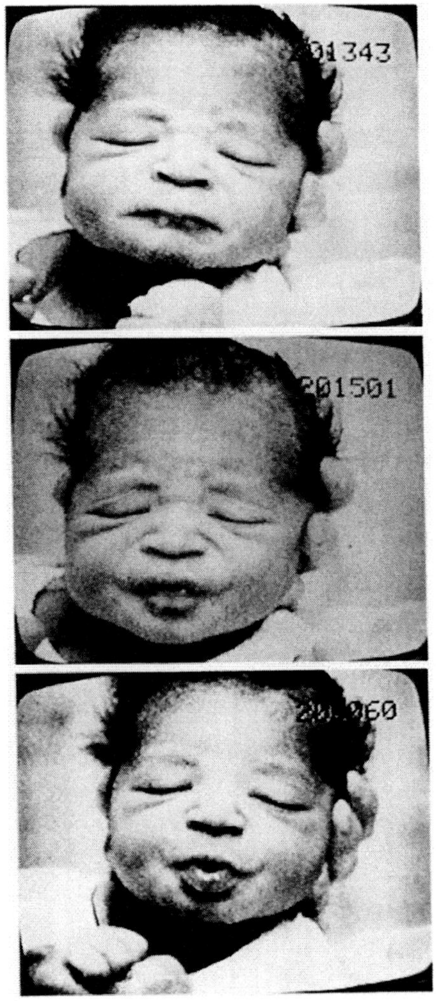

Figure 2a: Infant facial expressions in response to sweet taste; initial negative facial reaction followed by relaxation and sucking [43].

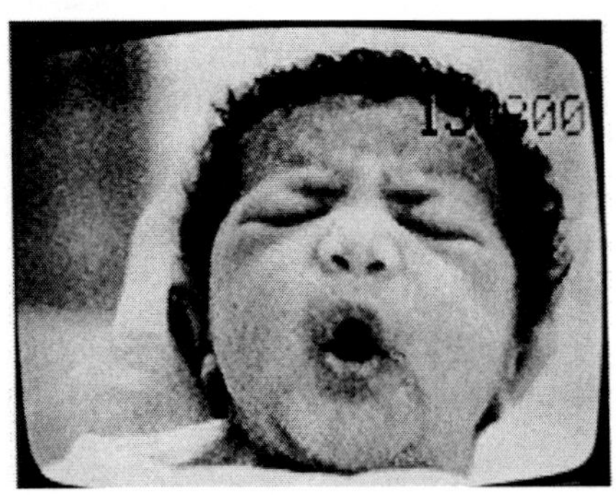

Figure 2b: Infant facial expression in response to sour taste [43].

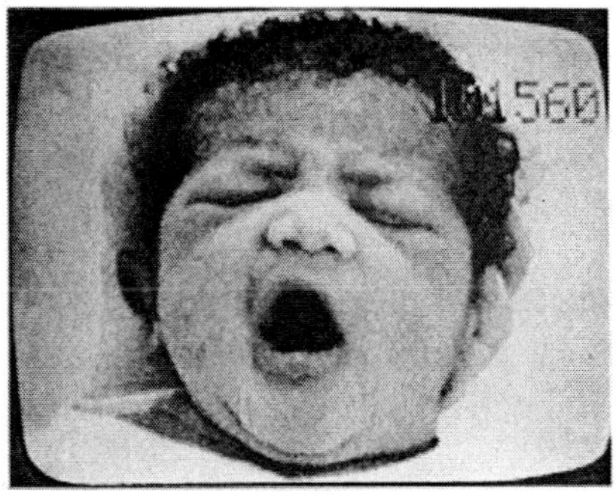

Figure 2c: Infant facial expression in response to bitter taste [43].

Infants. Infant facial expressions have been used to assess acceptance or rejection of taste stimuli in some of the earliest studies on human taste development [43, 44]. Infant facial expressions (Figure 2a-c) are fairly consistent in response to various taste stimuli such as the sweet taste of sucrose (facial relaxation and mouth gaping), the sour taste of citric acid (lip pursing and facial grimace), and the bitter taste of quinine and urea (tongue protrusion and facial grimace). There are no distinctive facial expressions associated with exposure to salty taste in infants [45].

Intake studies, which measure the amount of solution consumed during a brief time period, are most commonly used to assess taste preference in newborns. Intake studies typically use weaker concentrations of the taste solution compared to studies that measure facial expressions. Presumably, the volume of consumption may be indicative of the infant's preference for the taste solution [45].

Children. The most commonly used measure of child food preferences is a "taste and rate" procedure, in which children taste a food and describe how much they like the food on a 3-point scale (Figure 3). This method has produced reliable results in children as young as 3 years of age, but may not be practical to measure acceptance for a large number of foods. Guthrie et al. [46] tested whether food photographs or realistic food models could provide a reliable alternative to real foods in the evaluation of children's food preferences. Results suggest that high quality food photographs may provide a reliable alternative to real foods in the assessment of children's food preferences.

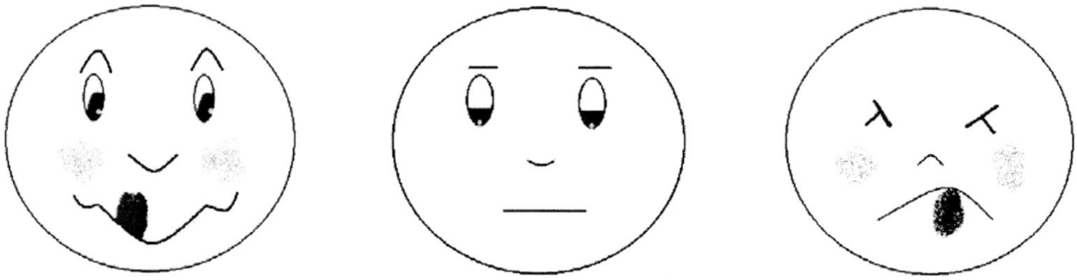

Figure 3: Three-Point Hedonic Scale

Summary

In summary, food preferences are learned in part through early exposure, exposure frequency, and experience with foods. Given the high prevalence of fast food restaurants, convenient marts, and the wide variety of snack foods, the present environment presents children overexposure to high-fat high-sugar foods that may become further preferred through learning. Once established, children's food preferences can be challenging to modify. Implementing behavioral techniques, such as role modeling and reinforcement for healthier food choices, in early childhood may help to establish healthier dietary choices by children that may be more sustainable.

References

[1] Mennella, J.A., A. Johnson, and G.K. Beauchamp, Garlic ingestion by pregnant women alters the odor of amniotic fluid. *Chemical Senses*, 1995. 20(2): p. 207-9.

[2] Mennella, J.A., C.P. Jagnow, and G.K. Beauchamp, Prenatal and postnatal flavor learning by human infants. *Pediatrics*, 2001. 107(6): p. E88.

[3] Mennella, J.A., Mother's milk: a medium for early flavor experiences. *Journal of Human Lactation,* 1995. 11(1): p. 39-45.

[4] Maller, O. and R.E. Turner, Taste in acceptance of sugars by human infants. *Journal of Comparative & Physiological Psychology,* 1973. 84(3): p. 496-501.

[5] Nisbett, R.E. and S.B. Gurwitz, Weight, sex, and the eating behavior of human newborns. *Journal of Comparative & Physiological Psychology*, 1970. 73(2): p. 245-53.

[6] Nowlis, G.H. and W. Kessen, Human newborns differentiate differing concentrations of sucrose and glucose. *Science*, 1976. 191(4229): p. 865-6.

[7] Jacobs, W.W., G.K. Beauchamp, and M.R. Kare, Progress in animal flavor research, in *Flavor chemistry of animal foods*, R.W. Bullard, Editor. 1978, American Chemical Society: Chicago. p. 1-20.

[8] Beauchamp, G.K. and M. Moran, Dietary experience and sweet taste preference in human infants. *Appetite*, 1982. 3(2): p. 139-52.

[9] Beauchamp, G.K. and M. Moran, Acceptance of sweet and salty tastes in 2-year-old children. *Appetite*, 1984. 5(4): p. 291-305.

[10] Beauchamp, G.K., B.J. Cowart, and M. Moran, Developmental changes in salt acceptability in human infants. *Developmental Psychobiology*, 1986. 19(1): p. 17-25.

[11] Kajiura, H., B.J. Cowart, and G.K. Beauchamp, Early developmental change in bitter taste responses in human infants. *Developmental Psychobiology*, 1992. 25(5): p. 375-86.

[12] Beauchamp, G.K. and J.A. Mennella, Sensitive Periods in the Development of Human Flavor Perception and Preference, in Annales Nestle, *Nestle Nutrition Workshop Series.* 1998, Nestec Ltd: Vevey, Switzerland. p. 19-31.

[13] Mennella, J.A. and G.K. Beauchamp, Developmental Changes in the Infants' Acceptance of Protein-Hydrolysate Formula and Its Relation to Mothers' Eating Habits. *J Dev Behav Pediatr*, 1996. 17: p. 386-391.

[14] Cook, D.A. and H.P. Sarett, Design of Infant Formulas for Meeting Normal and Special Need, in Pediatric *Nutrition: Infant Feeding, Deficiencies, Disease,* F. Lifshitz, Editor. 1982, Marcel Dekker, Inc.: New York, NY.

[15] Schiffman, S.S. and C. Dackis, Taste of nutrients: amino acids, vitamins, and fatty acids. *Percept Psychophys*, 1975. 17(140-146).
[16] Mennella, J.A., C.E. Griffin, and G.K. Beauchamp, Flavor programming during infancy. *Pediatrics*, 2004. 113(4): p. 840-5.
[17] Mennella, J.A. and G.K. Beauchamp, Flavor experiences during formula feeding are related to preferences during childhood. *Early Human Development*, 2002. 68(2): p. 71-82.
[18] Liem, D.G. and J.A. Mennella, Sweet and sour preferences during childhood: role of early experiences. *Developmental Psychobiology*, 2002. 41(4): p. 388-95.
[19] Birch, L.L. and D.W. Marlin, I don't like it; I never tried it: effects of exposure on two-year-old children's food preferences. *Appetite*, 1982. 3(4): p. 353-60.
[20] Pliner, P., The effects of mere exposure on liking for edible substances. *Appetite*, 1982. 3(3): p. 283-90.
[21] Sullivan, S.A. and L.L. Birch, Pass the Sugar, Pass the Salt: Experience Dictates Preference. *Developmental Psychology*, 1990. 26(4): p. 546-551.
[22] Birch, L.L., et al., Infants' consumption of a new food enhances acceptance of similar foods. *Appetite*, 1998. 30(3): p. 283-95.
[23] Zajonc, R.B., Attitudinal effects of mere exposure. *Journal of Personality and Social Psychology Monograph Supplement,* 1968. 9(2): p. 1-32.
[24] Borah-Giddens, J. and G.A. Falciglia, A meta-analysis of the relationship in food preferences between parents and children. *Journal of Nutrition Education*, 1993. 25(3): p. 102-107.
[25] Vereecken, C.A., E. Keukelier, and L. Maes, Influence of mother's educational level on food parenting practices and food habits of young children. *Appetite*, 2004. 43(1): p. 93-103.
[26] Skinner, J.D., et al., Toddler's Food Preferences: Concordance with family members' preferences. *Journal of Nutrition Education,* 1998. 30(1): p. 17-22.
[27] Hendy, H.M. and B. Raudenbush, Effectiveness of teacher modeling to encourage food acceptance in preschool children. *Appetite*, 2000. 34(1): p. 61-76.
[28] Birch, L.L., S.I. Zimmerman, and H. Hind, The influence of social-affective context to the formation of children's food preferences. *Child Development*, 1980. 51(3): p. 856-861.
[29] Hendy, H.M., Effectiveness of trained peer models to encourage food acceptance in preschool children. *Appetite*, 2002. 39(3): p. 217-25.
[30] Kremers, S.P., et al., Parenting style and adolescent fruit consumption. *Appetite*, 2003. 41(1): p. 43-50.
[31] Furnham, A., S. Abramsky, and B. Gunter, A cross-cultural content analysis of children's television advertisements. *Sex Roles*, 1997. 37: p. 91-99.
[32] Halford, J.C., et al., Effect of television advertisements for foods on food consumption in children. *Appetite*, 2004. 42(2): p. 221-5.
[33] Hart, K., J. Bishop, and H. Truby, Changing Children's Diets: Developing method and messages. *J Hum Nutr Dietet*, 2003. 16: p. 365-366.
[34] Wardle, J., et al., Increasing children's acceptance of vegetables; a randomized trial of parent-led exposure. *Appetite*, 2003. 40(2): p. 155-62.
[35] Liem, D.G., M. Mars, and C. De Graaf, Sweet preferences and sugar consumption of 4- and 5-year-old children: role of parents. *Appetite*, 2004. 43(3): p. 235-45.

[36] Fisher, J.O. and L.L. Birch, Restricting access to palatable foods affects children's behavioral response, food selection, and intake. *American Journal of Clinical Nutrition*, 1999. 69(6): p. 1264-72.

[37] Fisher, J.O., et al., Parental influences on young girls' fruit and vegetable, micronutrient, and fat intakes. Journal of the American Dietetic Association, 2002. 102(1): p. 58-64.

[38] Skinner, J.D., et al., Children's food preferences: a longitudinal analysis. *Journal of the American Dietetic Association,* 2002. 102(11): p. 1638-47.

[39] Rozin, P., The Selection of Food by Rats, Humans, and Other Animals, in Advances in the Study of Behavior, J.S. Rosenblatt, et al., Editors. 1976, Academy Press: New York. p. 21-76.

[40] Kalat, J.W. and P. Rozin, "Learned safety" as a mechanism in long-delay taste-aversion learning in rats. *Journal of Comparative & Physiological Psychology*, 1973. 83(2): p. 198-207.

[41] Cooke, L., J. Wardle, and E.L. Gibson, Relationship between parental report of food neophobia and everyday food consumption in 2-6-year-old children. *Appetite*, 2003. 41(2): p. 205-6.

[42] Gibson, E.L., J. Wardle, and C.J. Watts, Fruit and vegetable consumption, nutritional knowledge and beliefs in mothers and children. *Appetite*, 1998. 31(2): p. 205-28.

[43] Rosenstein, D. and H. Oster, Differential facial responses to four basic tastes in newborns. *Child Development*, 1988. 59(6): p. 1555-68.

[44] Bergamasco, N.H. and K.E. Beraldo, Facial expressions of neonate infants in response to gustatory stimuli. *Brazilian Journal of Medical & Biological Research*, 1990. 23(3-4): p. 245-9.

[45] Mennella, J.A. and G.K. Beauchamp, Early flavor experiences: research update. *Nutrition Reviews*, 1998. 56(7): p. 205-11.

[46] Guthrie, C.A., L. Rapoport, and J. Wardle, Young children's food preferences: a comparison of three modalities of food stimuli. *Appetite*, 2000. 35(1): p. 73-7.

[47] Birch, L.L. and S.A. Sullivan, Measuring children's food preferences. *Journal of School Health*, 1991. 61(5): p. 212-4.

In: Global Dimensions of Childhood Obesity
Editor: Richard K. Flamenbaum, pp. 169-198
ISBN: 1-60021-037-6

Chapter 9

OBESITY: CURRENT RESEARCH AND DILEMMAS

Roger J. Harris
Academic Centre for Child Health, Barts and The London School of Medicine and Dentistry, Queen Mary College, University of London and The Children's Department, Barts and The London NHS Trust, UK
Sophie Aubrey
Barts and The London NHS Trust, UK
Rebecca Gibbs and Ambreen Clement
Barts and The London School of Medicine and Dentistry, Queen Mary College, University of London,. UK

Abstract

There is a worldwide epidemic of obesity, with prevalence rates reaching alarming proportions in some western countries, but also in many parts of the developing world.

Hunger and weight gain are controlled by a complex group of interactions between the gut and brain. Recent advances have highlighted some of the main appetite control hormones, but these only help our understanding of the physiological processes controlling weight gain. Although there are a few extremely rare medical conditions causing childhood obesity, the main cause is a change in diet, with a high intake of energy dense, fatty and sugary food and drink, coupled with a dramatic decline in the amount of exercise being taken.

The long-term effect of this increase in obesity is likely to be an increase in cardiovascular mortality, as well as a massive rise in children with Type 2 diabetes, already being seen in many overweight teenagers from some racial groups.

A number of treatment strategies have been designed. Most are a combination of dieting, life style changes and family behaviour therapy. Medical and surgical interventions are reserved for those children who are morbidly obese, and likely to suffer life threatening events, such as sleep apnoea.

Unfortunately, intervention only has limited success, and the end result may well be a decline in the current increasing longevity, especially in the developed world.

"Thou seest I have more flesh than another man, and therefore more frailty"
Falstaff: Henry IV Part 1: III, 3

Introduction

It appears that as long ago as the late 16th century in England there was some anxiety about the consequences of obesity – William Shakespeare wrote the above words in 1596. However, overall the historical view of obesity is a jolly, devil may care person, loved by everyone and the life and soul of any gathering – in Victorian times, Mr Pickwick was a popular figure written about by Charles Dickens. However, although there has been increasing anxiety about obesity, particularly in the developing world for a number of years, it is only with the rapid rise over the past 10 years or so that anxiety about the long-term consequences of obesity has become more apparent. We now have to come to terms with the potential long-term effects of obesity, as it is going to impact significantly on use of medical services in the future, as well as perhaps effecting an individual's survival.

At long last governments in the developing world are beginning to address the problem of increasing obesity. In the UK obesity is now one of the British Government's main priority areas.

What Do We Mean by Obesity

There is still some debate on deciding what is meant by being obese in children. There is no simple way to measure fat mass in children other than skin fold thickness, which can be used as a screening tool in community paediatrics in the UK. It has been shown that triceps skin fold is correlated with fat mass, and if this is combined with Body Mass Index (BMI), gives a reasonably sensitive assessment of the percentage of body fat [1]. However, skin fold thickness measurements have poor reproducibility and are dependent on individual observers, and so can be considered as no more than a guide.

In the first 2 years of life, the traditional and probably still acceptable method of assessing obesity is by weight for length measurements. If weight is two centiles above that for length is over the 95th centile, then the baby is considered overweight. This is a purely statistical definition, and it is important to measure head circumference, as a large head will alter weight for length ratios.

BMI is more widely used, and is measured by weight in Kg/height in metre^2 and has for some time been considered the gold standard for assessing obesity in adults, and more recently in children. The accepted BMI for adults, both in the UK and internationally, for being overweight is 25-30 kg/m^2 and for obese is 30 kg/m^2 or greater [2]. Cole et al [3] extrapolated risk from adult experience to childhood by using data derived from six countries. Although BMI is a good measure of childhood obesity, it does not measure the amount of fat directly [4]. However, it has until recently been widely accepted as a guide in childhood.

One of the difficulties with BMI measurements is that it does not allow for the athletic and muscular individual, who may have a high BMI. In addition, a child's body fat depends on age, gender and pubertal stage. The BMI decreases from 2 until 5, and then increases again between the ages of 5 and 8. Ethnic variations, timing of growth spurts and higher normal fat levels around puberty can cause further difficulties with the measurement of BMI [3].

Waist circumference or waist to hip ratios are used as indirect measures of intra-abdominal adipose tissue. Although by no means clarified for children, there is some evidence that in adult waist circumference measurements above 95cms are associated with an increase in mortality from cardiovascular and metabolic problems [5]. Visceral or intra-abdominal adiposity does appear to be associated with similar risks in children. [6]. Of concern, however, is the data from the large INTERHEART study showing that Waist-to-hip ratio shows a graded and highly significant association with myocardial infarction risk worldwide. The authors suggest that a redefinition of obesity based on waist-to-hip ratio rather than BMI increases the estimate of myocardial infarction attributable to obesity in most ethnic groups [7]. At the moment there is very limited data on waist-to-hip measurements in children, and more is needed [8].

Other measurements of obesity such as DEXA scanning and imaging are expensive and not appropriate for routine assessment of obesity in childhood.

Figures 1 and 2 are BMI and waist measurement charts currently in use in the UK. The waist measurement charts are based on the data published by McCarthy et al [8]. There are at present no waist-to–hip charts available for children.

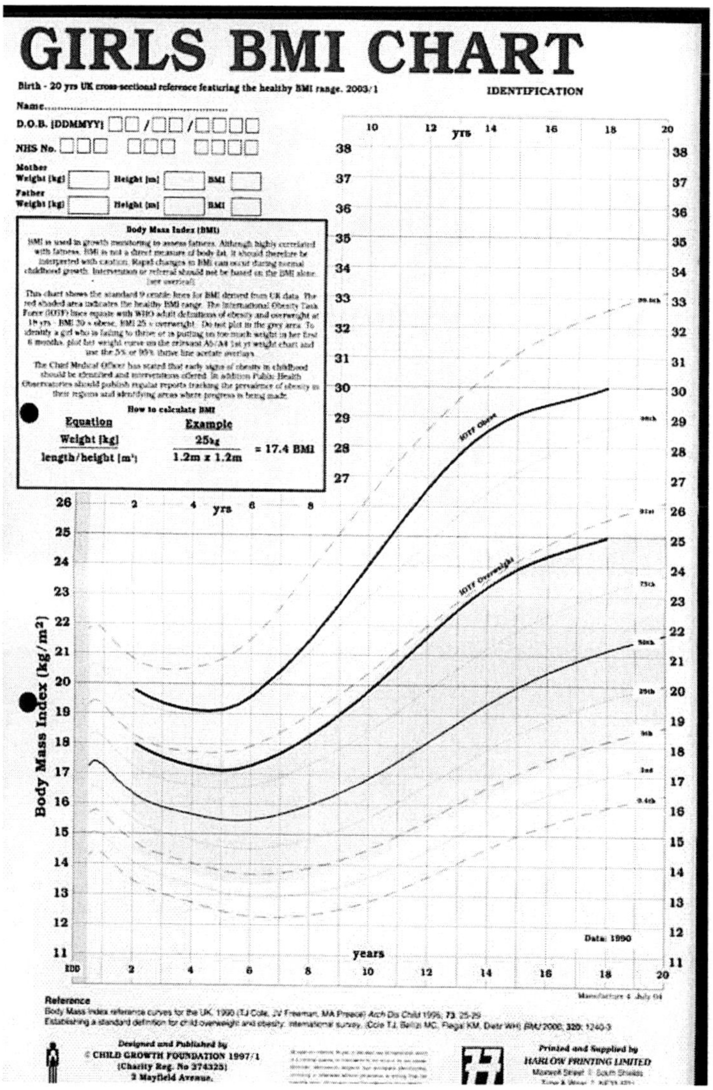

FIGURE 1. Girls BMI chart as used in the UK. Boy's charts are also available

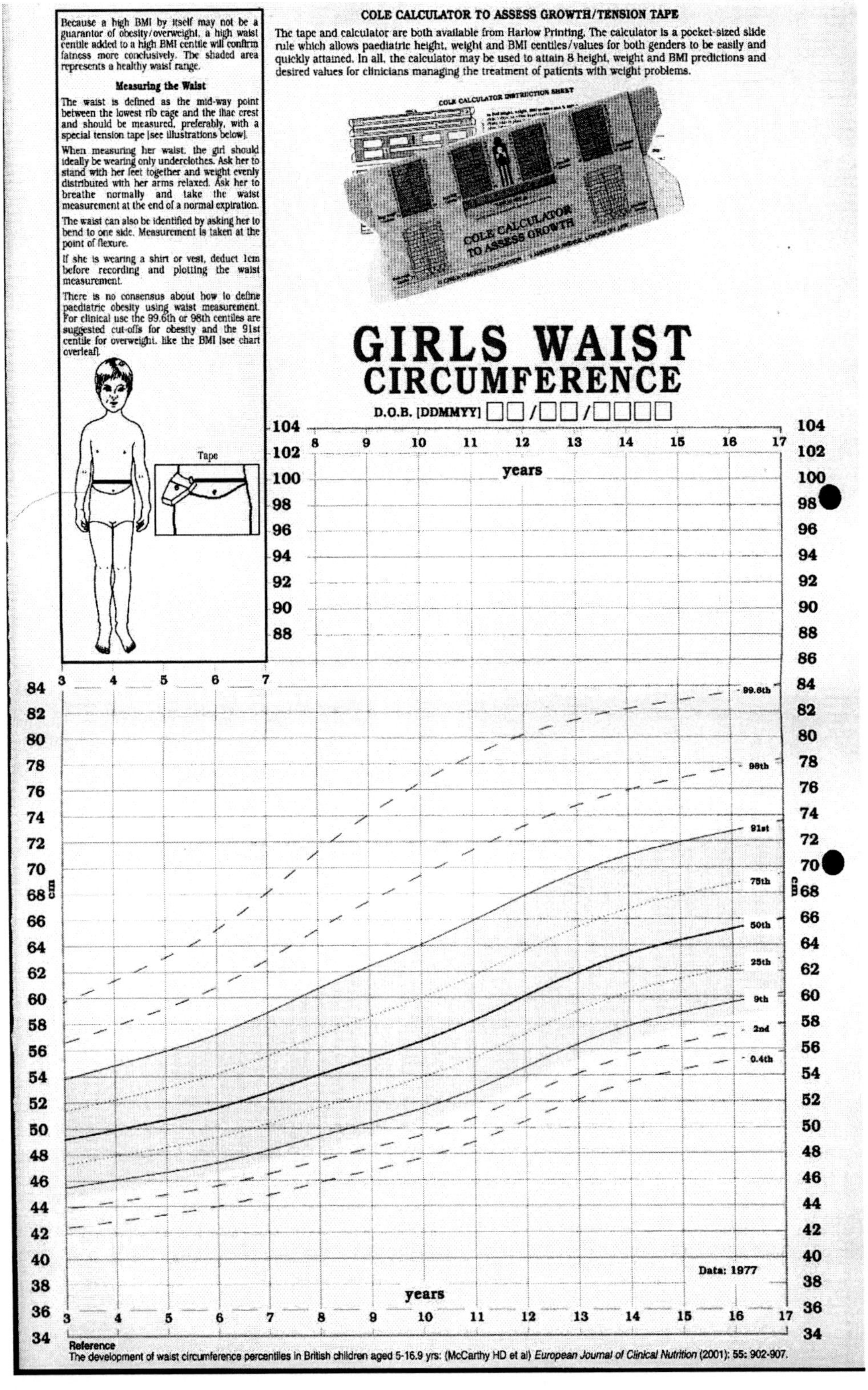

FIGURE 2. Girl's Waist circumference charts as used in the UK. Boy's charts are also available.

Obesity: A Worldwide Problem

Current estimates suggest that as many as 250 million people or 7% of the current world population are obese. Two to three times more people are overweight [9]. An estimated 22 million children worldwide are obese. Despite differing international opinions as to what constitutes obesity in children, the rate at which overweight and obesity have increased is alarming. In 2002 The Lancet suggested that rates had increased 2.3-fold to 3.3-fold over about 25 years in the USA, 2.0-fold to 2.8-fold over 10 years in England, and 3.9 fold over 18 years in Egypt [10]. Within these populations, rates vary between the sexes and racial groups.

Though obesity is usually seen as a problem of wealthy, first world countries, it appears that the risk varies dramatically between ethnic and social groups within any population; a problem of the affluent and of the indigent depending on which country is examined.

In developed countries it is the urban poor who are most at risk, possibly due to a nutritionally imbalanced, fast-food rich diet and less opportunity for physical activity [10]. In the USA the prevalence of childhood obesity has risen twice as fast among minority groups (including those of Hispanic origin, Pima Indians and other Native Americans)[9] as in the white population. A definite trend is that the distribution of body-mass index has shifted in a skewed fashion, i.e. the heaviest children have become even heavier [10].

In Australia there has been a similar rise in childhood obesity to the rest of the world. By 1995 15% of boys and 15.8% of girls were overweight and 4.5% boys and 5.3% of girls were obese [11].

However, in developing countries it is generally the children of the wealthy that are most at risk of becoming obese. China is a prime example of a developing nation with sharply rising levels of childhood obesity. In 2000 the prevalence rate reached 7.1% in Beijing and 8.3% in Shanghai, with an increased risk with age; 11.7% of six year olds were described as obese by the WHO. Among the predisposing factors for this trend are the increased availability and low price of fast food and high levels of physical inactivity amongst the children of financially well-off families [12].

However, certain countries display both a high prevalence of wasted or malnourished children alongside a burgeoning level of overweight and obesity. An example of this is in Northern Africa, where at 8%, the level of overweight children exceeds that of wasted children at 7%. A similar, though less extreme situation is found in the countries of Eastern Asia and South America. Whilst the term 'Childhood obesity' often conjures up the image of a child of wealthy parents eating convenience foods and engaging in little physical activity, this may be an outdated idea; the children of Egypt, Argentina, Malawi, Nigeria, Uzbekistan, Peru, Qatar, South Africa and Jamaica actually show a higher percentage of overweight children than that of the USA.

The widespread interest in the prevalence of overweight and obesity in children and young people across the world has produced many studies detailing these rising levels in more local populations, on both small and large scales. These studies use various methods of data collection and standards for defining obesity; the most commonly used being BMI and those of the International Obesity Task Force (IOTF) [13].

A study in which a stratified 10% random sample of school pupils from the United Arab Emirates were weighed and measured, allowing their BMI to be calculated. These results were compared with international reference data, and the conclusion drawn was that the frequency of obesity among UAE youth is 2 to 3 times greater than the recently published international standards [14].

Some studies focus on children in minority ethnic groups. A study of 'Ethnicity, socio-economic status, overweight and underweight in East London adolescents' published in 2005 suggested that whilst obesity was prevalent in all ethnic groups studied, Indian males appeared to be at risk of being both overweight and underweight [15].

In the United States, The National Center for Disease Statistics regularly publishes the results of the National Health and Nutrition Examination Survey (NHANES), which regularly records the heights and weights of American Children. Here, the standard for overweight is viewed as children with BMI figures at or above the 95th percentile of the sex specific growth charts. Table 1 shows a comparison of the results obtained across five decades of records. There is an apparent 45% increase in the prevalence of children with a BMI above the 95th percentile between 1988-94 and 1999-2002 [16].

TABLE 1. Percentage of children and adolescents with a BMI at or above the 95th percentile, ages 6-19 years, for selected years 1963-65 through 1999-2002

Age (years)[1]	NHANES 1963-65 1966 -70[2]	NHANES 1971-74	NHANES 1976-80	NHANES 1988-94	NHANES 1999-2002
6 to 11	4	4	7	11	16
12 to 19	5	6	5	11	16

[1]Excludes pregnant women starting with 1971-74. Pregnancy status not available for 1963-65 and 1966-70.
[2]Data for 1963-65 are for children 6-11 years of age; data for 1966-70 are for adolescents 12-17 years of age, not 12-19 years.

Adding sex and ethnic groups to this shows that it is the minority groups in the USA that display the highest levels of obesity. Non-Hispanic white children show lower rates of overweight and obesity in almost every category. These figures are shown in Table 2 [17].

TABLE 2. BMI for age greater than or equal to 95th centile, % prevalence ± SE

Sex	Age, years	All	Non-Hispanic White	Non-Hispanic Black	Mexican American
Both	2 to 5	10.3 (1.2)	8.6 (1.5)	8.8 (1.5)	13.1 (2.0)
	6 to 11	15.8 (1.1)	13.5 (1.5)†§	19.8 (1.4)‡	21.8 (1.7)‡
	12 to 19	16.1 (0.8)	13.7 (1.1)†§	21.1 (1.2)‡	22.5 (1.3)‡
	6 to 19	16.0 (0.8)	13.6 (1.1)†§	20.5 (0.8)‡	22.2 (1.1)‡
Male	2 to 5	9.9 (1.6)	8.2 (1.9)	8.0 (1.8)	14.1 (2.1)
	6 to 11	16.9 (1.3)	14.0 (1.5)†	17.0 (1.5)†	26.5 (2.2)‡§
	12 to 19	16.7 (0.9)	14.6 (1.3)†	18.7 (1.7)	24.7 (1.9)‡
	6 to 19	16.8 (0.8)	14.3 (1.1)†	17.9 (1.0)†	25.5 (1.3)‡§
Female	2 to 5	10.7 (1.5)	9.1 (2.0)	9.6 (1.8)	12.2 (3.4)
	6 to 11	14.7 (1.6)	13.1 (2.3)§	22.8 (2.5)‡	17.1 (2.0)
	12 to 19	15.4 (1.2)	12.7 (1.8)§	23.6 (1.8)‡	19.9 (1.9)
	6 to 19	15.1 (1.1)	12.9 (1.6)†§	23.2 (1.1)‡	18.5 (1.4)‡

*BMI rounded to the nearest 0.1; pregnant girls were excluded from the study
† significantly different from Mexican Americans at $P<0.05$, with Bonferroni adjustment
‡ significantly different from non-Hispanic Whites at $P<0.05$, with Bonferroni adjustment
§ significantly different from non-Hispanic Blacks at $P<0.05$, with Bonferroni adjustment

As a contrast to the USA and Western Europe, height and weight were measured among 2161 primary schoolchildren aged 6 - 13 in Hat Yai province in Thailand, which is described as a transitional society. The study suggested that 14.1% of the children in Hat Yai municipality were obese. Statistically significant associations with obesity were found for family history of obesity, low exercise levels and parental obesity. Significant trends of increased risk were associated with higher family income and smaller family size, factors that are illustrated almost universally when describing the 'Westernisation' of societies [18]

The problem of obesity is prevalent in both adults and children across Europe. Following the global pattern, rising rates are seen in children, with as many as one in four children affected in some regions. The European Association for the Study of Obesity currently suggests that Greece has the highest levels of obesity in Europe, with 30% of adult women described as obese. Figure 3 shows the data collected by the International Obesity Task Force on overweight in European Children [13]. It appears to be the children who live in the countries surrounding the Mediterranean who show the highest prevalence rates of overweight, at between 20-40%, whereas the children of Northern Europe show much lower rates [9].

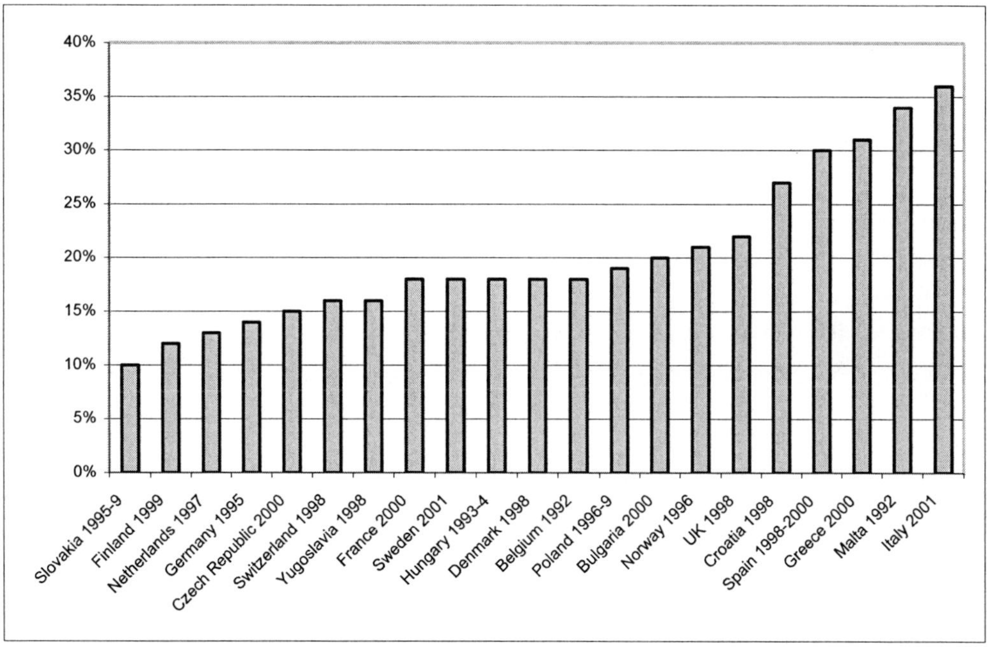

Source: IOTF collated data. (Overweight in children corresponding to BMI>25 at age 18 using IOTF assessment method)

Figure 3. Number of overweight children in European countries

The highest levels of childhood overweight are currently experienced in Italy. However, parental perception of a child's weight is important, and a study in Milan, using 569 mother and child pairs were weighed. 29% of the mothers and 35% of the children were found to be overweight or obese. Only 10% of mothers underestimated their own weight, yet 28% of women underestimated their child's weight. Similarly, whilst 37% overestimated their own weight, only 9% of mothers overestimated their child's weight. When told of their results,

57% of the mothers with an obese or overweight child were not concerned, and 44% of the women with overweight or obese children believed that their child was eating correctly [19].

The rising level of obesity seen in children in the UK has received widespread coverage in the national press, with Government reports and media headlines reinforcing the idea that obesity (amongst both adults and children) is becoming a serious problem, not only for the health of Britain's children, but also due to the potential burden that a generation of obese adults could place on the National Health Service. Seven years after the WHO described obesity as a 'Global Epidemic', the House of Commons Select Heath Committee has concurred with this by choosing 'epidemic' to describe the rapid rise in obesity throughout the United Kingdom [20].

In 2002, using the International classification of obesity, the Health Survey for England reported that for two to fifteen year olds 21.8% of boys and 27.5% of girls were either overweight or obese [21] An earlier study looking at the prevalence of overweight and obese children between 1989 and 1998, using population based cross-sectional studies suggested that from 1989 to 1998 the proportion of overweight children rose from 14.7% to 23.6% and that of obese children rising from 5.4% to 9.2% [22].

Childhood overweight and obesity prevalence trends in England have been studied between 1974 and 2003, using school based and a general population health survey. The prevalence of obesity in boys increased from 1.2% in 1984 to 3.4% in 1996 – 1997 and 6% in 2002 – 2003. In girls, obesity increased from 1.8% in 1984 to 4.4% in 1996 – 1997 and 6.6% in 2002 – 2003. Children from manual classes and low-income households had a greater increase in obesity than children from higher income households [23]. This may be related to difficulties in obtaining healthier foods due to financial constraints [24]. Between 1974 and 1984 there was little change in the prevalence of obesity [25], and it seems that the main increase in obesity started after 1984, accelerating more in recent years.

The rise in obesity is a worldwide phenomenon. In the developed world it is seen more commonly in the poorer strata of society, whereas in the developing world it is very much a reflection of the wealthy. Rates of rise are accelerating everywhere, and urgent action is needed.

Although obesity is the main subject, it must not be forgotten that inner city, poor areas in the developed world, as well as having a higher prevalence of obesity, also have high rates of other nutritional problems, such as poor growth, iron deficiency anaemia and rickets [26]. There is clearly a major problem of nutrition in poorer communities in the developed world, of which obesity is just one indicator.

The reasons for this preponderance of poorer and ethnic minorities are chiefly due to the non availability of healthy foods on cost grounds, meaning that cheaper, energy dense foods are eaten, coupled with a complete change of environment. Many immigrants come from a background of hardship, where physical activity needs to be much higher to survive, together with (often) poor sources of food. It is possible that in such parts of the world there is a genetic tendency to obesity, kept at bay by poor availability of food and increased physical activity. It may be a way of enabling populations to survive during periods of famine. When these groups arrive in the west, with the promise of better living, does the adaptation to a more comfortable lifestyle with more availability of inappropriate food and less opportunity for physical exercise, form an additional reason for the high rates of obesity seen in immigrant populations? This is an area that requires further research.

Causes of Obesity

Although the main causes of obesity are inappropriate diet, with increasing consumption of energy dense diets, poor in nutrients, with high levels of sugar and saturated fats, together with lack of exercise, which will be considered later, genetic and medical causes need to be looked at.

Genetic Influences

In the past, before the recent increase in the prevalence of obesity, there did appear to be children who ate voraciously and yet remained slim, and those who became obese despite a relatively low calorie intake. Until relatively recently these comments were considered as nothing other than folklore, and that the obese children were just lazy. However, recent advances in the genetic and hormonal understanding of appetite regulation and deposition of adipose tissue have shown a scientific basis for these observations. There are a myriad of small peptide hormones, mainly released from the gastro-intestinal tract that seem to stimulate various parts of the brain responsible for appetite control and fat deposition.

Early interest focussed on leptin, which was the first specific gene recognised as important in human body weight control. The leptin gene is an adipocyte hormone that is involved with a variety of hormones and neurotransmitters to control appetite [9]. It has important effects in regulating body weight, metabolism and reproductive function. It is known to have high levels in obese subjects, which indicates that obesity is not related to leptin deficiency, except in extremely rare cases.

Leptin is mainly found associated with adipocytes, which suggests that body weight is sensed as the total mass of fat in the body. Smaller amounts of leptin are also found in the stomach and placenta. Leptin receptors are known to be expressed in those parts of the hypothalamus associated with regulating body weight. Leptin is encoded by the obese gene (ob) and once encoded, this acts on the leptin receptors in the hypothalamus, providing information about the levels of fat reserves. It influences changes in feeding behaviour through suppression of appetite and an increase in metabolic activity and energy expenditure. It has been suggested that leptin also stimulates the rate of lipolysis and the expression of enzymes of the fatty acid oxidation in adipose and pancreatic cells, causing a reduction of triglyceride content. It is possible that differences in the fats production rate of leptin, resistance to leptin at its site of action, or a combination of these factors could influence eating behaviours and energy used to cause obesity [27].

Mice given recombinant mouse or human leptin led to a dramatic reduction in food intake and massive weight loss. It appears that weight loss resulting from administration of leptin in this case results from:

- Decreased hunger and food consumption, mediated in part at least through neuropeptide Y synthesis. Neuropeptide Y is a potent stimulator of feeding behaviour.
- An increase in energy expenditure, measured as increased oxygen consumption, higher body temperature and loss of adipose tissue mass [28].

Overall, however, it is not clear exactly how leptin expression is regulated and indeed how it interacts with the various other appetite regulating hormones now described. However, there are extremely rare cases described of leptin deficiency and other monogenic deficiencies that result in morbid obesity [29, 30]. Morbidly obese children given recombinant leptin significantly reduced weight [31].

Although there are many other hormonal influences on appetite and weight described, most interest has focussed on the peptide ghrelin and its more recently described opposite, obestatin.

Ghrelin was initially identified as the peptide that stimulated the release of growth hormone, but it was subsequently shown that ghrelin, together with several other hormones, has an effect on appetite and energy balance. It is mainly found in epithelial cells in the stomach, and is known to be derived from a prohormone usually referred to as proghrelin. Although growth hormone release remains its main physiological function, it stimulates appetite by acting on the arcuate nucleus area of the hypothalamus, which is known to control food intake. It circulates in high levels in a fasting state, which indicates that it transmits a hunger signal from the periphery to the hypothalamus [32].

Obese patients tend to have lower ghrelin levels than normal, but it is not clear whether that is cause or effect. Food fails to suppress ghrelin levels in obese patients. Patients with anorexia nervosa have high levels of ghrelin, which fall as the condition improves [33]. Humans injected with ghrelin exhibit a feeling of intense hunger [34].

Children suffering from the Prader-Willi syndrome (PWS), which is characterised by excessive appetite with massive progressive obesity, short stature and learning difficulties have been shown to have high levels of ghrelin [35]. Clearly, if PWS is in part related to the high levels of circulating ghrelin, then possible ghrelin blocking mechanisms could be used to try and improve the condition.

Obestatin has only recently been described and has caused much media speculation as to its commercial use in the future in the treatment of obesity. It was discovered by a bioinformatic prediction that another peptide derived from proghrelin existed. A ghrelin-associated peptide was discovered and named obestatin [36]. It appears to act in an opposite way to ghrelin, in that it decreases food intake and weight in laboratory animals, and in addition slows down gastric emptying, which is the opposite of ghrelin. It is clearly far too early to hail this peptide as the answer to obesity, as it has many as many of its effects appear a little contradictory [37], but it highlights the media desire for a "quick fix" for obesity.

Large numbers of other appetite regulating hormones have been described, and it is clear that much has yet to be learned about the interactions and the ways that they control appetite and weight. They are summarised by Speiser et al [9] and Farooq [29].

Another important factor in the aetiology of obesity is when to stop eating. Meal termination and satiety is believed to be controlled by another group of peptides. Peptide YY is released into the circulation from the distal bowel in proportion to the calories ingested. Administration of the active form of the peptide caused a marked inhibition of food intake [38]. Obese individuals have lower fasting levels of this petide, but remain susceptible to its inhibitory effects [39].

Glucagon-like peptide 1 and oxyntomodulin are also released into the circulation after food intake, acting on different parts of the brain, and again when administered to humans, cause a fall in food intake [40, 41].

This is a rapidly expanding area of research, and new petides are being discovered all the time [42]. Study of these peptides certainly adds to our understanding of the physiology of hunger, weight gain and satiety, but whether any will lead to a successful management of hunger and therefore obesity remains to be seen.

There have also been searches for possible genetic sites related to obesity, but most chromosomes seem to have obesity related genes. A human obesity gene map exists, and continues to expand as more genes and chromosomal regions are linked with human obesity. The most recent evidence has 430 genes, markers and chromosome regions associated or linked with human obesity [43].

The genetic and hormonal control of appetite regulation and obesity is a rapidly expanding field of research. As indicated earlier, several monogenic causes of obesity have been identified, and it is to be expected that the next few years will bring many more such children to our attention.

The medical profession may learn more in the future about the physiology of hunger, appetite and weight control, but what must never be lost sight of is the importance of maintaining a healthy eating pattern and increasing the amount of exercise.

Medical Causes

There are rare medical causes of obesity in childhood. There are some syndromes that have obesity as a component. PWS has already been mentioned; Bardet-Biedl syndrome is characterised by variable amounts of obesity, learning difficulties, pigmentary retinopathy, polydactyly and renal anomalies. Several chromosome regions, including genes involved in cilial and centriole function have been identified [44, 45].

One of the more difficult questions that patients ask is whether the cause of a child's obesity is due to his/her "glands". Endocrine causes are extremely rare, although growth hormone and thyroid deficiency, as well as cortisol excess are associated with obesity. All are associated with a combination of decreased energy expenditure and decreased growth.

However, increasingly the metabolic syndrome is being recognised in childhood and adolescence [46]. This is the result of obesity, not a cause. It consists of obesity, especially around the waist, elevated blood pressure, elevated lipids and cholesterol, and insulin resistance.

Obesity is seen secondary to severe brain injury and in children who have brain tumours, or following cranial irradiation. It is presumed that the cause is due to alterations in hypothalamic neuropeptides [47], but the cause remains unknown.

Some medications are also associated with obesity in children. The best known of these are corticosteroids, but also cyproheptadine, used often to stimulate appetite and sodium valproate, used in treating epilepsy.

These causes are summarised in Table 3.

TABLE 3. Medical cause of obesity

RARE SYNDROMES	ENDOCRINE CAUSES	NEUROLOGICAL CAUSES	MEDICATIONS
Prader-Willi	Hypothyroidism	Serious brain injury	Corticosteroids
Bardet-Biedl	Growth Hormone deficiency	Brain tumours and/or irradiation	Cyproheptadine
	Cushing's syndrome		Sodium valproate

What does a paediatrician do when confronted by a family insisting that their obese child has a "gland" problem? Fortunately all of the clinical conditions referred to have a fairly typical phenotype or other clinical features, and further investigation should seldom be necessary. It may take time and patience to explain this to anxious parents, but this time is well spent. In the obesity clinic at The Royal London Hospital metabolic rate is sometimes measured to show both the child and the parents they are normal.

It must also be remembered that obesity may be a finding in disturbed teenagers and younger children. Children who suffer neglect or emotional abuse often comfort eat, and as a result become seriously overweight.

Environmental and Social Causes

However, despite our increasing knowledge of the genetic factors affecting obesity and appetite, together with the rare medical conditions mentioned above, the overwhelming cause of the increase in obesity worldwide is inappropriate dietary intake and lack of exercise. There is clearly an association between environmental and genetic factors, but the genetic factor has always been there as far as we can tell, and so the difference now is food intake and lack of exercise.

The increasing BMI average of children is due to an imbalance between energy intake and energy expenditure. Significant influences on a child lifestyle are parenting, schooling, peers and the media.

Eating habits have changed significantly over the last 20 years. The total energy expenditure consists of metabolic rate, thermic effect of food and physical activity. There is no evidence to show the resting metabolic rate has changed in recent years nor has the thermic effect of food altered [48, 49]. Accordingly, the major cause of obesity is related to various aspects of lifestyle that have resulted in reduced physical activity.

The rapid rise in childhood obesity is mirrored by an increase in sedentary leisure pursuits for children such as computers, video games, and television watching [50]. The opportunity for physical activity has decreased with the increasing use of cars, television watching and lack of space for active games, etc.

In the UK, very few schools in the state sector still have athletic or sports activities. In fact, recently one of the best-known comprehensive schools in London has sold its sports ground for a housing development [51]. During the 1950's and 1960's, most schoolchildren played soccer, rugby football, hockey or cricket regularly and in addition had regular physical exercise sessions. All this has stopped in the majority of state schools, although it still exists in private sector schools.

Nowadays the "school run" is a feature of everyday life in British society. Parents take their children to school in the car, sometimes for a journey of a few hundred yards only, rather than children walking or cycling to school, as was the norm in the past.

The energy intake of preschool children has actually declined over the past 10 years, but this has been outstripped by an increase in inactivity [52, 53]. A British report found the growing percentage of obese individuals since 1950, paralleled with an increase in both television viewing and the number of cars per household [54].

The relationship between television viewing and obesity has three aspects:

- Decreased energy expenditure (excessive inactivity while viewing);
- Increased energy intake (consumption of high-energy density snacks rich in sugar and fat while viewing);
- Food advertisements

A cross-sectional US study found that children who did the least physical activity or watched the most TV tended to be the most overweight [50]. A study in Mexico City established that the obesity risk decreased by 10% for each hour per day of moderate to-vigorous physical activity, and increased by 12% for each hour per day of television viewing [55].

Another major factor in television viewing is the frequent advertisements for convenience foods, mostly fast food, soft drinks, sweets, and sugar-sweetened breakfast cereal. British children are exposed to about ten food commercials per hour of television time [56]. It has been suggested that exposure to 30 second commercials increase the likelihood that 3-5 year olds would later select an advertised food when presented with options. Healthy options, such as fresh fruit and vegetables are less likely to be advertised. A study of the effects of television viewing on obesity in two schools over an academic year showed that in the intervention school where there was a reduction of 40% in television viewing time, BMI of the children reduced significantly [57].

The Hastings Review [58], published in the UK by the Food Standards Agency in 2003, concluded that advertising to children had an adverse impact on food preference, purchasing behaviour and consumption. Unfortunately, its opinions were not widely shared, and an attempt to introduce a bill in the British parliament calling for a ban on advertising of food and drinks high in fat, salt or sugar during children's television failed after running out of parliamentary time. However, there is now a reduction in such advertising in the UK, in line with many other European countries.

The National Diet and Nutrition Survey found that 40% of boys and 60% of girls surveyed were failing to meet Health Education Authority physical activity recommendations. Young people should participate in physical activity of at least moderate intensity for one hour per day. The survey found that children's consumption of fruit and vegetables has been falling over the past 20 years, with more than half of those surveyed eating no fruit or vegetables in a given week [52].

Diet is an important area of research in the fight against combating childhood obesity. However, although diet is a contributing factor in childhood obesity, only a small reduction in energy intake is recommended for overweight children. This is due to the adequate need for both energy and nutrients required for normal growth and development.

Recently, research has looked at milk, the first and main source of energy intake at the start of life. Children who were bottle-fed seem to be more at risk of obesity later in childhood than those who were breast-fed. Formula fed infants were heavier than those who received no milk other than breast milk in the first 12 months of life, although they were of similar length and head circumference. It was also found that the energy intake of breastfed infants was lower than that of formula fed infants, even after the introduction of solids, and suggested that relatively low energy intakes are a due to the self regulation in breastfed infants [59]. In children aged 5 and 6 years a substantial, dose dependent, protective effect of breast feeding on obesity and overweight was seen: three to five months of exclusive breastfeeding was associated with a 35% reduction in obesity at the age of 5 to 6 years [60].

Fat has been the most topically and central to the dietary causes of obesity. Fat is the most energy dense macronutrient, using the energy intake plus energy expenditure argument, excessive consumption is often believed to cause weight gain. However, epidemiological studies have shown inconsistencies between dietary fat and adiposity in children and young adults. One study has shown the prevalence of obesity has greatly increased, despite an apparent decrease in proportion of total calories consumed as fat in the diet of US children [61].

Type of dietary fat could be of greater importance than total fat consumption in the cause of obesity related morbidities. Saturated fat has a well-known risk of cardiovascular disease in adults. Intake of partially hydrogenated Trans-fat, commonly found in commercial bakery products and fast foods increase risk for cardiovascular disease and in contrast unsaturated fats (from vegetables and marine sources) decrease risk of this [62].

The decrease in dietary fat has been accompanied by a compensatory increase in carbohydrate consumption, especially in the form of refined foods (e.g., breads, cereals, cakes, soft drinks). These foods have high glycaemic index and studies have shown consumption of these kind of foods induce a sequence of hormonal events that stimulate hunger and cause overeating in adolescents [63].

An additional problem with the change in dietary fat intake is the overall reduction in omega-3 fatty acids, and the higher intake of omega – 6 fatty acids. In evolutionary terms, it is believed that the ratio of omega-6: omega-3 fatty acids was around 1. Now it is of the order of 15:1. These high intakes of omega-6 fatty acids also predispose to cardiovascular disease, cancer, and inflammatory and autoimmune diseases, whereas a higher omega-3 intake protects against these. Even reducing the omega-6: omega-3 ratio to 4:1 significantly reduced the mortality from cardiovascular disease [64]. It follows that any dietary intervention must take note of this and adjust the diet accordingly.

Consequences of Obesity

Health Consequences

Many good quality cohort or case control studies have addressed the relationship between obesity in child and adulthood and adverse cardiovascular events. The main body of evidence is from the United States of America. The main cardiovascular consequences of childhood obesity that occur during childhood are sub clinical coronary artery disease and atherosclerosis. Healthcare professionals should be aware of the risk factors. Increased blood pressure, adverse lipid profiles, hyperinsulinaemia and changes in left ventricular mass. Coronary artery disease and atherosclerosis are relatively common in obese children and adolescents (SIGN, 2003) [65].

In addition, childhood obesity is associated with a range of medical conditions, mainly poor pulmonary function, advanced growth and early maturity, hepatic steatosis and cholelithiasis, and a wide range of less common polycystic conditions such as pseudotumor cerebri, sleep apnoea, polycystic ovary disease and orthopaedic complications [66]. Also the increasing incidence of type II diabetes previously unheard of in children is related to obesity. Obesity in childhood is known to be an independent risk factor for adult obesity. The risk of developing adult obesity (BMI >28) at age 35 is up to 80% in individuals who were obese when they were children (older than 9 years.) [67]. Figure 4 is a diagrammatic summary of the main complications seen.

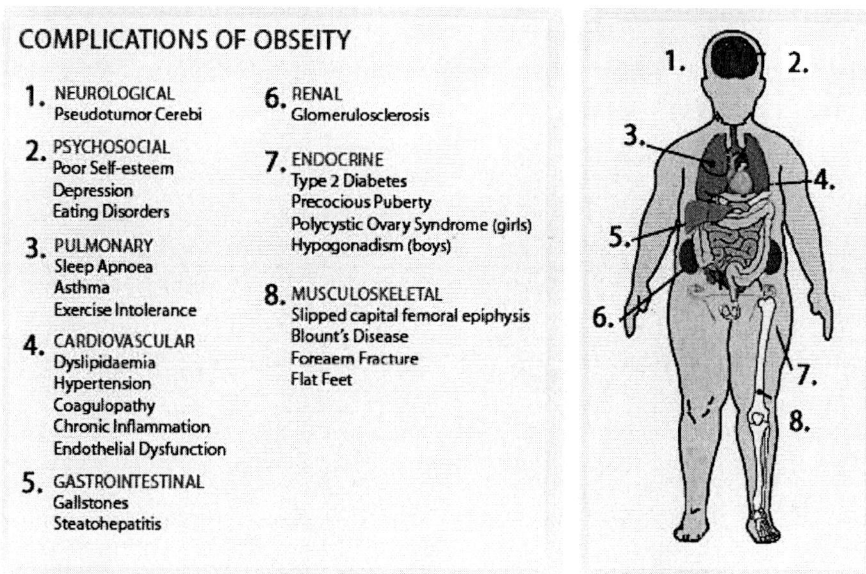

Figure 4. Main medical complications seen in obesity

The WHO has estimated the relative risks of a variety of complications associated with obesity. These are indicated in Table 4

Table 4. Relative risks associated with obesity

Greatly increased risk (relative risk x 3)	Moderately increased risk(relative risk x2-3)	Slightly increased risk (relative risk x 1-2)
Type 2 diabetes	Coronary Heart Disease	Cancer (breast, colon, endometrial)
Gallbladder disease	Hypertension	Reproductive hormone abnormalities
Dyslipidaemia	Osteoarthritis (knees)	Polycystic ovary syndrome
Insulin resistance	Hyperuricaemia and gout	Impaired fertility
Breathlessness		Low back pain
Sleep apnoea		Anaesthetic risks
		Fetal abnormalities

(**Source**: WHO 1998)

The most significant effect seen in children is the rise in Type 2 diabetes. In adults it has been estimated that 20% of adults from South Asia are diabetic, and rising levels of Type 2 diabetes in children are now reflecting this. In Tower Hamlets, a poor inner city suburb in East London, there is a very high population of Bangladeshi families, and many cases of Type 2 diabetes are now being seen in children as young as 10 and 11 years of age.

Many reviews have confirmed the rising prevalence of Type 2 diabetes in children. Most commonly the children are of South Asian, Hispanics and Black racial origins, with a lower rate in white Caucasians. All reports confirm the association with obesity [68, 69, 70]. There is a preponderance of females, and many show acanthosis nigricans. It should be mandatory as part of the management of obese children, especially those with acanthosis, to screen regularly for insulin resistance and Type 2 diabetes.

Psychological Consequences

Obese children are more likely to show evidence or psychological distress than are non-obese children and the effect is greater for girls than boys. Obesity in childhood and adolescence is also associated with poor self-esteem, being perceived as unattractive, depression, disordered eating, bulimia and body dissatisfaction [65]. Bullying is related in that obese pre-adolescents are more likely to be bullied, and conversely, many obese children become bullies, taking advantage of their superior physical size [71]. Therefore obese children showing signs of distress should be considered for referral for psychological assessment and treatment. Two good quality studies, from the UK and one from the USA show adverse associations between childhood obesity and educational attainment and income in women [72, 73]. Girls overweight at age 16 were compared with their lean peers 7 years later. They were found to have completed fewer years of school, earned less, had higher rates of household poverty and were less likely to be married. The same adult financial penalties of adolescent overweight have been found in British women.

Children at High Risk of Developing Obesity

There appears to be a significant relationship between degree of deprivation and increased prevalence of childhood obesity [72]. Obesity appears to be more prevalent with increasing age in British children. There does, not appear to be a difference of obesity rates between different genders. If one parent is obese there is a 3.4 fold increased risk of a child becoming obese this increases to 8 fold if both parents are obese. [74]

Management of Obesity

Treatment is time consuming and can be very difficult both for the child, the parents, and the professionals looking after obese children. Before considering the various treatment strategies, prevention of obesity is clearly the most cost-effective way of management.

Prevention starts before birth. Low birth weight, the result of maternal under nutrition, cigarette smoking or placental insufficiency, or a high birth weight, often associated with diabetes mellitus in the mother, are both associated with obesity in later childhood and early adult life [75]. It is possible that restricted fetal growth, accompanied by rapid postnatal growth, may be an important factor. Prevention means rigorous assessment of fetal growth, pregnant mothers trying to maintain a normal BMI, meticulous glucose control for diabetic mothers, encourage moderate exercise, and strictly no smoking in pregnancy. After birth, breast-feeding may offer some protection and should be encouraged, even if the baby is small- or large- for gestational age. Weaning should not be until 6 months of age, as earlier introduction may well be associated with the development of obesity.

Prior to going to school, families should be encouraged to eat together at fixed times avoiding fatty foods and sweet or fizzy drinks; television should not be allowed at mealtimes, and should be rationed at other times. Advertisements for convenience foods and sugary drinks should not be allowed. Even young children should be encouraged to walk or run rather than travelling everywhere in a car.

When it comes to school, much work needs to be done and is indeed being done to encourage schools to provide healthy meals rather than convenience foods, and to ban drink vending machines and other tempting snacks. Games and PE to be encouraged and compulsory for all except those with significant medical problems. Table 5 summarises the main area of prevention required

Table 5. Summary of measures to prevent childhood obesity

Before Birth	1st year of life	Pre-school	School
Normalise BMI	Breast feed	Avoid fatty and sweet foods	Avoid vending machines
Avoid smoking	Avoid sugary drinks	Ration television and video games	No sweets or convenience foods available
Moderate exercise	Don't wean before 6 months	Eat as a family at fixed times	Encourage healthy eating
Rigorous fetal growth assessment		Don't skip meals	Games and PE to be compulsory
Strict glucose control		Sensible amounts of exercise	Walk or cycle to school where possible

However, despite prevention being encouraged, there will still be many obese children, and treatment has to be offered.

Four major evidence reviews of treatment have been recently published. These help examine the evidence for treatment. [59, 76, 77, 78] The focus of this section is primarily nutrition, however, behavioural and exercise approaches are also discussed as the evidence dictates an approach with nutrition and exercise / reduction of sedentary behaviours and a psychological component are most effective. Despite much recent work in the area there still remains a lack of clarity in the evidence base to some of these recommendations. Where this is the case consensus guidelines from a group of professionals who treat obese children and adolescent have been consulted [66].

Advice should be considered where the child is defined as overweight or obese by the Child Growth Foundation BMI charts (see Figures 1 and 2). The child and family should be ready and willing to make necessary lifestyle changes.

There are many tools in the literature available to assess readiness to change [79, 80]. It is vital that a child / family is ready to change before embarking on a treatment programme. A weight management programme for a parent or an adolescent who is not ready to change may not only be futile but also harmful because an unsuccessful programme diminishes the child's self esteem and impairs future efforts to improve weight [66].

Barts and The London obesity clinic assesses readiness to change by 3 simple questions:

a) Is the child / family concerned about the child's weight?
b) Do they feel weight loss / maintenance is possible?
c) What practices need to be changed to achieve Wt loss/ maintenance?

Treatment Advice

The Scottish Intercollegiate Guidelines Network [65] published guidelines for treatment of childhood obesity in the community (Table 6). The SIGN guidelines also give guidance on which children may need referral to a hospital or community paediatric consultant (Table 7).

Table 6. Treatment of the obese child in the community

- Treatment should only be considered when a child has a BMI $\geq 91^{st}$ centile, and the child and family are perceived to be ready and willing to make the necessary lifestyle changes.
- In the UK, no drug is currently licensed for the treatment of obesity in children.
- For most obese children, maintaining their present weight but not increasing it is an acceptable goal. As the child grows taller their weight becomes right for their height. This can be demonstrated to parents by charting weight over time on BMI centile charts.
- Weight maintenance can only be achieved by sustained behavioural changes to improve activity levels and eating habits. This involves:
  - Increasing habitual physical activity to a minimum of 30 minutes/day
  - Reducing physical inactivity (e.g. TV viewing and computer games) to less than two hours per day.
  - Eating a well-balanced and healthy diet.
- Possible approaches to implementing behavioural changes include:
  - Encouraging children and families to make a few small, permanent changes in behaviour at a time.
  - Developing family awareness of eating, activity and parenting behaviours.

Encouraging the family to monitor eating and activity habits.

Source SIGN, guidelines (SIGN 2003)

Table 7. Which obese or severe overweight children should be referred to a Consultant Paediatrician or Physician in hospital or the community

• Any child who may have serious obesity-related morbidity such as sleep apnoea, obesity hyperventilation syndrome, orthopaedic problems or psychological morbidity. • Children with a possible underlying medical cause (suspect this if children are also short for their age), including all children under 24 months old who are obese (BMI $\geq$ 99.6th centile). All children who are severely obese.

Source SIGN guidelines (SIGN, 2003)

Family Involvement

It is beneficial if the family and clinician can agree goals together. The family and all carers should be involved in the treatment programme. If the child is the only family member who changes eating habits or who must exercise the child may feel deprived, scapegoated or resentful, and relapse is more likely. Involvement of the entire family and all carers will create new family behaviours consistent with the child's new eating and activity goals [66].

For children of primary school age there is evidence to support parents taking the primary responsibility for the behaviour changes in the treatment of their child's obesity [81] In practice this means that in children under 13 years of age the parents need to ensure that crisps / sweets / biscuits are ideally kept out of the house and only given in limited amounts. Children are ideally given only healthy choices at mealtimes. Sugary drinks are substituted with diet / sugary free drinks or water. Five portions of fruit and vegetables a day are taken etc. All the family and children should be encouraged to eat the same healthy food. On a practical level we find this is a key message to give to parents in our clinics. Therefore when a parent asks us to tell their child not to eat so many crisps we will reiterate to parents that they must take control of the child's intake - really younger children do not have the will power given the choice. It is very important for primary school age children (and younger) that parents (not children) are given the responsibility for ensuring sensible food choices are made.

Assessment

Before giving advice to a family some assessment of current lifestyle / risk factors as well as anthropometry is useful. Families must be treated sensibly with compassion and conviction that obesity is an important medical problem that can be treated. Questions about food consumption and activity should be framed in objective, non-accusatory language [66].

History

To try and identify any possible 'Trigger Factors' it is useful to ascertain when the obesity commenced. Children who are short for their age and any children who are obese under 24 months (BMI > 99.6^{th} centile) should be referred to a paediatrician to exclude an underlying medical cause.

Activity

As the treatment is likely to include an increase in activity it is important to assess current levels of activity and sedentary activities. We find it useful to ask how many hours per day are spent watching television. In the USA children are thought to spend more time watching television than at school.

A careful history of physical activity will uncover opportunity to increase energy expenditure. Deterrents or barriers to increasing activity should also be recognised. These include unsafe neighbourhoods and lack of adult supervision.

Previous Experiences with Weight Loss

Many families may have tried to control their weights or that of their children. It is useful to find out if any tactics in the past have worked. If diets have not worked – why not?

Current Diet

It is often found patients tell health professionals what they think they want to hear; therefore food diaries are useful to identify current dieting patterns and have the benefit of encouraging self-monitoring. Otherwise general questions around whether regular meals are taken, where meals are taken and what the parent / child feels the main problem are useful.

Psychological Factors

There is a greater incidence of binge eating disorders in the obese [82] it is therefore important for the health professional to exclude any eating disorders. Also to try and elucidate psychological triggers to eating. i.e. does the patient eat more when happy or sad?

Dietary Treatment

Counting calories can be tedious, difficult and inaccurate. Other strategies are easier and therefore often more likely to succeed. Reduction or elimination of specific foods may reduce calories without making children feel hungry or deprived. For example the family can eliminate from the diet one or two high calorie foods, such as chips, chocolate or fried foods, or they can replace all sugary drinks with diet / low calorie drinks. Other practical ways to reduce calorie intakes are shown in table 8.

For some children however a Calorie deficit diet (generally 600 kcal /day below requirements) can prove useful. Adult literature has shown this treatment to be effective [83] and for children it is also equally useful to have treatment options. It may be necessary to hospitalise a child if this is considered until the diet is well established and the family educated thoroughly.

Table 8. Practical ways to reduce calorie intake

• Ensure breakfast and regular meals are taken. • Eat only at mealtimes and recognised snack periods. • Eat if possible as a family. • Discourage eating in front of the television or snacking when playing / working on the video/computer. • It is more time consuming to eat whole foods for example apples compared to apple juice or puree. This helps satisfy as does eating slower and higher fibre foods. • Drink water or low calorie drinks only. • Recognise that fruit juices are energy dense - There has been a link established between soft drinks consumption and obesity. • Use low fat margarines and spreads but still use sparingly, they are still energy dense. • Avoid sugared or chocolate-coated cereals - but remember some breakfast is better than no breakfast. • Avoid eating late at night. • Discuss school dinners with the child and ideally the school, remember the plate model. Aim for meat, carbohydrate and vegetables but avoid chips and fried foods. Fresh fruit and yoghurts are useful as puddings. • Avoid using food as a reward. • Encourage the family and child to persist in dietary modification but supportively.

Plate Model (figure 1)

This is a useful concept for families. The DoH has suggested the ideal plate should be covered two fifths by vegetables or salad (not including potatoes / without added butter or high fat sources). Two fifths should be covered by a starchy / carbohydrate food such as bread / pasta / rice / potatoes and only one fifth covered by meat, fish, cheese, etc which tend to have a high fat content.

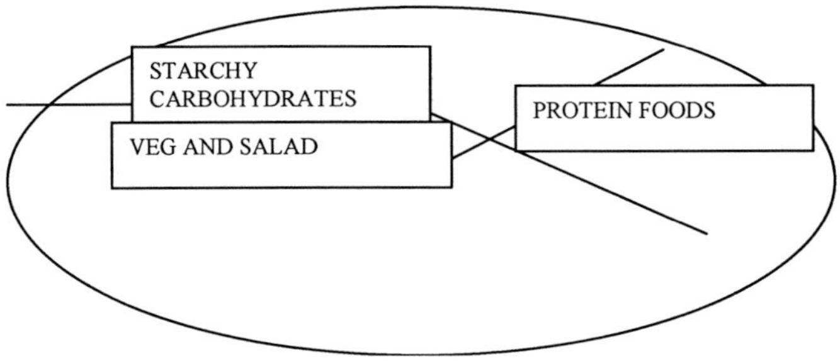

Figure 1. Plate model

Snacking

Snacking appears to be a major factor in childhood obesity. It is important to ensure that children are eating enough at mealtimes to reduce the need to snack. Watch out for crisps, chocolate bars and biscuits at break and other times. Changing snacks maybe the most difficult aspect of the whole slimming effort and needs handling sympathetically, particularly since peer group pressure to eat, or unkind teasing may accompany snack avoidance. Fruit is the ideal snack - but toast, yogurts, breakfast cereals, plain popcorn and raisins are other options.

Reduction of Sedentary Behaviours / Increase in Exercise

There is evidence supporting the use of laboratory based exercise programmes in the treatment of childhood obesity. These programmes consisted of walking, jogging, cycling, high repetition resistance, exercise combinations within a laboratory setting, as opposed to free-living lifestyle activity interventions [80]

One school based RCT showed a reduction in television viewing corresponded with a decreased BMI and triceps skin fold thickness. However 2 school based RCT's showed an exercise only intervention failed to change BMI. In childhood there is increasing evidence that restricting time spent doing sedentary activities is important in treating obesity. Two RCT's compared exercise advice versus reduction of sedentary behaviour advice both with diet at 1 year follow-up all groups lost weight however one study showed the reducing sedentary behaviours group had a more significant reduction in percentage overweight [81].

The SIGN guidelines [65] and the Barlow and Dietz [66] recommendations both suggest obesity in children may be prevented and treated by making lifestyle changes such as increased physical activity and decreasing physical inactivity (e.g. TV watching). Time spent doing sedentary behaviours should be under 2 hours / day.

Only 55% of boys and 39% of girls meet the Health Education Authority Recommendation of 60 minutes of moderate activity a day. By the age of 15 just under half (48%) of boys and around a fifth (18%) of girls attain the recommended levels.

Behavioural / Parenting Interventions

Behavioural treatments have been the most studied approach to paediatric obesity. A Cochrane review identified 10 family based behaviour modification programmes. These included behaviour modification, dietary and exercise education, with a mix of sessions involving the child parents and in some cases the entire family. The review concluded that while some of findings appear promising, the small size of some of the studies and the disparate advice of the interventions mean there is at present insufficient evidence to recommend any specific programme [77]. The SIGN guidelines recommend lifestyle change involving making small gradual changes to behaviour. Family support is usually necessary for treatment to succeed.

Parents should be a role model and try to improve their own eating habits and lack of activity. Parents should be consistent, determine what food is offered and when. The child should then decide whether to eat. The parents should only offer healthy options - parents can ask the child to choose between an apple or an oatcake not an apple or a cookie. Food should never be used as a reward.

It is of interest that one study has shown that there is sometimes a better weight loss in an obese child if the parents alone are targeted for intervention, both dietary and life style [84].

The reviews of obesity prevention and treatment all indicate that multifaceted treatment is most effective.

Very Low Calorie Diets

Very low calorie diets provide 800 Kcal/ day or fewer [85].

The protein sparing modified fast (PSMF) is a high protein diet, which is supposed to spare lean body, mass and has been the most widely used and reported very low calorie diet in children. These may be followed for 2-3 months and then patients are advised onto diets gradually returning to normal balanced diets [86]. Comparisons of the efficiency and safety of these diets are hard to make as studies vary and particularly important long term follow up data often does not exist, in practice these diets are rarely used in the U.K. Practically with the morbidly obese child a short admission to hospital following a normal calorie diet – i.e. (1500-2000kcal/d) will often induce rapid weight loss – it needs to be remembered that very obese children often have very high calorie requirements to maintain that level of weight.

In all of the dietary interventions, it must be kept in mind that it is equally important to adjust the balance of omega-3 and omega-6 fatty acids as discussed earlier. No reduction in weight brought about by increasing activity will be successful in the long-term unless the quality of food is also improved. A continuing high intake of omega-6 fatty acids will still result in significant mortality and morbidity from cardiovascular disease.

Medical Treatment

There is rarely need for drug treatment of obesity as by far and away the most important management is life style changes and appropriate food intake. However, for some of the rare medical conditions there may be a case for a pharmacological approach, and also for those obese children who suffer from potentially life threatening episodes such as sleep apnoea.

In the past stimulant drugs such as amphetamines, fenfluramine were used, but these are now known to have many dangers and are no longer used.

Sibutramine is a nonselective inhibitor of neuronal reuptake of serotonon, noradrenaline and dopamine. It acts as an anorectic drug, and caused an initial fall in weight over 6 months in a series of 43 obese adolescents, but no further weight loss following its use [87]. It has a relatively limited use due to its side effects, especially rises in blood pressure and should always be used in conjunction with lifestyle changes and diet. It is rarely used in adolescents in the UK.

Orlistat inhibits pancreatic lipase and increases faecal losses of triglyceride. A trial in Sweden to try and prevent diabetes showed a 37% reduction in Type 2 diabetes following the use of orlistat [88], and a 3 month trial in another study caused significant falls in weight and lipid levels [89]. This drug does appear to be effective in selected individuals, and is currently the drug of choice in the UK for use in those very severe life threatened obese children.

Metformin acts by increasing glucose uptake in the liver, decreases gluconeogenesis, and reduces hepatic glucose production. It does appear to result in reduced food intake, weight loss, an improvement in lipid profiles and to delay the onset of Type 2 diabetes. In the United Kingdom Prospective Diabetes Study (UKPDS), patients on metformin showed weight maintenance but not weight loss over a 15-year period; more importantly long-term there was a reduction in myocardial infarction mortality (90). However, whereas the metformin use in this programme reduced the development of diabetes by 31%, lifestyle intervention reduced it by 58% (91). Other trials have shown a weight reduction with metformin [92].

Metformin clearly has a use in the prevention of Type 2 diabetes, and as such would be the medication of choice in overweight children who have a strong family history. This is of particular relevance in East London, where the large Bangladeshi community has a very high genetic risk of developing Type 2 diabetes.

Surgery

There is seldom if ever a place for bariatric surgery in childhood or adolescence. Gastric banding or a gastric bypass has been used, but there are complications from the procedure. It is more useful in extremely obese adults with severe co-morbid conditions, although has on rare occasions been used in adolescents. It is suggested that it should only be used on those children who have reached skeletal maturity and who have a BMI > 40 (defined as very severely obese); in addition they should have co-morbidities associated with obesity that might be remedies with a sustained weight loss [93]. However, its use in adolescence is highly controversial, and in the UK it is extremely rarely performed.

The above treatments must never be used without lifestyle and dietary changes. The danger is that many desperate parents will learn about them and may even be tempted to seek them to self medicate their children, with potentially devastating effect. All of these treatments should only be considered in a multi-professional setting where all other attempted measures have failed. Under no circumstances should they be used indiscriminately by paediatricians or general practitioners without reference to a specialist obesity service.

Summary of Main Conclusions

The core principles appear to be reduce energy intake and encourage healthy eating, decrease sedentary behaviours to less than 2 hours / day, increase activity to 60 minutes / day and give primary responsibility for the behaviour change to the parents rather than the children in under 13 year olds. Guidance for health professionals has been developed by four major evidence reviews ([59, 76, 77, 78]. More good methodological quality research is needed to improve treatment of paediatric obesity further.

Conclusion

Unless there is a major change in diet and lifestyle, the current epidemic of obesity will continue to rise, with all its associated morbidity. Many governments are now beginning to realise the economic cost and consequences of the obesity epidemic, and are taking measures to improve matters.

A first step would be the total banning of convenience food adverts on television and on advertising hoardings. The food industry must put its house in order by reducing the amount of refined sugars and saturated fats in their food, in addition to a reduction in salt. Some of the worldwide chains are beginning to offer healthy alternatives, but much more needs to be done. Strenuous efforts should be made to provide all children with healthy school meals, and to educate both children and parents about healthy eating.

Major attempts must be made to re-introduce compulsory PE and games sessions at all schools. In London, as we are going to host the 2012 Olympic Games, it is to be hoped that a major result of this will be to encourage younger people to take more exercise.

At present survival rates in the western world are high – but with this legacy of rising obesity in our population, can we be sure that the survival rates of our current children will be as good in the future? It has been estimated that obesity reduces life expectancy by an average of 9 years (WHO figures), and so it is essential that all health professionals work together to try and defeat this rising tide.

References

[1] Sardinha LB, Going SB, Teixeria PJ, Lohman TG. Receiver operating characteristic analysis of body mass index, triceps skinfold thickness, and arm girth for obesity screening in children and adolescents. *Am J Clin Nutr* 1999; 70: 1090-1095

[2] Cole TJ, Freeman JV, Preece MA. British 1990 growth reference centiles weight, height, body mass index and head circumference fitted by maximum penalised likelihood. *Stat Med* 1998; 17: 407-29

[3] Cole TJ, Bellizzi MC, Flegal KM, Dietz WH. Establishing a standard definition for child overweight and obesity worldwide: an international survey. *BMJ* 2000;320: 1-6

[4] Wells JCK. A Hattori chart analysis of body mass index in infants and children. *Int J Obes* 2000; 24: 325-329

[5] Bigaard J, Tjonneland A, Thomsen BL, OvervadK, Heitmann BL, Sorensen TAI. Waist circumference, BMI, smoking, and mortality in middle aged men and women. *Obes Res* 2003; 11: 895-903
[6] Maffeis C, Pietrobelli A, Grezzani A, Provera S, Tato L. Waist circumference and and cardiovascular risk factors in prepubertal children. *Obes Res* 2001; 9: 179-18
[7] Yusuf S, Hawken S, Ôunpuu S et al (2005). Obesity and the risk of myocardial infarction in 27000 participants from 52 countries: a case-control study. *Lancet* **366**: 1640-1649.
[8] McCarthy HD, Jarrett KV, Crawley HF. The development of waist circumference percentiles in British children aged 5 – 16.9 years. *Eur J Clin Nutr* 2001; 55: 902-907
[9] Speiser PW, Rudolph MCJ, Anhalt H et al. Consensus statement: Childhood obesity. *J Clin Endocrinol Metab* 2005; 90: 1871-1887
[10] Ebbeling CD, Pawlak DB, Ludwig DS. Childhood obesity: public - health crisis, common sense cure. *Lancet* 2002, 360: 473-82
[11] Magarey AM, Daniels LA, Boulton TJ. Prevalence of overweight and obesity in Australian children and adolescents: reassessment of 1985 and 1995 data against new standard international definitions. *Med J Aust* 2001; 174: 561 - 564
[12] Cheng TO. Obesity in Chinese children. *J R Soc Med* 2004; 97: 254
[13] International Obesity Task Force and the European Association for the Study of Obesity. Obesity in Europe; London: International Obesity task Force 2002
[14] Al-Haddad FH, Little BB, Abdul Ghafoor AG. Childhood obesity in United Arab Emirates school children: a national study. *Ann Hum Biol* 2005; 32:72-9
[15] Taylor SJ, Viner R, Booy R et al. Ethnicity, socio-economic status, overweight and underweight in East London adolescents. *Ethnic Health* 2005; 10: 113-28
[16] CDC 2005. Prevalance of overweight among children and adolescents ages 6 – 19 years, for selected years 1963-1965 through 1999-2002. http://www.cdc.gov/nchs/products/pubs/pubd/hestats/overwght99.htm#Table%20
[17] Hedley AA, Ogden CL, Johnson CL et al. Prevalence of overweight and obesity among US children, adolescents, and adults 1999 – 2002. *JAMA* 2004; 291: 2847 – 2850
[18] Mo-suwan L, Geater AF. Risk factors for childhood obesity in a transitional society in Thailand. *Int J Obes Relat Metab Disord* 1996; 20: 697 - 703
[19] Genovesi S, Giussani M, Faini A et al. Maternal perception of excess weight in children: a survey conducted by paediatricians in the province of Milan. *Acta Paediatr* 2005; 94: 747 – 752
[20] House of Commons Select Health Committee: Obesity. Third report of session 2003 – 2004. London; House of Commons 2004
[21] Health Survey for England 2002: the health of children and young children. London, Department of Health 2002
[22] Bundred P, Kitchiner D, Buchan I. Prevalance of overweight and obese children between 1989 and 1998: population based series of cross sectional studies. *BMJ* 2001; 322: 326 – 328
[23] Stamatakis E, Primatesta P, Chinn S et al. Overweight and obesity trends from 1974 – 2003 in English children: what is the role of socioeconomic factors? *Arch Dis Child* 2005; 90: 999 – 1004

[24] Drewnowski A, Specter SE. Poverty and obesity: the role of energy density and energy costs. *Am J Clin Nutr* 2004; 79: 6 – 16
[25] Chinn S, Rona RJ. Prevalence trends in overweight aand obesity in three cross-sectional studies of British children. *BMJ* 2001; 322: 24 - 26
[26] Harris RJ. Nutrition in the 21st century: what is going wrong. *Arch Dis Child* 2004; 89: 154 – 158
[27] Palou A, Serra F, Bonnet ML, Pico C. Obesity: molecular bases of a multifactorial problem. *Eur J Nutr* 2000; 39: 127-144
[28] Pelleymounter MA, Culler MJ, Baker MB et al. Effects of the obese gene product on body weight regulation in ob/ob mice. *Science* 1995; 269: 540-543
[29] Farooqi S, O'Rahilly S. Monogenic obesity in humans. *Annu Rev Med* 2005; 56: 443 - 458
[30] Krude H, Biebermann H, Gruters A. Mutations in the human proopiomelanocortin gene. *Ann NY Acad Sci* 2003; 994: 233-239
[31] Farooqi IS, Matarese G, Lord GM et al. Beneficial effects of leptin on obesity, T cell hyporesponsiveness, and neuroendocrine/metabolic dysfunction of human congenital leptin deficiency. *J Clin Invest* 2002; 110: 1093 – 1103
[32] Kojima M, Kangawa K. Ghrelin: structure and function. *Physiol Rev* 2005; 85: 495 – 522
[33] Soriano-Guillen L, Barrios V, Campos-Barros A, Argente J.Ghrelin levels in obesity and anorexia nervosa: effect of weight reduction or recuperation. *J Pediatr* 2004; 144: 36-42
[34] Wren AM, Seal LJ, Cohen MA. Ghrelin enhances appetite and increases food intake in humans. *J Clin Endocrinol Metab* 2001; 86: 5992 – 5995
[35] DelParigi A, Tschop M, Heiman ML et al. High circulating ghrelin: a potential cause for hyperphagia and obesity in Prader-Willi syndrome. *J Clin Endocrinol Metab* 2002; 87: 5461 – 5464
[36] Zhang JV, Ren P-G, Avssian-Kretchmer O et al. Obestatin, a peptide encoded by the Ghrelin gene, opposes Ghrelin's effects on food intake. *Science* 2005; 310: 996 – 999
[37] Nogueiras R, Tschop M. Separation of conjoined hormones yields appetite rivals. *Science* 2005; 310: 985 – 986
[38] Batterham RL, Cowley MA, Small CJ et al. Gut hormone PYY(3-36) physiologically inhibits food intake. *Nature* 2002; 418: 650 – 654
[39] Batterham RL, Cohen MA, Ellis SM et al. Inhibition of food intake in obese subjects by peptide YY 3-36. *N Eng J Med* 2003; 349: 941 – 948
[40] Wynne K, Stanley S, McGowan B et al. Appetite control. *J Endocrinol* 2005; 184: 291 – 318
[41] Cohen MA, Ellis SM, Le Roux CW et al. Oxyntomodulin suppresses appetite and reduces food intake in humans. *J Clin Endocrinol Metab* 2003; 88: 4696 – 4701
[42] Druce M, Bloom SR. The regulation of appetite. *Arch Dis Child* 2006; 91: 183 - 187
[43] Snyder EE, Walts B, Durand E et al. The human obesity gene map: the 2003 update. *Obes Res* 2004; 12: 369- 439
[44] Grace C, Beales P, Summerbell C et al. Energy metabolism in Bardet-Biedl syndrome. *Int J Obes Relat Metab Disord* 2003; 27: 1319 – 1324

[45] Kim JC, Badano JL, Sibold S et al. The Bardet-Biedl protein BBS4 targets cargo to the pericentriolar region and is required for microtube anchoring and cell cycle progression. *Nat Genet* 2004; 36: 462 – 470

[46] Weiss R, Dziura J, Burgert TS et al. Obesity and the metabolic syndrome in children and adolescence. *N Engl J Med* 2004; 350: 2362 – 2374

[47] Lustig RH, Post SR, Srivannaboon K et al. Risk factors for the development of obesity in children surviving brain tumours. *J Clin Endocrinol Metab* 2003; 88: 611 – 616

[48] Hill JO, Prentice AM. Sugar and body weight regulation. *Am J Clin Nutr* 1995; 62: 264S – 273S

[49] Lissner L, Heitmann BL. Dietary fat and obesity: evidence from epidemiology. *Eur J Clin Nutr* 1995; 49: 79 – 90

[50] Anderson RE, Crespo CJ, Bartlett SJ et al. Relationship of physical activity and television watching with body weight and level of fatness among children. *Third National Health and Nutrition survey* 1998

[51] London Evening Standard, 8th November 2005

[52] Anon. *National Diet and Nutrition Survey: children aged 4 to 18, Vol 1. report of the Diet and Nutrition Survey.* London HMSO 2000

[53] Pullinger J. *Social Trends.* London. HMSO 1998

[54] Prentice A, Jebb S. Obesity in Britain: gluttony or sloth. *BMJ* 1995; 311: 437 – 439

[55] Hernandez B, Gortmaker SL, Colditz GA et al. Association of obesity with physical activity, television programs and other forms of video viewing among children in Mexico City. *Int J Obesity* 1999; 23: 845 – 854

[56] Lewis MK, Hill AJ. Food advertising on British children's television: a content analysis and experimental study with nine year olds. *Int J Obesity* 1998; 22: 206 – 214

[57] Robinson TN. Reducing children's television viewing to prevent obesity: a randomised controlled trial. *JAMA* 1999; 282: 1561 – 1567

[58] Hastings G, Stead M, McDermott L et al. Review of Research on the Effects of Food promotion to children. *Food Standards Agency*, November 2003

[59] Dewey KG, Heinig MJ, Nommsen LA et al. Growth of breast-fed and formula-fed infants from 0 to 18 months. *Pediatrics* 1992; 89: 1035 - 1041

[60] Von Kries R, Koletzko B, Sauerveld T et al. Breast feeding and obesity: a cross sectional study. *BMJ* 1999; 319: 147 – 150

[61] Troiano RP, Briefel RR, Carroll MD et al. Energy and fat intakes of children and adolescents in the United States: data from the National Health and Examination Surveys. *Am J Clin Nutr* 2000; 72: 1343S – 1353S

[62] Hu FB, Stampfer MJ, Manson JE et al. Dietary fat intake and the risk of coronary heart disease in women. *N Engl J Med* 1997; 337: 1491 – 1499

[63] Ludwig DS, Majzoub JA, Al-Zahrani A et al. High glycemic index foods, overeating and obesity. *Pediatrics* 1999; 103: e26

[64] Simopoulos AP. The importance of the ratio of omega-6/omega-3 essential fatty acids. *Biomed Pharmacother* 2002; 56: 365 - 379

[65] SIGN (2003) Management of obesity in children and young people. A national clinical guideline 69. Scottish Intercollegiate Guidelines Network.

[66] Barlow SE, Dietz WH. Obesity Evaluation and Treatment: Expert Committee Recommendations. *Pediatrics* 1998; 102: e29

[67] Guo SS, Churnlea WC. Tracking of body mass index in children in relation to overweight in adulthood. *Am J Clin Nutr* 1999; 70: 145S-148S.
[68] Ehtisham S, Barrett TG, Shaw NJ. Type 2 diabetes mellitus in UK children – an emerging problem. *Diabet Med* 2000; 17: 867 – 871
[69] Kiess W, Bottnet A, Raile K et al. Type 2 diabetes in children and adolescents: a review from a European perspective. *Horm Res* 2003; 59, suppl 1: 77 – 84
[70] Zdravkovic V, Daneman D, Hamilton J. Presentation and course of Type 2 diabetes in youth in a large multi-ethnic city. *Diabet Med* 2004; 21: 1144 – 1148
[71] Griffiths LJ, Wolke D, Page AS et al. Obesity and bullying: different effects for boys and girls. *Arch Dis Child* 2006; 91: 121 - 125
[72] Gortmaker SL, Must A, Perrin, JM et al. Social and Economic consequences of overweight in adolescence and young adulthood. *N Engl J Med* 1993; 329:1008-12.
[73] Sargent, JD, Blanchflower DG. Obesity and stature in adolescence and earnings in young adulthood . Analysis of a British birth cohort. *Arch Pediatr Adolesc Med* 1994; 148: 681-7.
[74] Parsons TJ, Power C, Logan S, Summerbell CD. Childhood predicators of adult obesity: a systematic review. *Int J Obes Relat Metab Disord* 1999; 23 (supp 8) S1-S107.
[75] Hediger ML, Overpeck MD, McGlynn A et al. Growth and fatness at three and six years of age of children born small- or large- for gestational age. *Pediatrics* 1999; 104: e33
[76] Summerbell CD, Kelly S, Campbell K. The prevention and treatment of childhood obesity. *Effective Health Care* 2002; volume 7: no.6.
[77] Summerbell CD, Ashton V, Campbell KJ et al. Interventions for treating obesity in children. *Cochrane Database Syst Rev* 2003; 3: CD001872
[78] Mulvihill C, Quigley R. The management of obesity and overweight, an analysis of reviews of diet, physical activity and behavioural approaches. Evidence briefing. 1st edition 2003;. London: Health Development Agency.
[79] Bundy C. Changing behaviour:using motivational interviewing techniques. *J Roy Soc Med* 2004; 97(supp44):43-47
[80] Zimmerman GL, Olsen CG, Bosworth MF. A 'stages of change' approach to helping patients change behaviour. *Am Fam Phys* 2000; 61: 1409-1416.
[81] Golan M, Weizman A, Apter A, Fainaru M. Parents as the exclusive agents of change in the treatment of childhood obesity. *Am J Clin Nutr* 1998; 67:1130-5.
[82] Burniat W, Cole T, Lissau I, Poskitt E. Child and Adolescent Obesity. Causes and consequences, prevention and management. Cambridge University Press, 2002.
[83] Leslie WS, Lean ME, Baillie HM, Hankey CR. Weight management: a comparison of existing dietary approaches in a work-site setting. *Int J Obes Relat Metab Disord* 2002; 26: 1469 - 1475
[84] Golan M, Crow S. Targetting parents exclusively in the treatment of childhood obesity: long term results. *Obes Res* 2004; 12: 357 - 361
[85] Wadden TA, Stunkard A J, Brownell, KD. Very low calorie diets: their efficacy , safety, and future. *Ann Int Med* 1983; 99: 675-84
[86] Caroli M, Chiarappa S, Borrelli R Martinelli R. Efficiency and safety of using protein sparing modified fast in pediatric and adolescent obesity treatment. *Nutr Res* 1992; 12:1325-34.

[87] Berkowitz RJ, Wadden TA, Tershakovec AM, Cronquist JL. Behaviour therapy and sibutramine for the treatment of adolescent obesity: a randomized controlled trial. *JAMA* 2003; 289: 1805 – 1812

[88] Torgerson JS, Hauptman J, Boldrin MN et al. XENical in the prevention of diabetes in obese subjects (XENDOS) study: a randomized study of orlistat as an adjunct to lifestyle changes for the prevention of type 2 diabetes. *Diabetes care* 2004; 27: 155 – 161

[89] McDuffie JR, Calis KA, Uwaifo GI et al. Three-month tolerability of orlistat in adolescents with obesity-related comorbid conditions. *Obes Res* 2002; 10: 642 - 650

[90] Clarke P, Gray A, Adler A et al. Cost-effectiveness analysis of intensive blood-glucose control with metformin in overweight patients with type II diabetes (UKPDS No. 51). *Diabetologia* 2001; 44: 298 – 304

[91] Diabetes Prevention Program research Group. Reduction in the incidence of type 2 with lifestyle intervention or metformin. *N Engl J Med* 2002; 346: 393 – 403

[92] Freemark M, Bursey D. The effects of metformin on body mass index and glucose tolerance in obese adolescents with fasting hyperinsulinemia and a family history of type 2 diabetes. *Pediatrics* 2001; 107: E55

[93] Inge TH, Krebs NF, Garcia VF et al. Bariatric surgery for severely overweight adolescents: concerns and recommendations. *Pediatrics* 2004; 114: 217 - 223

In: Global Dimensions of Childhood Obesity
Editor: Richard K. Flamenbaum, pp. 199-254
ISBN: 1-60021-037-6

Chapter 10

Childhood Obesity: Caregivers' Perceptions, Attitudes and Behaviors Related to Physical Activity and Inactivity

Mozhdeh B. Bruss
Department of Family and Consumer Sciences,
Western Michigan University,USA
Timothy J. Michael
Department of Health Physical Education and Recreation,
Western Michigan University, USA
Joseph R. Morris
Department of Counselor Education and Counseling Psychology,
Western Michigan University, USA
Linda L. Dannison
Department of Family and Consumer Sciences,
Western Michigan University, USA
Jackie A. Quitugua
Public School System, Commonwealth of the Northern Mariana Islands
Rosa T. Palacios
Division of Public Health, Commonwealth of the Northern Mariana Islands

Abstract

The purpose of this study was to investigate primary caregivers' perceptions, attitudes and behaviors related to physical activity and inactivity among 6-10 year old children in order to better understand factors related to childhood obesity. This exploratory study used qualitative methods to identify sociocultural and familial factors related to physical activity and inactivity among different Asian/Pacific Island groups resident in the Commonwealth of the Northern Mariana Islands. Results suggest that among caregivers there are distinct sociocultural beliefs, attitudes, and behaviors related to physical activity and inactivity.

Gender differences were observed with relation to caregivers' perceptions of physical activity. Benefits and disadvantages of physical inactivity were highlighted by the caregivers. An important finding was the view held by caregivers that children need other children to stay physically active. Additionally, different ethnic groups gave different meaning to weight normalcy, physical activity and inactivity. Familial differences were also observed among ethnic groups, with regards to preventive strategies related to childhood obesity and factors that influence their understanding of weight status. With regards to community support for the prevention of childhood obesity, caregivers perceived environmental changes as a necessary condition for increasing physical activity among families. In addition, caregivers identified the need for nutrition education programs that offer awareness and skill-building workshops in bringing about food-related behavior modification among families.

Introduction

There is a growing concern globally for the increase in childhood obesity, a risk factor for adult obesity (Guo, Roche, Chumlea, Gardner, & Siervogel, 1994). Childhood obesity is increasing in many populations around the world (Drewnowski & Popkin, 1997; Troiano, Flegal, Kuczmarski, Campbell & Johnson, 1995; O'Loughlin, Paradis, Meshefedjian & Gray-Donald, 2000). The etiology of the increase has been studied in a number of different populations and both genetic and environmental factors have been established as major contributors with in these populations (Bouchard, 1997; Whitaker, Wright, Pepe, Seidel & Dietz, 1997; Drewnowski et al., 1997; Whitaker, Pepe, Wright, Seidel & Dietz, 1998). In the US, between 1991 – 1994, overweight and obesity among 9-year old children showed an increase from previous studies (Dwyer, Stone, Yang, Webber, Must, Feldman, Nader, Perry & Parcel, 2000). In a recent five-year Canadian study, an annual percentage increase of 0.5 - 1.7 in the prevalence of overweight and obesity was observed as compared to earlier studies that showed a 0.8% annual increase. The Canadian study shows that the rate of increase was most dramatic in the 1990s (O'Loughlin et al., 2000).

At the international level, urbanization has played a major role in the lives of children growing up in the city, who may have fewer opportunities to engage in exercise (Drewnowski & Popkin, 1997). BMI decreases were observed in children with higher baseline aerobic activity and increased leisure activity (Klesges et al., 1995). In a study that examined television viewing and vigorous activity among 8-16 year old children, BMI and index of trunk fat measurements were more closely related to television viewing than vigorous physical activity (Andersen, Crespo, Bartlett, Cheskin & Pratt, 1998).

In children, genetics and environment both influence body weight (Goran, 2001; O'Loughlin, Paradis, Meshefedjian, Gray-Donald, 2000). There is a need for a better understanding of familial and sociocultural perception, attitude and behavior related to physical activity and inactivity among different ethnic groups. Research on the genetic origins of obesity suggests that environment plays a major part in its development. With obesity among children and adults increasing dramatically throughout the world over the past two decades, a period of time too short to suggest that genetic changes might be responsible, environmental causes become a likely cause (International Obesity Task Force, 1997). In some communities there has been a more dramatic increase than others, especially among the ethnic minority groups in the US, such as Hispanics (Goran, 2001). The changing US demographics requires building a body of literature that provides an insight into the different ethnic groups and to help establish differences and similarities in the sociocultural values, beliefs and practices related to childhood obesity in each of these cultures. This knowledge is needed to build specialized programs that can effectively address individual needs rather than generic prescriptions that may be ineffective for populations most at risk of childhood obesity. There is limited empirical information about parental behaviors and sociocultural factors that are associated with the development of childhood obesity among various ethnic populations.

The purpose of this study was to explore primary caregivers' perceptions, attitudes and behaviors related to physical activity and inactivity among 6-10 year old children. In order to explore these physical activity and inactivity behaviors associated with obesity, a stable multi-ethnic population with distinct ethnic groups and high rates of obesity would be ideal. The Commonwealth of the Northern Mariana Islands (CNMI) was selected because it has many of these elements making it suitable for investigating factors related to childhood obesity. Caregivers, primary contributors to environmental factors, play a major role in the care and supervision of school-aged children. CNMI is a multiethnic society with two distinct indigenous populations namely Chamorros and Carolinians with high rates of adult obesity (CNMI Food and Nutrition Policy and Ten Year Plan of Action, 1996). Childhood obesity has been linked to physical activity and inactivity (Klesges et al., 1995; Janz, Levy, Burns, Torner, Willing & Warren, 2002). This exploratory study identified sociocultural and familial factors related to physical activity and inactivity among these groups and the largest immigrant population resident in the CNMI, namely Filipinos.

This study looked at behavior, value, and belief systems with regards to physical activity and inactivity. It examined physical activity and inactivity among 6-10 year old children from an ethnographic perspective. It investigated childcare giving practices within the social context of families influenced by the social milieu of cultures. There are culturally based characteristics including care giving perceptions, attitudes and practices that may influence weight status of children. This study sought to identify these characteristics specifically in regards to physical activity and inactivity among three identified ethnic groups. A review of the literature suggested that there is insufficient empirical data in regards to sociocultural and familial factors related to physical activity and inactivity in the prevention of childhood obesity.

The CNMI was a suitable place for such a study. It offered a multiethnic population with minimal migration, high rates of childhood obesity, a strong US food supply system and economic resources. This study investigated cultural influences on the physical activity and inactivity as it relates to childhood obesity. Because of the CNMI's status as a US commonwealth, the public health nutrition intervention strategies are often modeled on US community health education programs. These programs have faced numerous challenges in influencing behavioral change in this sociocultural setting. The strong connectedness of the individual to cultural ways, beliefs and values may be a stronger influence on diet than the knowledge of nutrition information disseminated through the formal health sector (Bruss, Morris & Dannison, 2003).

According to the CNMI Food and Nutrition Policy (1996) thirty-three percent of the school-aged children are considered overweight based upon body mass index (BMI). Understanding the sociocultural characteristics of these children in relation to the maintenance of normal BMI is necessary for designing effective intervention programs. Primary care givers are most intimate with their children's physical activity and inactivity habits, therefore this study used focus groups with primary care givers in the CNMI to identify characteristics that are related to childhood obesity.

Qualitative research methodology (Krathwohl, 1998) was used to explore complex, wide-ranging questions in order to create a framework for how care giving beliefs, attitudes, and practices are related to physical activity and inactivity in a multi-ethnic community. In addition, the study investigated and defined specific characteristics that are related to weight status among 6-10 year old children. This method did not test specific hypotheses. Methods used in this study can aid other researchers in investigating sociocultural and familial factors in other ethnic groups especially those affected by high rates of childhood obesity.

Background Information

Sociocultural Factors

Social scientists have long been involved in the study of culture. Scott Coltrane (1998), a sociologist has written, "Depending on personal histories, individual characteristics, social experiences, environmental contexts and many other factors, people tend to 'see' the world differently" (P. 1). According to Bubolz and Sontag (1993), "When studying a family ecosystem, one must make explicit the values and goals that each individual holds, those that are shared by the family as a unit, as well as those operative in the social-cultural environment" (p. 436). Lee Cronk (1999), anthropologist, separates culture from behavior, but describes the interaction of the two elements by offering this analogy, "Culture is neither the act of baking a cake nor the cake itself, but the recipe, the socially transmitted information that tells a person how to bake a cake" (P. 12). Therefore depending on the environment and resources, the information may be modified to ensure cultural preservation. Dohrenwend & Smith (1962) postulated two levels of cultural change; preservation or loss of traditional cultural ways and adoption of new cultural behavior. This may be influenced by knowledge of one's group membership and emotional significance associated with it (Tajfel, 1981).

Familial Factors

A person's ability to associate and dissociate develops in the first decade of life and increases with age (Aboud and Christina, 1970). This ability instills a sense of family membership which supports the transmission of knowledge, attitudes and behaviors. For instance, families may develop consensus around food, eating and exercise. Additionally, parenting styles may influence dietary habits. In one study, parents endorsing authoritarian style of parenting, one that uses control, prohibitive and anxiety inducing strategies reported more frequent availability of sweets in the home (Gabel and Lutz, 2000).

Interaction between Sociocultural and Familial Factors

In order to live in a cultural context, individuals often retain certain aspects of their culture while gaining skills and/or traits that allows them to function in the parameters of the dominant culture. This is described as ethnic identity coupled with acculturation. Hraba (1979) describe ethnic identity as a multidimensional and subjective construct. It is a psychological experience that may be articulated or demonstrated in any display of identity. Individuals develop ethnic identity based on ethnic origin and evolving personal cultural components. This process usually begins in childhood with parents socializing their children and instilling a sense of group membership. Anchored in this group identity, children learn cultural values and behaviors facilitating their self-definition (Rosenthal & Cichello, 1992) and reinforcing group membership.

The development of ethnic identity, which is not merely transfer of ethnicity from parents to children (Phinney, 1990) requires the presence of two or more competing ethnic groups. In addition, because a person's ability to associate and dissociate develops during the first decade of life and increases with age (Aboud & Christina, 1970) development of ethnic identity may be seen as a process that begins in childhood, but continues until self-definition has been achieved. Maslow's hierarchal theory of Belonging (1954) may be used to explain the development of ethnic identity within the context of the family and community. Frideres and Goldenberg (1982) suggest that ethnic identity helps members of a group recognize acceptable behavior, while being aware of the outsiders' behavior as either correct or incorrect. Schonpflug (2001) in a study of 200 Turkish adolescent males living in Germany and Turkey found that cultural transmission defined as social learning requires transmission belts (conditions that are favorable for transmission of values). Relational indicators such as; parenting styles and marital quality, and socio-developmental conditions, such as; father's education, adolescent developmental phase and sibling position were found to interact with transmission of values.

Sociocultural and Familial Factors: Examine Weight Normalcy, Diet, and Physical Activity/Inactivity

Ethnic minority groups comprise more than 20% of the US population. As a group they are experiencing increasing rates of overweight and obesity. The prevalence of obesity in the different ethnic groups can range from 2 - 52%, which may suggest that obesity is more acceptable in some populations than others. This attitude coupled with certain feeding practices may increase the risk of childhood obesity (Kumanyika, 1993). Moreover, family similarities in fatness suggest attitude toward food, eating, and physical activity habits may be learned and reinforced within the home (Garn & Clark, 1976). Also, mothers' personal experience with obesity may influence parenting interactions in regards to weight, diet and physical activity (Anjali et al., 2001).

Using sociocultural and familial factors to examine weight normalcy, diet and physical activity/inactivity will provide a better understanding of the increasing rates of childhood obesity among different ethnic groups in the US (Bruss, Morris & Dannison, 2003). The three environmental mediators of weight normalcy, diet, and physical activity/inactivity are described in the context of sociocultural and familial factors.

Weight Normalcy

Sociocultural Factors Related to Weight Normalcy

Perception of "weight normalcy" may be influenced by cultural beliefs and practices. There are conflicting images of female attractiveness influenced by traditional culture and mass media. Weight normalcy varies by socioeconomic status and dietary habits (Powdermaker, 1997). Among Mexican and White Americans in Texas, a positive association between overweight and age, marital status, and social positioning of women was observed (Ross & Mirowsky, 1983). In this study of Mexican and White American population resident in Texas,

Ross & Mirowsky found that there is a positive association between overweight, older age, marital status and social class positioning for women. Gender differences related to overweight were observed among the two groups. White American women weighed less than White American males, while Mexican women weighed more than the Mexican men (Ross & Mirowsky, 1983).

In Guam, a multiethnic Pacific Island community, overweight and obesity are an acceptable social norm. Pinhey et al. (1997) looked at the interaction between ethnicity, BMI and happiness among Filipinos, Asians, Chamorros and Micronesians residents of Guam. BMI levels for Chamorros of Guam and the Micronesian migrants to the island is 26.6, where as it is 23.5 for Filipinos and 23.6 for Asians. When variables such as ethnicity, age, gender, education, and income were included in the analysis, overweight Asian and Filipino respondents expressed a significantly lower level of happiness than their Chamorro and Micronesian counterparts. Among the Chamorros and Micronesians overweight and obesity is less stigmatized and a more acceptable social norm (Pinhey et al., 1997).

Familial Factors Related to Weight Normalcy

In a longitudinal study boys with both overweight parents were more at risk for increased BMI, while girls whose fathers were overweight demonstrated a BMI gain of 0.4 kg/m^2 (Klesges et al., 1995). In another study, heavier mothers tended to have heavier daughters; and a positive correlation was found between the daughter's overweight status and maternal disinhibition (Cutting et al., 1999). In this study, maternal disinhibition defined as the level to which eating was prompted by emotional and environmental influences was studied in relation to overweight and eating behaviors in seventy-five preschool children. Parents' BMI, dietary restraint and eating disinhibition along with children's weight-for-height were measured. Cutting et al., (1999) found that overweight parents were more likely to report the influence of palatable foods or emotional factors on eating.

Familial influences associated with overweight in children were also observed in relation to parent and child's gender. The degree of overweight for mothers and children were associated with mother's dietary disinhibition. The results showed that heavier mothers had heavier daughters and that there was a positive relationship between maternal disinhibition and daughter's overweight status. Higher maternal disinhibition was associated with higher free access to food by daughters. This study confirms previous studies that mothers influence their daughter's eating habits and weight status. Researchers also indicated that further investigation is needed in looking at the influence of parenting styles along with parental beliefs, attitudes and eating behaviors on childhood obesity (Cutting et al., 1999).

Also, larger studies have found a relationship between parental weight and child weight, showing that two lean parents tend to have lean children, while two obese parents tend to have obese children. One obese and one lean parent also affect the child's weight (Garn & Clark, 1976). For both obese and non-obese children younger than ten years of age, parental obesity defined as BMI ≥ 27 was found to double the risk of adult obesity. By age seventeen, children of obese parents are three times as fat as the children of lean parents (Whitaker et al., 1997).

In a qualitative study of eighteen participants in the Women, Infant and Children (WIC) Program, mothers were found to use their own perception to determine their child's weight condition (Anjali et al., 2001). Researchers found that mothers' definition of overweight and obesity was not based on height and weight measurements or growth chart classification. In general mothers disregarded the weight status information offered by health professionals in the WIC clinic and used their own perception to determine their child's weight condition. Indicators such as limitation in physical activity and/or being teased by others were signs associated with being overweight. The mothers did not consider children who were active and those with a healthy diet and/or good appetite as overweight. Furthermore, mothers saw genetic factors as an influence on weight status regardless of environmental conditions. The results of this qualitative research indicate that mothers' experiences strongly influence their belief, attitude and practices with regards to their children's diet and weight status. Related to weight normalcy, participants reported the following views and attitudes (a) dislike and distrust for growth charts, irrelevance of growth charts in assessing children, (b) genetic predisposition to a certain body size, (c) cultural acceptance of large frames, (d) overweight status a contributing factor to inactivity in children, and (e) definition of obesity. Most mothers felt that their children's overweight status was out of their control with the exception of some that recognized parental diet and activity habits as factors that may influence a child's behavior. Also, most mothers in this study were considered obese by BMI definition. They shared views regarding strengthening children's self esteem as a way to buffer the effects of being teased about their weight. This suggests personal experience with obesity may influence parenting interactions related to weight, diet and physical activity (Anjali et al., 2001).

Low maternal education has also been associated with failure to perceive preschool aged children as overweight. In a study of 622 children 2-5 years, 79% of the mothers did not perceive their overweight children as overweight. Even when controlling for maternal BMI, low maternal education was associated with a failure to perceive their children as overweight. Mothers believed that a heavy infant was an indicator of a healthy infant and successful parenting (Baughcum et al., 2000).

Sociocultural and Familial Factors Related to Weight Normalcy

In a prospective cohort study of 447 African Americans, anthropometric measurements and socioeconomic data was collected at birth. The following variables studied at birth showed independent association with adiposity or body fatness in young adulthood; pre-pregnancy BMI, female sex of the baby, and first born status. When these three variables were controlled, no relationship was seen for birth weight for gestational age and socioeconomic status to adiposity in young adulthood. First-born status among African Americans was identified as a risk factor for increased adiposity in adulthood. An association between maternal BMI and female gender in increased adiposity in adulthood was also observed (Stettler, Tershakovec, Zemel, Leonard, Boston & Katz, 2000).

According to Bruss & et al. (2003) cultural differences among Asian/Pacific Island caregivers were observed in their attitude toward children's overweight and underweight status. These differences may positively or negatively influence the caregiver's behavior toward their child's weight status. These differences were reported to create conflict within families. In a study of predominantly Hispanic parents, researchers found that more than one-third of those interviewed did not believe that their obese child was overweight. This belief coupled with certain feeding practices may put children at increased risk for obesity (Myers & Vargas, 2000).

Physical Activity and Inactivity

Childhood obesity has been linked to physical activity and inactivity (Klesges et al., 1995; Janz, Levy, Burns, Torner, Willing & Warren, 2002). Furthermore, the environmental changes in society are increasing the likelihood of physical inactivity in populations around the world (Stephens, 2002). For instance, on average American children watch 25-27 hours of television per week, while spending only 14 minutes per day in physical activity (Stephens, 2002). In addition, Utter, Neumark-Sztainer, Jeffery & Story (2003) found high television/video use with increased intake of soft drinks, fried foods, and snacks. They also observed gender differences in physical inactivity in children. For instance, television/video use and time spent reading/doing homework was positively associated with BMI for boys, while television/video and computer use was positively associated with BMI for girls. Similarly, Crespo, Smit, Troiano, Bartlett, Macera, & Andersen (2001) found that females who watch television are most at risk for obesity. Crespo, et al. (2001) examined NHANES III data from 1988 – 1994 for 4,069 children between the ages of 8-16 years. Findings of this study showed that children who watch one or less hours of television had the lowest prevalence of obesity, while those with four or more hours of television viewing had the highest prevalence of obesity. Non-Hispanic White males had the highest reported number of physical activity sessions per week. Compared to males, females consumed fewer calories and were less physically active.

In a review of 54 studies, Sallis, Prochaska, & Taylor (2000) identified five categories of variables as correlates of physical activity among 3-12 year old children. These include eleven demographic and biological variables, fifteen psychological, cognitive, and emotional variables, eighteen behavioral variables, twenty-one social/cultural variables, and eleven physical environment variables. For each category, researchers found individual variables that are potential correlates with physical activity. For instance, within the context of the demographic and biological variable category, boys were more active than girls and there were no ethnic differences in activity level between non-Hispanic Whites and other groups. In the psychological variable category, perceived barriers were negatively related to physical activity, while preference for physical activity and intention to be active had positive association. In the behavioral variable category, healthy diet and previous physical activity were positively associated with physical activity. Results of the social/cultural variable category analysis suggested that slightly over a third of the studies showed positive association between parental physical activity and children's physical activity. Finally, in the physical environment variable category, there was a positive relationship between children's physical activity and access to facilities/programs and time spent outdoors. Sallis et al. (2000) found that in general physical activity studies are limited in their analysis based on differences in ethnicity, socioeconomic status, and urban/rural dwelling.

Sociocultural Factors Related to Physical Activity and Inactivity

In a study of television viewing among 8-16 year old children, 26% of all children reported four or more hours of TV/day. Ethnic and gender differences were observed in television use. Girls (23%) watched less TV than boys (29%), while 43% of Black girls and boys reported watching four or more hours of TV/day. In this study BMI and index of trunk fat measurements were highest for those who reported 6-8 sessions of vigorous activity/week and lowest for those who reported three or less sessions of vigorous activity/week. Boys and girls with highest BMI watched four or more hours of TV, while those with the lowest BMI watched less than 1 hour of TV. In this study BMI and index of trunk fat measurements were more closely related to TV watching than vigorous activity (Andersen, Crespo, Bartlett, Cheskin & Pratt, 1998).

Familial Factors Related to Physical Activity and Inactivity

In a study of 219 families, decrease in BMI was observed in 3-5 year old children with higher baseline aerobic activity and increased leisure activity (Klesges et al., 1995). In addition, Trost, Sirard, Dowda, Pfeiffer & Pate (2003) found no relationship between parents' overweight status and parental influence on 3-5 year old children's physical activity behavior. In another study of 65 parent-child pairs using parent-completed surveys and children's BMI, parental control of child eating showed a positive association with amount of TV viewing and negative association with children's involvement in extracurricular activities. Researchers also found that children who eat more junk foods and sugars tend to watch more television (Gabel & Lutz, 2000).

In a national representative sample of 7-11 year old Canadian children (n=7,216), organized and unorganized sports and physical activity were negatively associated with children's BMI (parental reporting). However, television viewing and video games were positively correlated to overweight and obesity. In fact, physical activity reduced the risks of overweight by 10-24%, while physical inactivity increased the risks of overweight by 17-44%. Additionally, physical activity reduced the risk of obesity by 23-43% and physical inactivity increased the risk of obesity by 10-61%. Physical activity and inactivity partially contributed to the relationship between high socioeconomic status and two-parent household and risk of childhood overweight and obesity (Tremblay & Williams, 2003).

In a population of 9-12 year old American military dependents, Arluk, Branch, Swain & Dowling (2003) found a significant relationship between childhood obesity, maternal BMI, and physical inactivity. Measures of physical inactivity included computer use, television viewing and total hours spent in sedentary activities. In addition, fathers' participation in children's physical activity and the presence of parents at home when the child arrives from school were also related to children's weight status.

Sociocultural and Familial Factors Related to Physical Activity and Inactivity

Lindquist, Reynolds, & Goran (1999) examined ethnic differences in childhood physical activity with an attempt to study sociocultural predictors of children's physical activity and fitness levels. Television viewing used as an indicator of inactivity was measured as hours per day reported by the subjects' parents. Results showed that the only significant predictor of television viewing was single parent home status. Hours per week of exercise were strongly influenced by gender. Days per week of exercise were relatively uninfluenced by sociocultural characteristics. Only single-parent home status emerged as a significant correlate. Single-parent home and African American children reported less time in physical education (PE) program exercises. Older children were more likely to participate, but children with a higher stage of pubertal development were less likely to participate on a sports team. Single-family children, males and Caucasians had higher levels of physical fitness. This study shows the multidimensional nature of childhood physical activity and the influence of sociocultural factors on children's activity patterns (Lindquist et al., 1999).

Researchers have also shown that physical activity levels among children declines with increasing age (Kimm, Glynn, Kriska, Barton, Kronsberg, Daniels, Crawford, Sabry & Liu, 2002) mainly due to changes in children's preference for physical activity and frequency of parents transporting children to activity locations (Sallis, Alcaraz, McKenzie & Hovell, 1999). These changes call for reinforcers (incentives) that encourage children to engage in physical activity, especially vigorous or high-intensity activities (Sallis et al., 1999). Also, these findings suggest the need for identifying intrinsic and extrinsic motivation to increase physical activity among children in different ethnic populations. Examining sociocultural and familial factors related to physical activity that focus on intrinsic and extrinsic motivation becomes increasingly important in childhood obesity prevention.

Csikszentmihalyi's flow theory suggests that physical activity environments can be created to support flow state experience, which is a state that can motivate children to decrease their physical inactivity and increase physical activity (Mandigo & Thompson, 1998). Mandigo and Thompson (1998) suggest six strategies that promote flow state for increasing physical activity. These include 1) recognizing developmentally appropriate activity for children, 2) creating fun-filled activity, defined as balance between individual skill and challenge of activity, 3) giving children a sense of control, by permitting them to change the activity, 4) setting clear goals and objectives that can be evaluated through feedback from the children, 5) avoiding giving negative feedback to the children or putting pressure to achieve tasks, and finally, 6) promoting intrinsic versus extrinsic motivation. Limited information was found in the literature with regards to ethnic and/or familial differences in intrinsic and extrinsic motivation of children and the other above-mentioned strategies for promoting physical activity among children.

Rationale for Study

Recommendations for Physical Activity/Inactivity

A number of different national and international organizations recognize and promote physical activity in children through specific recommendations. The focus of these recommendations is mainly to help the development of life-long health promotion and disease prevention behavior. With regards to childhood obesity prevention, the reduction of physical inactivity along with diet and increased vigorous physical activity is often recommended. A review of the recommendations by four national and international organizations suggests that they are varied with regards to their focus on younger children and their caregivers in promoting physical activity and limiting physical inactivity. This is especially important in light of studies which show that physical activity patterns in older children is strongly associated with previous physical activity experiences and episodes (Sallis, 2000). Additionally, the Youth Risk Behavior Surveillance System (YRBSS), a major U.S. monitoring system mainly, collects and reports physical activity/inactivity data for 9th -12th grade students. A recent paper from the Journal of Pediatrics (Strong, W.B., Malina, R. M., Blimkie, C.J.R., Daniels, S.R., et al. 2005) discusses recommendations for physical activity for school age youth based upon a systematic literature review. The stated purpose was to develop recommendations for the appropriate amount of physical activity needed to ensure adequate health and behavior outcomes. Many organizations have their own recommendations that are slightly different from one another (National Association for Sport and Physical Education (NASPE), The World Health Organization (WHO), Pan American Health Organization (PAHO), and Center for Disease Control (CDC). However, this paper written by a panel of experts in the areas of physical activity, children and obesity explored not only the research evidence, but organizational and governmental recommendations such as the previous ones and came to a consensus as to what the recommendation should be based on the best evidence. The recommendations state that children and youths should accumulate 60 minutes of moderate to vigorous physical activity daily. The panelists' further state that what physical activities are participated in should be based upon the age and motor ability of the child. In addition, for those children and youth that are not habitually physically active the "10% rule" should be followed in terms of increasing the amount of physical activity each week.

Body Fatness and Physical Activity/Inactivity

In December 2000, the President's Council on Physical Fitness and Sports published a report entitled Physical activity protects against the health risks of obesity. The report identified the role of physical activity and inactivity in obesity and suggested examining obesity as a multi-factorial problem (Welk, 2000). Janz, Levy, Burns, Torner, Willing & Warren (2002) conducted a study of 4-6 year old children. Results suggest that physically active children on average had 1 kg less fat mass as compared to inactive children. In this study children had 4% less body fat when they had thirty-five minutes or more of vigorous physical activity as compared to those who had seventeen minutes or less. Children whose parents reported one or less hours of television had 3% less body fat than those with more than three hours of TV viewing. Researchers in this study investigated the relationship between physical activity/inactivity and body fatness in children. Specifically, they looked at the relationship between type of physical activity and excess adiposity and estimate of effect size among 4-6 year old children. Parental reports of television viewing, accelerometry-measured physical activity, body mass index, and body composition measures derived from Dual-Energy X-Ray Absorptiometry (DEXA)were collected on 467 healthy 4-6 year old children DEXA provided fat mass, total body mass, percentage of body fat (fat mass/total body mass), fat-free mass (sum of bone mineral and lean mass), and trunk fat mass (predominantly abdominal fat). Physical activity was measured using accelerometry, which accumulates movement values over a period of time, such as movement counts per minutes. Children wore the accelerometer for four consecutive days including 1 weekend day. From the raw data the researchers constructed three variables, 1) volume or total daily physical activity (total movement counts/total minutes or time of measurement), 2) daily minutes spent in moderate through vigorous physical activity (counting number of minutes in which accelerometry movement count readings were $\geq$615 and $\leq$2,972 counts equivalent to 3-6 metabolic equivalents or MET), and 3) daily minutes spent in vigorous physical activity (counting number of minutes in which accelerometry movement count readings were $\geq$2,972).

The criterion variable was body composition measures and predictor variables were age, height, vigorous activity and TV viewing. After adjusting for age and height, there was a linear trend for vigorous physical activity and percent body fat, fat mass, and trunk fat mass. There was an inverse relationship between physical activity and fatness and positive relationship between fatness and TV viewing. The study concluded that there is observed positive relationship between vigorous physical activity and percent body fat, fat mass, and trunk fat mass. For girls, television viewing was inversely related to body fat, fat mass, and trunk fat mass, while for boys TV viewing was inversely related to percent body fat. Gender differences were observed with regards to physical activity. In general, boys were found to have greater levels of total physical activity, more moderate/vigorous physical activity and more vigorous physical activity. No gender differences were found with regards to television viewing.

Prevention of Childhood Obesity

The benefits of physical activity in children are well documented, especially the long-term protective effect that it has on body fat in childhood (Moore, Gao, Bradlee, Cupples, Sundarajan-Ramamurti, Proctor, Hood, Singer & Ellison, 2003). Moore et al. (2003) in a prospective study of children that they followed from preschool to early adolescence found that by age 11, the most active children had the lowest BMI and less subcutaneous fat. Additionally, adiposity rebound (AR) was delayed in the more active children, reducing their risk of obesity. Considering the benefits of physical activity, there are limited physical activity interventions that have examined mediators of physical activity behavior in children (Lewis, Marcus, Pate & Dunn, 2002). However, there are increasing numbers of intervention studies that have looked at the impact of reducing physical inactivity on school aged children's BMI. One-hundred and ninety-two children in grades three and four in two socio-demographically and scholastically matched public elementary schools in California, participated in a study that targeted reduction of physical inactivity. The study was setup to assess the effects in the reduction of TV viewing, videotape, and video game use on changes in adiposity, physical activity, and dietary intake. Children in the experimental elementary school received an eighteen-lesson, six-month classroom curriculum to reduce TV, videotape and video game use. Changes in measures of height and weight, dietary behaviors and parental report were measured. Compared with controls, children in the intervention group had significant decreases in BMI. This study demonstrated that reducing sedentary activities, maybe a promising, population-based approach to preventing childhood obesity (Robinson, 1999). In another school-based intervention study that involved classroom diet and physical activity lessons gains in knowledge were significant among the treatment group (Gortmaker, Cheung, Peterson, Chomitz, Cradle, Dart, Fox, Bullock, Sobol, Colditz, Field & Laird, 1999). In this study, although researchers reported dietary behavioral changes with regards to intake of fruits and vegetables and decrease in percentage of total energy from fat, no change was measured in vigorous physical activity between the control and treatment groups.

These intervention studies suggest that although children may be influenced cognitively to adopt dietary changes and reduce physical inactivity, they are less likely to increase vigorous physical activity. Findings from the study by Sallis, Prochaska, & Taylor (2000) suggest that in children the intention to be physically active may be positively correlated with physical activity, even though in adults, knowledge of physical activity or health or the intention to be active does not translate to physical activity behavior (Sallis & Owen, 1999). Results of studies by Sallis et al. (2000) and Gortmaker et al. (1999) suggest that adopting vigorous physical activity behaviors in children may need other factors beyond cognitive influences. These important findings suggest the need to further explore sociocultural and familial transmission of messages related to physical activity and inactivity among different ethnic populations such as the Asian/Pacific Islanders who are affected by increasing rates of childhood obesity.

The literature establishes that childhood obesity is multi-factorial with sociocultural and familial factor mediators such as weight normalcy, diet, and physical activity/inactivity. Because, weight normalcy and diet of Asian/Pacific children have been examined and reported in previous studies, this study mainly examined physical activity/inactivity among this population. This study explored sociocultural and familial factors related to physical activity/inactivity of 6-10 year old children so as to better understand childhood obesity from the perspective of Asian/Pacific Island care givers. Findings from this study will be used to develop intervention programs intended to target childhood obesity prevention.

Methods

Demographics

The Commonwealth of Northern Mariana Islands (CNMI) is an archipelago consisting of 14 islands in the Western Pacific Ocean with a total land area of 176.5 square miles. The three main populated and developed islands of the CNMI are Saipan, Tinian, and Rota. It has a multiethnic population of 69,221 (CNMI 2000 Census) consisting of distinct ethnic groups of Pacific Islanders and Asians. Chamorros and Carolinians are indigenous to the CNMI, while Filipinos, Chinese, and other Micronesians (Palauans and Chuukese) are recent immigrants (Table 1).

Table 1. Population of the CNMI by Ethnicity

Ethnicity by Ethnic Category	Number	Percent of Total
Pacific Islander		
Chamorro	14,749	21.3
Carolinian	2,652	3.9
Chuukese	1,394	2.0
Palauan	1,685	2.4
Pohnpeian	640	0.9
Yapese	205	0.3
Marshallese	112	0.2
Kosraean	56	0.1
Other Pacific Islanders	509	0.7
Asian		
Filipino	18,141	26.2
Chinese	15,311	22.1
Korean	2,021	2.9
Japanese	952	1.4
Bangladeshi	873	1.3
Nepalese	300	0.4
Other Asian	1,012	1.5

Table 1. Continued

Ethnicity by Ethnic Category	Number	Percent of Total
Other		
White	1,240	1.8
Black	41	0.1
Other Race	474	0.7
Mixed Ethnicities†		
Chamorro and Other	4,383	6.3
Asian and Other	3,016	4.4
Carolinian and Other	2,124	3.1

Source: CNMI 2000 Census

† People claiming 2 or more ethnic backgrounds

School System

The CNMI public school system enrolls 76% of all K-12 grade students in the CNMI. There are thirteen elementary and junior high public schools in the three CNMI islands of Saipan, Rota and Tinian. According to the CNMI Statistical Yearbook (1999), a total of 6,596 K – 8th grade students were enrolled in 13 public schools. Majority of the private schools are independently-run parochial systems with affiliation to different Christian denominations, such as Catholics, Baptists, Seventh-Day Adventists, Protestants, and others.

Approach to Data Collection

Qualitative methods were used to collect and analyze data, which included four in-depth focus groups and writing samples from each of the study participants. Validation of data was performed utilizing triangulation methodology. Triangulation methodology provides the researcher with the opportunity to verify data from multiple perspectives. Based on the review of the literature and professional experience in the CNMI, this qualitative study utilized a set of nine research objectives. These were developed and used to create culturally and theoretically relevant questions. The objectives were explored in the focus group interview protocol and the writing samples. These are (a) a culturally relevant definition of primary care giver, (b) definition of weight normalcy, (c) knowledge of "weight control measures", (d) definition of weight control measures in regards to physical activity and inactivity, (e) attitude towards "weight control measures", (f) level of involvement in weight control measures, (g) perception of child's experience in relation to weight control measures, (h) views on childhood obesity preventive interventions, and (i) understanding (perception, knowledge, attitude and behavior) of weight in children.

Data Collections Methods

Study Participants

Selection of Schools and Ethnic Groups

Local CNMI collaborators from the Saipan Public School System assisted in the selection of four schools for participation in this study, three of which were public and one parochial. Although, all ethnic groups were included, majority of the study participants came from three ethnic groups, Chamorro, Carolinian, and Filipino. Chamorros and Carolinians are the two indigenous groups of the CNMI. Filipinos are the largest resident Asian group (Table 1) in the CNMI and have considerable interaction within the community.

Selection of Study Participants

The local CNMI collaborators, through the school principals at the selected schools, invited the children's adult care givers to learn more about the research project. A general call was made to the parents and other adult care givers. Thirty-two participants from three public elementary and one private elementary school responded to the invitation to participate in the study project. All thirty-two participants decided to participate in the study. Each participant reviewed and signed the consent form at the beginning of their focus group sessions.

Study Group Composition

A total of four groups were formed for the study. Participants were all primary care givers consisting of mothers, grandparents, and fathers. Ethnicity was recorded based on individual self-report. Each participant had at least one school-aged child or grandchild (6-10 years of age) in the household. The groups had the following makeup: Group 1 - majority Filipino caregivers, Group 2 - majority Carolinian caregivers, Group 3 - majority Chamorro female caregivers, and Group 4 - majority Chamorro male caregivers.

Focus Groups

As noted earlier at the beginning of each focus group session, each participant reviewed and signed the consent form. Those who chose to sign the consent form to participate in the focus group were assured of confidentiality. Participants in the focus groups were advised to keep confidential all information about other participants in the study. A number was assigned to each participant as an identifier to further protect confidentiality.

The focus group interview protocol was developed based on the review of the literature, first author's experience working in the CNMI and discussion with the last two authors who served as local collaborators. Three researchers with previous experience conducting focus groups used a semi-structured interview protocol to collect the data. Interviews were in English, the common-spoken language in Saipan. The protocol included a set of eighteen culturally relevant questions that were formulated based on the above-mentioned research objectives. Care was taken in developing research questions that took into consideration cultural intricacies of the community and would not be a potential risk to the focus group participants. Participants were invited to answer questions as it related to their personal experience, their children's experience, and behaviors that influence weight status among school-aged children. Sessions were limited to ninety minutes.

Writing Sample

The writing sample protocol was developed based on the review of the literature. The protocol asked participants to interpret and write their meaning for a set of words based on the following specific objective: Primary care giver's definition of weight control measures with regards to physical activity and inactivity. Participants were presented with a list of words and asked to write meanings for these words that are related to the different weight control measures. These included but were not limited to (a) physical activity, (b) television viewing, (c) computer games, (d) physical inactivity, and (e) school physical education program. The consent form signed by the participants covered the use of data from both the focus groups and the writing samples.

Data Analysis

Qualitative methodology was used to analyze the data from both the focus groups and the writing samples, using methods described by Bogden and Biklen (1998). Focus group interviews were audio taped and transcribed by a local Saipan agency that was not associated with the study, but had familiarity with the local accents. The content of the transcripts were verified for accuracy against the audiotapes by the researchers. The focus group transcripts and the writing samples were read and a system of coding was developed. Initially a coding system was developed that involved coding categories for all responses; making a list and assigning each one a number; marking each comment with the appropriate number(s); and adding new codes as needed. The next step involved identifying the major concepts as a result of the coding system. From the major concepts important themes were developed using frequently mentioned ideas. Subsequently comparison of responses was made across the four groups. Similar responses for the groups were combined and the main points of view within each theme were highlighted with the use of direct quotation. Results are reported by focusing on the distinctive areas of discussion from the groups, i.e. beliefs and attitudes related to physical activity and inactivity, behaviors related to physical activity and inactivity influencing weight status among school-aged children, and community support of families in the prevention of childhood obesity.

Methods for Triangulation

As indicated earlier, triangulation or verification is a process used by qualitative researchers to ensure authenticity through multiple methods of data collection and extensive interaction time with the subjects (Creswell, 1998). This study employed two methods. The first method involved conducting focus groups using questions that are were culturally relevant. The second method was to obtain writing samples from each of the study participants using words identified in the literature related to weight control measures. This method was used to obtain caregivers' views related to physical activity and inactivity using a different methodology.

For this purpose, two types of data were used to support or contradict the interpretation of findings (Creswell, 1998).

Interpretation of Data

Qualitative research methods were used to develop a system of categories. The goal was to ensure that the analysis and categories are as close to the material as possible. This process of inductive category development which is reductive in nature and has been used in psychology was used for the analysis of the data. As a result of the literature review a set of criterion or objectives were developed which guided the formulation of the study questions used in the focus groups and the writing samples. Additionally, the framework that uses a sociocultural and familial factor lens to examine physical activity and inactivity was used to analyze the data. The content of the transcripts of the focus groups along with the writing samples provided by the participants were analyzed looking for possible categories. When the research question suggested quantitative analysis of the data such as frequency of coded categories, then the data were analyzed and reported in that manner.

Additionally, when categories were defined, typical passages were found from the transcripts and the writing samples to provide rich meaning for the categories. According to Patton (1990), inductive analysis allows for categories to emerge followed by generating a hypothesis, which can then be tested and examined for other possible explanations or additional hypothesis. The data were differentiated based on categories that related to the literature and those that emerged from the original data. This inductive and deductive process was repeated with each step of the analysis. Inductive analysis which is usually post-hoc and is based on the data was used to explore new ideas not previously considered, but were identified by the study participants, while deductive analysis which was based on the literature was used to examine the data looking for confirmation.

Because this study asks the parents to report physical activity and inactivity, it was important to determine reliability of this information. With regards to physical inactivity, research has shown that parental reporting of children's television viewing has high reliability when correlated with automated time-lapse video observations (Andersen, Field, Collins, Lorch & Nathan, 1985). Although, parental reporting of children's physical activity is the most feasible community-based source of data, it is subject to parents' bias and may not be as reliable as logs and diaries (Sallis & Saelens, 2000). Also, different age children may engage in different patterns of physical activity. For instance, 2-5 year old children are found to engage in short 10 minute bouts of spontaneous physical activity with frequent rest periods (Bailey, Olson, Pepper, Porszaz, Barstow, & Cooper, 1995).

Results

The findings from this study are from two data sources, which include results from four focus groups and individual writing samples. The findings are organized according to the themes that emerged from the data. These themes are broadly divided into four main topics: (a) Physical Activity, (b) Physical Inactivity, (c) Weight Status, and (d) Intervention Strategies. The first two topics will be presented in detail according to the following sub-categories: (a) caregiver's views and perceptions of physical activity or physical inactivity, (b) caregiver's attitudes toward physical activity or inactivity, and (c) caregiver's behavior toward physical activity or inactivity. Views and perceptions include the caregiver's definition and meaning of research terminology, their determination of what adequate amounts of activity are and appropriate limits of physical inactivity, their description of the patterns of physical activity and inactivity, their assessment of these activities, and their explanation of children's need for other children being present to stay physically active. Additionally, a theme that emerged from the data was the perceived benefits and disadvantages of physical inactivity for children. This along with behavior related to physical activity and inactivity which include practice of each along with parental involvement are presented. The third topic (weight status) presented in detail is according to the following sub-categories: (a) perception of physical activity and inactivity in relation to overweight and obesity, (b) factors influencing understanding of weight status, and (c) cultural perceptions of weight normalcy. Finally, intervention strategies as offered by the caregivers will be presented in three main sub-categories: (a) physical activity intervention used by parents to normalize child's weight, (b) physical activity and dietary intervention in chronic disease prevention, and (c) community support of families in the prevention of childhood obesity.

Findings suggest that among caregivers there are distinct sociocultural beliefs, attitudes, and behaviors related to physical activity and inactivity. Gender differences were observed with relation to caregivers' perception of physical activity. Benefits and disadvantages of physical inactivity were highlighted by the caregivers along with children needing other children to stay physically active. Additionally, different ethnic groups gave different meaning to weight normalcy, physical activity and inactivity. Familial differences were also observed among ethnic groups, with regards to preventive strategies related to childhood obesity and factors that influence their understanding of weight status. Finally, caregivers' perception of community support for the prevention of childhood obesity was investigated. Results indicated that caregivers perceived environmental changes as a necessary condition for increasing physical activity among families. Additionally, a need for nutrition education programs that offer awareness and skill-building workshops resulting in food-related behavior change targeting families were identified.

Initial analysis of the data investigated culturally-based definition of primary caregiver among the study participants. Among all groups, mothers were identified as the primary caregiver. Participants in the Chamorro group indicated that the caregiver is also the one who stays at home. The Carolinian group added that the caregiver is the person who makes the decision and/or takes care of the children, while the Filipino group also identified fathers and friends as the primary caregiver. Of interest is that the fathers identified aunts, uncles, older siblings, and the entire family as caregivers, but did not identify themselves as the primary caregiver, although they clearly saw the mothers as the one who has a distinct power and responsibility within the family structure. As one father stated, *"Mom, you don't argue with mom, we are just soldiers, they're the admiral. Even up to now, my mom calls the shots you know."*

Physical Activity of Children

Perceptions of Physical Activity

Participants indicated that children are usually engaged in some sort of active play, whether it is playing outside or indoors. Although, sometimes parents may have to ask their children to go and play especially when the child is sitting around, the common perception is that children only sit around when they are sick. Caregivers see illness as the only obstacle to movement otherwise children are naturally seen as active. Additionally, Table 2 presents direct quotes from participants regarding their views and perceptions of physical activity. These data were derived from the content analysis of the writing samples. Individual caregivers in all the groups emphasized the benefits of physical activity associating it with health and/or strength, as indicated in these comments.

Table 2. Perceptions of Physical Activity and Types of Physical Activity

Focus Groups	**Participant Comments**	
	Perceptions of Physical Activity	**Types of Physical Activity**
Chamorro	(n=6) *"Child is very active in physical education"* *"Amount of exercise one exhibit"* *"Very active, healthy"* *"Means an activity that I do out of my normal schedule each day"* *"Doing something that would make you sweat"* *"The activities for all parts of our bodies"*	(n=4) *"Walking, playing with kids, house work"* *"Running, jogging, jumping, walking"* *"Sports, biking any extra curricular (physical)"* *"Playing sports, bike riding"*
Fathers	(n=3) *"Spontaneous or moved a lot"* *"Important, need to stay healthy"* *"To stay fit"*	(n=2) *"Daily movement, walking up/down stairs, riding bike, baseball practice"* *"Playing bike with dad"*
Filipino	(n=6) *"Good for your health"* *"Healthy exercise"* *"Physically healthy and strong"* *"Make our body more strong and healthy"* *"Is for the exercise"* *"Exercise"*	(n=2) *"Daily exercise such as playing ball, running, swimming, etc."* *"Basketball"*
Carolinian	(n=6) *"Body movements, exercising, sports"* *"Exercise"* *"Playful, actions in some kind of sports, and habits"* *"Healthy, well balanced, daily routine activities that are fit"* *"Things we do by moving our whole body"* *"Able to do a lot of things at this age, child that is not always sick, move, run, jump, etc. all the time"*	(n=1) *"Playing sports and exercise"*

Gender Differences in Perceptions of Physical Activity

Gender differences were observed among the focus group participants with regards to perception of physical activity. Male participants differentiated between the various types of physical activity such as team sports, dance programs, and outdoor play. Male participants also emphasized the difference between sports program versus outdoor play indicating that children do more when involved in sports program. The female participants on the other hand did not make these distinctions and grouped all physical activity together including playing outdoors, basketball, dancing, and even supervised Boy Scout activities. Female participants focused on patterns of physical activity, such as children around the age of nine engage more in play than any other activities, with some children being more active than others in their age group.

Appropriate Levels of Physical Activity

Familial differences were observed among caregivers with regards to perceived appropriate levels of physical activity for children. Participants reported that appropriate levels depends on the child and is driven by the child's nature and physical ability, as indicated by one mother, "*some children they do more than their age level*". Others had specific time limits for appropriate levels of physical activity. These included thirty minutes of daily outdoor racing recommend by the doctor for weight control for an overweight child, forty-five minutes of running around and playing basketball, and one-hour of biking for a ten year old child. However, in the case of very active children, caregivers suggested that appropriate levels may be defined by the child's tolerance, although there is a need to prevent children from being worn out or overly tired. Among the participants, the general perception of physical activity for children was positive, as reflected in one mother's comment, "*The more the better*".

Types of Physical Activity

The types of physical activity for children were identified as supervised Boy Scout programs, dancing, outdoor playing, and basketball. Caregivers indicated that although there are formal activities such as team sports, boys and girls scouts program, and informal activities such as neighborhood play, team sports for females in this age group are limited,

> Like here, there are a lot of people on the beach side. It's good. We always swim and walk on the beach. There are a lot of sports going around, which we put our kids into, but here, there is not much for girls.

Table 2 presents data from the content analysis with regards to the participants' responses related to types of physical activity.

Patterns of Physical Activity

Patterns of physical activity were reported to be unique to each child when compared with other children within the neighborhood or immediate and extended family, as indicated by the these comments,

> My son is more active than our neighbors. He can run, he can play all through [the] evening until shower time.

> I have a neighbor son, he's 6 years old and I will tell him he's doing more than my 8 and 9 year old daughters doing. He's more active.
>
> I have my brother in law, he has kids too, three girls, their age from 6 to 10, between there. Their kids always sitting down, but my daughter climb, running around and them they just sitting down so I think my daughter is doing more.

Caregivers also identified gender differences related to patterns of physical activity. Specifically, girls that enter puberty were observed to present a tendency to be less active and a desire to be different than younger children who are perceived as being interested in play and toys.

Children Need Other Children to Stay Physically Active

Across all the cultures caregivers discussed the need for children to have other children to stay physically active and to reduce television viewing. Caregivers noted the difficulty that single children have with no one to play with, which impacts their activity levels, as indicated by one mother,

> See that is my problem, when my son doesn't have anybody to play with and he watches a lot of TV and I try to make him stop watch TV and go play, but nobody to play with all he does is kill the plants outside, and throw rocks. It is kind of hard because he has nobody to play with and we have a play station, he couldn't wait to play with it, but I have boxed it up, because I think what I should do is to try to find friends for him. It is my problem.

The benefit of having siblings to engage children in play was noted by the fathers. One father reported that during the weekends the children want to play with their cousins and other playmates, which reduces their TV viewing, while another father noted that when he takes his children out of the house, he notices the rest of the children follow.

One parent indicated that her child gained a lot of weight watching TV and staying indoors. She tried to distract him by engaging him in the house chores. She indicated that she is hopeful that her child will be more physically active because recently children have moved into their neighborhood, and this seems to excite her son. Another parent indicated that her son's only activity is at school, since he is an only child and has no friends at home. In response to the question of what caregivers do to help their children be more active, one parent indicated having children around in the neighborhood helps. Caregivers recognize their children's natural desire for play and their readiness to always join other kids for outdoor play, as reflected in one Chamorro mother's comment,

> She loves to play when it comes to play she can get up in the morning and play ball. Once she hears the voice outside of the children, she's all ready. If you don't pull her to come and eat lunch, she will just stay out all day.

One mother reported that her child is disinterested in watching TV, prefers to play outdoors, only watches TV when she is alone and when there are no kids to play with her. Another mother is challenged with the problem of her son watching a lot of TV when he has no playmates and sees the solution as finding friends for her child. This parent stays after school for her child to play in the playground instead of coming home and watching TV. One mother sighed and said my son could play computer games for 8 hours on average per week when there are no kids to play with. Another Mother reported that her 6 year old son is an only child and gets bored fast and waits for the parents to come home to play with him.

Assessing Physical Activity Levels

With regards to assessing children's activity, caregivers reported that they monitor their activity by questioning the children or by observing them, as reflected in this mother's comment,

> My oldest son is slim and he loves to dance. And mostly I always see him calling the neighbors and they would take the player and plug it and put it out to the yard where the big tree is and they will dance. But I don't mind for him to dance because you know, dancing is also exercise.

Additionally, caregivers report children's physical activity by day of week and time of day, as indicated by one Carolinian mother,

> During the week, it's about a total of an hour, an hour and a half and then during the weekends, like they have activities in the morning and then in the afternoon, yeah, maybe they'll watch about two hours in the afternoon, you know, some shows and then they'll go out and play again when it's cool. You know, it depends on the time of the day and what day it is. Sometimes it's raining, so they stay inside ---- if somebody's on the game, and then the other one would watch TV.

Caregivers' Perception of School-Based Physical Education (PE) Programs

Table 3 presents direct quotes from participants regarding their views and perceptions of school physical education programs. The participants mainly focused on types of activities and content of physical education programs. With regards to the latter, some caregivers focused on the perceived learning components of physical education programs as reflected in their comments.

Table 3. School Physical Education (PE) Program Themes and Responses

Focus Group	Participant Comments
	Activities and Content of Physical Education
Chamorro (n=7)	*"Any program that involves physical activity"* *"Any program involving physical and mental alertness"* *"Schedule PE activity for children"* *"Stretching, exercising, extracurricular activities"* *"Sports"* *"Learning about health, sports and healthy food"* *"Playing kick ball"*
Fathers (n=3)	*"Physical activities"* *"Regular physical training; activities that require lots of movement and exerting energy"* *"School takes care"*
Filipino (n=7)	*"Program designed for kids for them to learn" "Healthy body and mind"* *"Should be taken at least three times a week"* *"Yes basketball"* *"We need PE programs in the school for our exercise"* *"For physical needs that I or we need at least 30 minutes a day"* *"Activity"* (expressed independently by 2 participants)
Carolinian (n=6)	*"Physical activity at school - sports, etc."* *"Playing sports and exercising in school"* *"Exercise"* (expressed independently by 2 participants) *"Exercise the body and evaluate"* *"Activities done at school"*
	Attitude toward Physical Education
Chamorro (n=3)	*"Good for our kids"* *"Good for the children"* *"Best for the kids"*
Fathers (n=2)	*"Important for kids"* *"To stay fit"*
Carolinian (n=1)	*"Is important everyday, to exercise for children"*

Missing Information for Physical Activity Filipino (n= 1)

Behavior Related to Physical Activity

Practice of Physical Activity

Current practice of physical activity includes children's involvement in outdoor play and sports programs. Children's outdoor play takes place in school playgrounds and away from the school. Caregivers were varied on their reporting of children's physical activity. Fathers reported that children are more active during the weekends with their relatives and when involved in organized sports, *"On the weekend, with the cousins, they want to play, so less*

TV". Although, neighborhood outdoor play was reported by mothers, *"After drawing, he just go out and play with the neighbors"*, children's physical activity is likely to take place in school playgrounds, as reflected in one Filipino mother's statement,

> Some of his physical activity he gets at school. It will be my husband, son, and I at the house, there are no friends, so whatever activity he does is at school, after school actually. He runs around on the playground until it is time to go, and that's about it, then we go home, he watches TV and does his school work.

Care giving Practices in Promoting Physical Activity

The role of parents in promoting physical activity was delineated by caregivers in all groups. Participants from among the fathers group reported that parent involvement in physical activity is likely to occur on the weekends, *"the weekends you go to the beach. We love the beach, but weekdays, we have nothing to do. He's got to ride his bike."* Additionally, participants in this group reported an observed increase in physical activity opportunities for children in the CNMI over the past two decades and suggested that children's lack of involvement in such activities may be due to parents' lack of support. One suggested reason for this lack of support was the family's socioeconomic status as expressed by one father,

I think in general, our kids are doing more than the average child does. The average child would probably be in the house more. I think with us parents, we are around to have our kids participate. And finish drop his kid at the other end of the island where the swimming is taking place, but not some parents, like they can't afford for their children to join some programs. We try to go one step further.

Because, caregivers perceived children to be inherently active, they indicated that children require active parental involvement mainly to keep them occupied and to organize structured and unstructured activities for them,

> Dancing every night is not enough. As soon as you sit down, they run around. They go around, running around. We're going to have to pick a time of activity and for how long and then next day we're going to have this. Try to make them busy with any kind of activity that a parent can participate with them. So you try to keep them busy and sometimes you do things with them and sometimes you just have them do things on their own or walk with them at the pathway.

Engaging children in household chores was reported to be a common practice among the caregivers. In some families, boys are also expected to engage in household chores before they can play outdoors as reflected in one Carolinian mother's comments,

> He does house chores for me because I got only three boys, I don't have daughters. They get to help me out. So after school, that's when I give him time to play outside.

Among the participants in the Chamorro group, strategies used by caregivers to help children be more active were identified. These include racing outdoors with one's children and ensuring that children go out biking, walking in the park, or playing catch.

Physical Inactivity in Children

Perceptions of Physical Inactivity

With regards to caregivers' perception of physical inactivity, with the exception of one caregiver who defined physical inactivity as *"Not engaged in any outdoor activity"* majority of the participants in the Filipino group either offered irrelevant responses such as *"Basket ball"*, *"P.E."*, or *"Exercise"* or no response for physical inactivity, indicating unfamiliarity with the word "physical inactivity". Among all the other three groups, words such as "couch potato" and "lazy" were associated with physical inactivity. Although more frequently expressed by the participants in the Carolinian group, individual caregivers in the other two groups also saw physical inactivity as a health-related condition, as indicated in these comments, *"Lack of energy, unhealthy"*, *"Become fat and lazy"*, *"Child that is not eating right"*, *"Sick, not well fit"*, and *"Not normal"*.

Types of Physical Inactivity

With regards to types of physical inactivity direct quotes derived from content analysis of the writing samples indicated that caregivers perceived physical inactivity as *"Watching TV"*, *"Playing TV games"*, and *"Sitting playing game"*. Additionally, participants offered their perception of these two types of physical inactivity, i.e. (a) television viewing, and (b) computer games presented in Table 4.

Table 4. Television Viewing and Computer Games

Focus Group	Participant Comments
	Television Viewing
Chamorro (n=5)	*"Watching a movie/video rental"* *"Watching favorite show"* *"Viewing cartoons or any other programs"* *"Sitting down watching TV programs"* *"Flipping through channels until you find what you like"*
Fathers (n=3)	*"Watching television"* *"Cartoon"* *"CNN"*
Filipino (n=3)	*"No television viewing"* *"Watching television"* (expressed independently by 2 participants)
Carolinian (n=7)	*"Watching TV"* (expressed independently by 4 participants) *"Habit of watching TV"* *"To scheme through a television program"* *"To watch for a few minutes"*
	Computer Games
Chamorro (n=4)	*"Nintendo 64, computer software"* *"Nintendo, Sega, x-box, game by advanced"* *"Electronic games such as Nintendo (Mario) play station, Sega, etc."* *"Any type of electronic games children/adults play"*
Fathers (n=2)	*"Playing Nintendo, PS2 and arcade games"* *"Play station and Nintendo 64"*

Table 4. Continued

Focus Group	Participant Comments
Filipino (n=3)	*"Yes computer games"* *"Games that you played in the computer or TV sets/ video"* *"To play games like machines"*
Carolinian (n=5)	*"Arcade or video games on the computer"* *"Playing games"* *"Nintendo or anything on computer that has games"* *"Games with control, I don't have a computer at home"* *"Any remote type of games"*

Missing Information for television viewing and computer games Chamorro (n=1), Filipino (n=2)

Appropriate Limits of Physical Inactivity

With regards to appropriate limits of television viewing and computer use, majority of the participants did not seem to have formulated restrictive views on this matter, although some suggested one or two hours per day. Fathers suggested two hours of television and computer use daily during the week. Although, reported use of television and computer was varied. In general, participants reported one to two hours of television and computer use daily during the week and as much as four hours on a weekend day.

Patterns of Physical Inactivity

Patterns of physical inactivity seem to depend on the child's preference and culture of the household. In regards to child's preference, caregivers either reported that their children are intensely interested in television and computer use or that they prefer to be physically active or engaged in outdoor play,

> Our neighbors come and watch TV in our house with our kids and play computer. Whenever they come, my kids are outside. She's not interested in computer and TV. Only seldom, sometimes she just watches and then that's it. She's not into it. But sometimes if the neighbor's kids come over, instead of watching TV, she watches them.
>
> During the week, [watch TV] for about one hour, once a day, because she likes to go out and play.

In response to what parents do to limit television use, one mother expressed that she does not have a problem with TV viewing, since her kids are disinterested in TV. Caregivers also reported that children, who are usually disinterested in television, seem to have higher use of TV when they don't have playmates. In general, children seem to set their own limit for television viewing. Factors that limit children's television viewing and influence their choice to engage in outdoor play is personal preference for outdoor play, personal preference for other activities such as reading or math work, playmates, and weather conditions, as indicated by one Filipino caregiver, *"She rather read or draw, we give her math, she rather enjoy doing that than watching TV."*

For school aged children weekends seem to be a challenge with regards to television viewing and computer use. One Chamorro mother said that weekday's use of computer games is different than weekend days. Her children are not allowed to play computer games or Nintendo during weekdays but there are no rules for the weekend days and evenings. One Filipino mother indicated that she allows her child one-hour of daily use of computer games following the child's routines of homework, dinner and shower. With regards to the culture of households, some families reported the use of discipline and structure to discourage television viewing, as reflected in this mother's comments,

> Even me, I'm not working I just stay home and I have four children, I have two daughters and two sons and they're all going to school. They don't watch TV on the weekdays, only on the weekends. It's their choice. So if they want to watch TV, they can watch TV. But usually I don't allow that. Even me, I don't like to watch TV. I rather do something else than sit down and just watch TV. I know I'm not going to learn something from the TV, especially since there's too many violence on the channels. And usually in my house there's a schedule for my children. My six years old daughter will also do chore in the house. It's a simple chore. They can go out and play. So my kids are not interested in watching TV. Every night I do the same thing that I want my children to do. At eight o'clock, I switch off the light and that's what I do everyday.

Attitude Related to Physical Inactivity

Benefits and Disadvantages of Physical Inactivity

From among all the groups, Carolinian participants seemed to focus more on the advantages and disadvantages of television viewing than any of the other groups. Caregivers seemed concerned with excessive periods of time spent watching television, indicating that it may not be healthy for children,

> I got three kids at home. One is in sixth grade, and two haven't gone to school yet. The youngest one will rather play outside, he doesn't bother. The second one, he can watch TV like three hours in the morning rather than doing anything. And I guess that's not healthy, and in the afternoon again, watch like two hours. And the one at school, when he finishes school, like three o'clock will be home, he can stay on the computer for four hours.

Majority of the participants discussed the disadvantages of television viewing with the exception of few caregivers, who focused on the benefits of television viewing,

> A lot of kids who watch TV, you can tell that their language is very good, too. It improves. But it depends on what they watch. Especially being here in Saipan, you know, we're not English speakers, English is our second language but you can really tell by the children who watch a lot of TV.

> I think they get more appetite, you know, if they sit down. The food commercial, oh, I'm hungry, you know, I'll go get me a snack, or mom, can you get me that. I want to go to McDonald's.

With regards to the disadvantages of television viewing, caregivers in this group felt that television may affect their child's attention span, decrease their appetite, expose them to violence, and teach them inappropriate words,

> I think sometimes when kids watch too much TV, it affects their attention span. Sometimes you'll be talking to them and they can't hear anything because they just are focused on the show.

> They could also loose their appetite.

> Maybe the kids learn something we don't want them to see, like some war, or some actions.

> You hear all those words, those bad words, but now, even in the cartoons, you can hear.

Across all the groups, the one advantage of television viewing was in regards to the issue of safety and supervision. Among the Filipino caregivers, it was noted that the culture indicates that children need to be indoors before dark and therefore it is not unusual to have them watch television in the evenings. Caregivers who expressed concern with safety and supervision, believed that it is easier to have the children at home watching television so they can keep track of them and offer parents peace of mind,

> Before when I had only one child, I have control of him and now that I have four kids, I rather them sit in the house and watch TV than one would go on one side and one would go on the other side.

> I go to work maybe about seven thirty, come home twelve O'clock for lunch, he is still watching cartoons. Go back to work; come back in the evening, still there watching TV. I mean they watch TV all day. But, at the same token, I prefer them doing that than, you know my head is more comfortable knowing that they are in the house doing something than outside playing with I don't know what. It's difficult, but you know I feel more comfortable knowing that they are in a house playing, all of them. And I go to work, thinking that, oh, one is in on the road.

Table 5 presents participants' responses from the content analysis of the writing samples related to conditions associated with television use

Table 5. Condition Associated with Television Use

Focus Group	Participant Comments
Chamorro (n=4)	*"Child's extra curricula to keep her sitting still, couch potato"* *"Too much of anything is bad for you. Therefore controlling the length of time watching TV is essential"* *"Something I do if I do not have a good book"* *"To put your whole self into it and not do the things that needs to be done"*
Fathers (n=2)	*"Leisure time"* *"Like to do, however need to control amount"*
Filipino (n=3)	*"Watching to get information and entertainment"* *"One way of relaxing and influences our children"* *"To learn some thing that happening around you"*

Regarding computer games a similar theme emerged from the data that highlighted caregivers' perception of computer use. Table 6 presents participants' responses related to perception of computer use which focuses on views and attitudes toward this type of physical inactivity.

Table 6. Perceptions of Computer Games

Focus Group	Participant Comments
Chamorro (n=5)	*"Can be an addiction"* *"Entertaining, challenging"* *"Too much of anything is bad for you. Therefore controlling the length of time watching TV is essential"* *"Fun, but I have put it away until school is out for summer"* *"You play with it, but you can get hooked by it."*
Fathers (n=3)	*"Extra activity"* *"Important, changing times requires you to have"* *"for fun"*
Filipino (n=3)	*"Brain exercise"* *"One way our children spend their time during their idle time"* *"It helps to my children especially they just started to learn to use"*
Carolinian (n=2)	*"Activities on the computer that don't help much in learning"* *"Exercise of the mind"*

Behavior Related to Physical Inactivity

Practice of Physical Inactivity

Among the Filipino group, caregivers reported one to two hours of television use daily during the week, with higher weekend and holiday usage. However, based on observation, caregivers reported that children's TV use is within the purview of each family dynamic, *"It depends on the parents, some children watch more, and they stay late to watch TV, because their life is watching TV."* Caregivers in the Chamorro group reported two or more hours of television and computer use daily during the week. Additionally, caregivers noted that during weekdays children are governed by different limits with regards to computer use than during the weekends, *"At my house, Monday through Thursday no computer games, no Nintendo, Friday, Saturday, and Sunday they could play."*

Among the Carolinian group TV and computer use was reported as one hour during the week, with more time on the weekends. Fathers reported that during weekdays, children typically watch about one hour of television. Additionally, it was noted that because of the recent increased access to television and computer games there may be an increase in physical inactivity among children, as observed by one father,

> My brother's kids who come over to the house, they do the same thing. You go to my brother's house, same thing, I mean you go to their house, there are computer games, I mean, every household.

Caregivers reported that they find it difficult to limit their children's television viewing when away from home. Additionally, participants shared their concern with their children's use of internet and chat rooms, especially when children indicate that they are working on their homework, as reported by one mother,

> And my son has his own computer and it's very hard, because sometimes when we check him, he said, oh mom, I'm doing my homework, but I don't know if he's doing something else.

Care Giving Practices in Limiting Physical Inactivity

The role of parents in limiting physical inactivity was delineated by caregivers in all groups. With regards to activities that are physically inactive such as television viewing and computer use, Carolinian participants along with the fathers reported that they try to maintain a schedule during weekdays to control these activities. Participants also reported different rules and limits for weekdays than weekends, as indicated by one Carolinian mother,

> During school days, you know, I don't make my children watch TV. But they watch the news, of course we turn on the TV during news time and then they watch the news with us and then after that we turn it to an educational learning channel or sometimes they have an assignment from school, they have to watch biographies about some people and they have to take notes or they have to watch Discovery channel and just like an hour a day. But during the weekends they can watch, as much as they want, or nowadays that they have computer games and those handheld Nintendo and play stations.

Because children may have the tendency to watch television during their get-togethers, there is a perceived need for parental intervention in limiting children's viewing and encouraging outdoor play as reflected in one mother's comment,

> If I would have visitors to come home and visit us, they will not sit in front of the TV. My children is to call the children that came to visit, to go outside and either play baseball or ride a bike or walk on the beach because we live by the beach.

Additionally, caregivers also reported that either their children are disinterested in television which does not require any action from them, "*I don't think I have many problems with TV because my kids are not really into TV*", or that they are intensely interested in television and will need very restrictive limits, "*I rarely let them play now, because he could play for eight hours a day, there is no way he can just turn it off after ten minutes*".

Although, caregivers recognize their role in limiting television viewing, they reported their challenges with this task. Among the Carolinian participants, it was noted that working parents may have difficulty in supervising their children's television viewing,

> It's hard if the parents are working. I really know what my daughter is doing and we keep track of where she goes or what she does. So I know what her daily activities are and what she's doing. For other parents, maybe they really don't know how their kids are with the TV because they are working.

Other issues raised were (a) children not following parent's directions, (b) caregivers having to take care of more than one child at a time, or (c) children in the same household having different preferences and tendency for physical inactivity. Caregivers also reported that they use different strategies to get compliance from their children with regards to television viewing. These include (a) encouraging children to engage in other activities such as reading books, or playing board games with siblings, (b) raising one's voice, (c) setting limits with monitoring to ensure compliance, (d) using rewards, or (e) spending time with the children, as reflected in these comments,

> Every night at eight o'clock in the evening, if it is 7:30, I tell them to stop watching TV. I tell them to sleep before eight o'clock.

> If they listen, then they get something. We give rewards, like we promise to buy them a bike, because they really wanted a bike. Say a doll or watch a movie, or go swimming, go picnic, family picnic.

Weight Status: Overweight and Obesity

Perception of the Relationship between Physical Activity and Weight Status

Caregivers recognized the psychological and physiological consequences of childhood obesity and the need for medical referral and weight control measures. Participants identified different environmental and societal factors related to overweight status among children. Frequent social gatherings, time spent at school, food availability and accessibility, media, cultural beliefs and practices, and physical activity are among factors that are perceived to interact with childhood obesity. The relationship of weight and activity were emphatically reported by all the focus group participants, indicating that more active children are less overweight, "*That boy is more overweight and my son is just the right weight, you know, more active.*" Fathers also noted the relevance of children's activity in maintaining their weight, especially with the changing time. Sociocultural beliefs regarding the importance of physical activity in childhood obesity was expressed by participants, as reflected in one mother's comment,

> When you look at a child that is fatter, then our parents will tell us that your child should exercise more, because he would not live longer.

Overall analysis of the data across all groups showed that participants recognized the role of physical activity and inactivity in maintaining normal weight status. For instance, Filipino participants identified a set of factors related to children maintaining normal weight status which emphasized physical activity and inactivity. These include (a) genetics, (b) fondness for activities, (c) ability to burn body fat, (d) higher activity level, (e) parental involvement in ensuring that children play for at least 2 hours per day, (f) child's preference for swimming, (g) food choices, and (h) eating the right amount and type of food. In addition, caregivers in the Carolinian group noted their observation of factors that may contribute to childhood obesity. Specifically, the need for more attention and active parental involvement with regards to increasing physical activity was indicated, as reflected in one Carolinian mother's comment,

> Maybe they think there is nothing for them to do, they just sit around and eat and watch TV. But if they have more attention and have someone to play with, I think that's what I mean when I say encourage them more, be involved as a parent. But here, usually mostly parents are working.

However, with regards to underweight status among children, Carolinian participants suggested that caregivers should seek medical assistance in diagnosing the problem. Specifically, it was suggested that the following issues be carefully examined, quantity of food consumed, genetic make-up, and/or potential health problems.

In addition to physical activity and inactivity caregivers also recognized the role of diet in overweight and obesity. Among the Chamorro group, caregivers reported that medical recommendations regarding the management of overweight children indicate limiting certain foods and increasing physical activity, "*limit soft drinks and do a lot of activities*". Similarly, prevention strategies of childhood overweight among the Filipino participants included the role of diet and exercise, as indicated by one mother, *"Diet and exercise. At least fifteen minutes per day."* Participants in this group also delineated the role of caregivers in controlling the child's food.

Factors Influencing Understanding of Weight Status

In general the extended family, health care providers, community members, and personal experience all seemed to influence caregivers' awareness and understanding of children's weight status. In understanding factors related to children's weight status, it was noted that caregivers are most intimately involved with their children's issues and in the position to assess their status, as reflected in one mother's comments,

> Only you, the person, the caregiver of the child knows whether the child is healthy or not because they know what food they give them and they know how often they get sick, so you know you can't judge other children because we don't know what their problem is.

There is a common belief that children's individual characteristic determines their weight status. This is reflected in one father's perspective, "*I have a son, and he eats a lot; but he don't get fat. I didn't know why, but I didn't eat that kind of a food when I was his age.*" Although, parents believe that individual characteristics determine their child's weight status, most recognize specific factors that interact with these characteristics. These include genetic makeup, physiology and metabolism, as expressed in these comments,

> Sometimes it runs in the family, like genes, you know.
>
> So they tell me, oh your daughter takes after you and then your son takes after the dad's family because they are big.

You will see, you will compare, and some of those children eat a lot. They don't really observe the basic food groups, but still they're normal. The body is normal, looks normal, you know, not overweight. Just sometimes it is the genes.

Individual weight differences influenced by activity level were also reported by the caregivers. These included children who are predisposed to being active or inactive, those who are generally interested in activities, and those whose parents ensure daily play, as indicated in these comments,

> My daughter is also very thin, I think she is overactive.
>
> I have an eight year and ten year old daughters and they're like total opposite. The ten year old would rather just sit and read and read and read and read all the way until she sleeps. But the other one, she'd rather get up and move around, so I notice their weight difference, too. The one that reads is bigger than the one that moves around.
>
> They're fond of activities, they like to swim, they like to play and that's why they're burning their fats.

Caregivers' perception of dietary factors related to weight status was varied by the weight status of the children and the parents' views on diet. With regards to normal weight status one mother stated, "*Food makes a lot of difference. You eat the right food, right amount, then that's good*", while underweight status among children was seen as a result of food restrictions in response to medical advice specifically in regards to management of chronic diseases.

Cultural Perception of Weight Normalcy

Sociocultural beliefs with regards to weight normalcy among participants were observed. Although, fathers did not identify wealth as a reason for fatness, female participants in the Chamorro group indicated that fat is perceived as wealth and being fat and large is a representation of it. As for children, both Chamorro and Carolinian participants indicated that culturally people prefer to see them as being fat. Underweight status among children seems to be a more sensitive issue than obesity. One Carolinian mother in response to communicating with a friend about their child's weight status, stated,

> It would be easier to tell a person or your friend that their child is obese than to tell a friend who has a child that's healthy and fit. You can be surprised; maybe the child is very sick.

Analysis of data also suggests that different groups within the community reinforce caregivers' perception of weight normalcy. Differences were seen among the different ethnic groups in communicating acceptable weight status. Informal network which involves the immediate and extended family through a socially constructed conception of weight communicate weight normalcy messages to caregivers. Moreover, certain ethnic groups rely on the formal network which involves the doctors and nutritionists for weight status information. Filipino participants recognized the doctor as a more accurate source of information on appropriate weight status and advice than another parent. In addition to doctors, Filipino participants also rely on nutritionists and regular annual medical check up to learn about the child's weight status. Grandmothers, aunts/uncles, and spouses were reported as individuals that influence fathers' perception of their child's weight status. Additionally, fathers reported that within the Chamorro culture there is a familial hierarchy that allows them to feel comfortable in advising their nieces and nephews with regards to weight control measures. However, advising their friends was seen as an intrusion. Carolinian participants identified both the family and doctors in influencing their perception of their child's weight status. Among the Carolinians, husbands were also seen as influencing primary caregivers' perception of child's weight status. Chamorro female participants reported that their mother-in-law and their husbands also influence their perception of their child's weight status. Carolinian and Filipino participants also identified their own personal judgment in this process. Visual assessment of child's weight, height and weight charts, personal feeling, and child fitting into clothes were used by caregivers to formulate personal judgment on child's weight status.

Intervention Strategies

Intervention Used by Caregivers to Normalize Child's Weight

Physical activity as an intervention in helping children normalize their weight was indicated by caregivers, "*If he's big, then tell them to make him move more.*" Among the participants in the father's group, the need to tell children to participate in physical activity, enrolling them in gyms so they can be encouraged to be active, and promising them a reward for engaging in physical activity were reported. In this group, participants also enquired as to whether the sports programs for children in the island teach them to prevent from becoming overweight. Caregivers reported to use different strategies for overweight and underweight children. Specifically in preventing a normal weight child from becoming underweight caregivers indicated that they need to stay close to the child and play with him, while in preventing children from becoming overweight caregivers need to monitor the child and tell him to control his intake.

Participants in the Carolinian group, focused on parental involvement in increasing children's activity. Among the Chamorro group participants, intervention strategies included encouraging overweight children to go to the gym to work out, and telling the child to do more activities like jogging, running and walking. Caregivers in this group also delineated the role of the parents in supporting children's physical activity. However, when using medical recommendations to help overweight children, adjustments were made to meet individual family needs, as reported by one Chamorro mother, "*Thirty minutes I think the doctor told me. I can't drive all the way from work to home and then take them over to walk. I just do it around the house.*" In addition to engaging children in sports to help children from becoming overweight, caregivers also reported that they try to encourage children who are slightly overweight to get into sports and work out. They encourage children to go out biking, limit their dietary intake and offer them dinner far in advance of bedtime,

> We try to encourage him to get into sports, work out, encourage him to go out biking with his friends, limit his intake, and try to make sure he has dinner before six o'clock so that he doesn't go straight to bed.

Physical Activity and Dietary Interventions in Chronic Disease Prevention

With regards to chronic disease prevention, physical activity and dietary intervention were also noted. The importance of exercise was emphasized by the participants in all the groups, especially because physical activity was seen as a more culturally acceptable behavior to adopt than restricting foods through dietary changes, "*Give them something fun to do, like take them to the beach, swim, and play some sports.*" Among the fathers, strategies in the prevention of chronic diseases focused on restricting children's diet and monitoring overweight children in families with a history of diabetes. Participants in this group also indicated that everyone should take responsibility for this matter and work together to support the child, "*Another thing is cultural, stop bringing it all to them. Everybody be responsible. Set an example.*" The role modeling of adults in this regard was noted by another participant in the Carolinian group, "*I think that when we educate too, we should also practice what we educate.*"

Differences among fathers and mothers were observed with regards to instructing children and helping them adopt health related behaviors especially in the prevention of childhood obesity and chronic diseases. Fathers reported to use social control through verbal messages and injunctions, while mothers reported to obtain compliance by active involvement, control and training. Although, verbal messages were the primary manner in instructing children, fathers also saw a role for older children in setting examples for their younger siblings and engaging overweight children in more activities around the house.

Fathers also reported that parents need to inform their overweight children about their weight and teach them about the consequences of being overweight, "*Educate; let him realize that going from overweight to obese there is consequences in that. You have to let them know it could be death or heart disease.*" Mothers believed that overweight children would benefit from parental involvement especially with regards to reducing the purchase of fatty foods. In addition to diet, mothers also identified the role of caregivers in monitoring dietary intake and promoting physical activity in preventing childhood overweight and obesity,

> I think they need to watch what their child eats and to maybe do some activities with their child, maybe exercise, or take a walk along the beach, just to encourage the kids other than eating.

Community Support of Families in the Prevention of Childhood Obesity

Caregivers identified ways that the community might support them in preventing childhood obesity. Specifically, the focus of these strategies was on education and environment. With regards to environment, caregivers mainly focused on increasing physical activity opportunities for families. These included (a) more public exercise places, such as gyms and outdoor places that promote family activity, (b) government's assistance with village-based community centers specifically with obtaining donated exercise equipments from local gyms, (c) making physical activity programs accessible and free to the public, and (d) ensuring adequate advertisement of such activities for the public. Additionally, caregivers focused on challenges faced with food related issues. One such issue was the perceived higher cost of purchasing healthier foods, *"I notice where I go out to the stores the healthy food is a lot like three times more expensive and it is hard for families who can't really afford it."* Another issue related to food was the sociocultural characteristic of the community which offers frequently held social gatherings (parties) that involve generous food offerings and hospitality. One Chamorro mother suggested a strategy to address such gatherings, "*stop the parties*".

In addition to making physical activity more accessible to the families, caregivers identified the need for nutrition education topics related to children. These include (a) food substitution, (b) amount of food needed by children, (c) additional knowledge of foods, (d) nutrients, (e) strength building foods, and (f) food preparation. Furthermore, with regards to education of families, caregivers identified four potential sources of information, (1) community-based education sessions, (2) media, (3) published literature, and (4) health care professionals. The venue and format of the community-based sessions were discussed by the participants. The village-based community centers were identified as a place where classes could be offered to families. Caregivers found the focus group format effective and suggested using it in conducting nightly classes for the families in the village as indicated by one mother,

> I know that some of the parents will feel uncomfortable when the first time they tell them to come but as soon as they sit down, those that were very quiet won't stop talking.

For those unable to leave their home, it was suggested that educational programs be offered on cable station. Participants in the Chamorro group also reported accessing nutrition education information through US broadcast radio programs, while learning about community-sponsored workshops through the local radio stations. Among the Filipino participants nutrition information was accessed through newspapers, books, and government programs.

Caregivers suggested offering free magazines with practical useful information for parents such as information about vegetables and foods that are beneficial for health. It was reported that such materials are currently distributed by the public health agency and may only be available in the hospital for patient care. The need to make such published information accessible to the community outside of health care clinics was identified by the participants. Caregivers suggested churches, grocery stores and office waiting areas as places were such information can be made accessible to families. Also, the schools were identified as a place where information can be sent home to the children, as suggested by two mothers, "*Like a newsletter every month*" and "*I think it will help when it is given out to the kids in the schools*".

Filipino participants emphasized the importance of the health care professionals as a reliable source of information for the families, as indicated by one mother, "*I think when it comes from your pediatrician it stands out stronger than others.*" Because, doctors are perceived as more accurate on diagnosing appropriate weight status and providing medical advice, physicians were identified as sources of information for families who have concerns with their children's weight status. Additionally, participants stated that one way families might access health care professionals is through community-based workshops that are offered by the public health agency. Caregivers indicated that they find the information from the public health sector helpful and accessible.

Finally, because of the devastating consequences of chronic diseases such as Type II diabetes, families in the CNMI are facing major lifestyle choices. Over the past two decades the CNMI community has become more aware of these issues, as one mother recalled,

> You know, a long time ago, I used to remember when I was small; nurses used to come to the house and talk about what kind of food the old people at the house should cut down on. That's when they just found out, I guess, about diabetes. So they told them, you know, the disease is coming here, you know, we're receiving a lot of these diseases and you want to avoid that.

Today, there is a general concern in the community regarding the effect of these nutrition problems on individuals and families. Results of this study suggest that families may be aware of the role of diet and activity in chronic diseases. However, they may need other interventions, such as making home visits as indicated by one mother, "*I think the best way to reach out to the community is to visit them at their house.*" Caregivers also recognized that information and awareness may not be adequate for bringing about lifestyle changes and suggested the need for skill building and repeated follow-up activities,

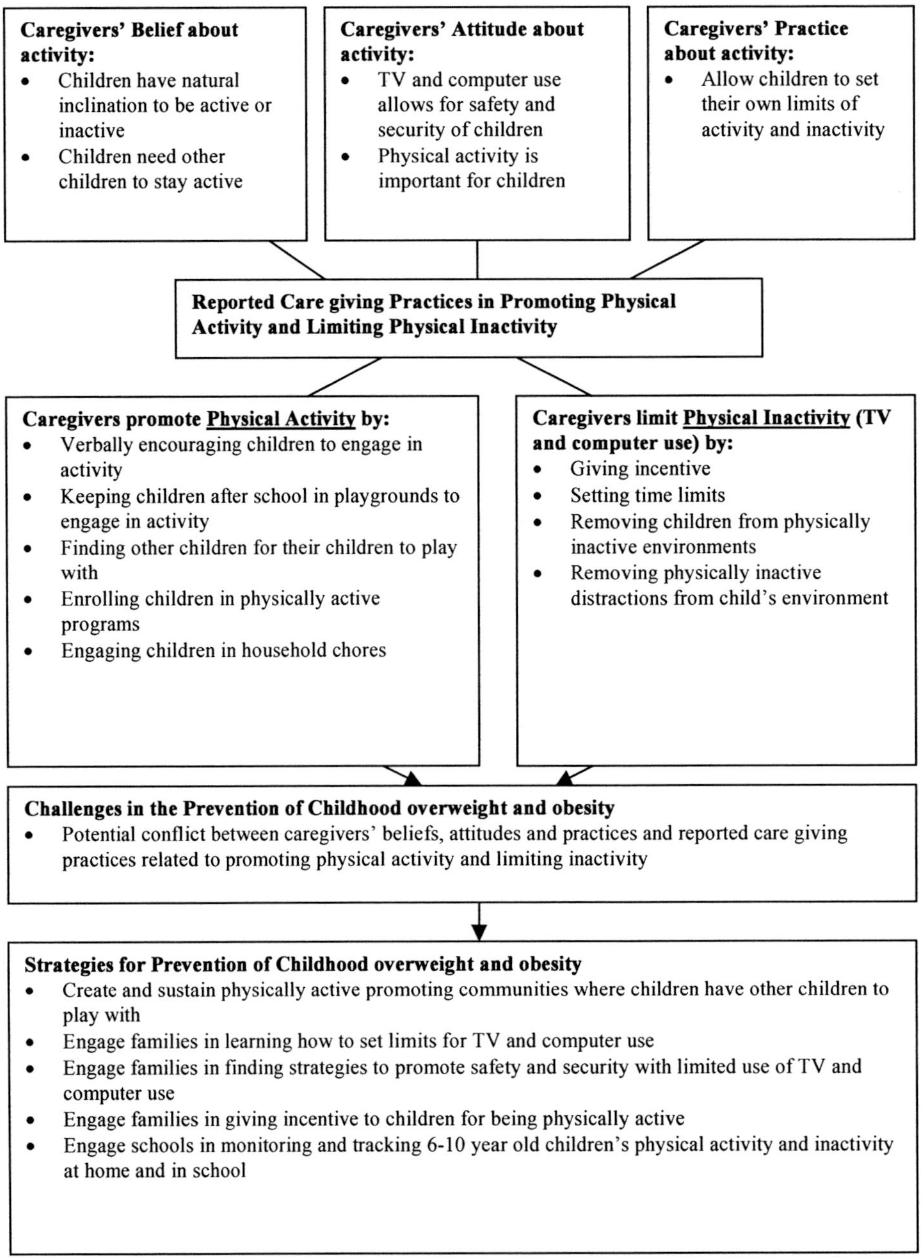

Figure 1. Framework for Interpretation

I think they're just educating, but I think if there's a workshop to help them prepare every meal, how to cook this kind [of food], maybe it's going to be more than just going around educating without action. Like, we're just here, I'm going to do that, but there's no follow up on it. People will just go back to their old habit. But if you go up and check what they're doing, are they coming up with some changes or what, instead of just talking, talking, talking and no movement, maybe there's no change. Go around and bring them together and bring somebody who knows how to cook to teach them that. We start doing that, change our bad habits of cooking with oil, fats or whatever, then we have to start and like if we have a lot of people to go visit to just evaluate and how to keep this menu going. It's going to be very hard at first.

Other education considerations identified by caregivers were to offer information in the vernacular. This was indicated by the participants in the Filipino group. Additionally, the need for visiting schools and training the school community was also identified by caregivers.

Framework for Interpretation

Figure 1 presents a framework for interpretation of the data. This framework presents (a) the general perception of caregivers related to activity, (b) reported care giving practices in promoting physical activity and limiting physical inactivity, (c) challenges in the prevention of childhood overweight and obesity, and (d) strategies for prevention of childhood overweight and obesity.

The framework helps with understanding care giving beliefs, attitudes and practices related to activity of 6-10 year old children and ways in which caregivers promote physical activity and limit physical inactivity. Additionally, results of the study presented in the framework suggest that beliefs, attitudes, and practices related to activity may have potential challenges for achieving physical activity outcome for children. For instance, caregivers' attitude of the role of television and computer in promoting safety and security for children may present a conflict with the ongoing practice of limiting physical inactivity. Caregivers' strategies in the prevention of childhood obesity are also presented in the framework, which suggests that within each community there lie the answers to problems indicating the need to engage the stakeholders in the process of investigation.

Discussion

Overview

The benefits of physical activity in children are well documented, especially the long-term protective effect that it has on body fat in childhood (Moore et al., 2003). An increasing number of intervention studies have looked at the impact of reducing physical inactivity on school aged children's BMI. Studies have demonstrated that reducing sedentary activities, maybe a promising, population-based approach to preventing childhood obesity (Robinson, 1999). School-based intervention studies have also found significant gains in knowledge from classroom diet and physical activity lessons among treatment groups (Gortmaker et al., 1999). However, in such studies no actual change was measured in vigorous physical activity as a result of the classroom lessons. Other studies have found that in children the intention to be physically active may be positively correlated with physical activity (Sallis et al., 2000). Results of these and earlier studies suggest that adopting vigorous physical activity behaviors in children may need other strategies beyond cognitive influences (Gortmaker et al., 1999; Sallis et al., 2000).

Based on these important findings and the limited information that is available on Asian/Pacific Island populations, this study examined caregivers' perceptions, attitudes, and behavior related to physical activity and inactivity of 6-10 year old children in the CNMI. Although, a number of objectives were developed and a set of questions were created, the exploratory design of this study allowed for the emergence of several themes that provide a better understanding of the issues related to the problem under study. Analysis of the data suggested that there are distinct sociocultural beliefs, attitudes, and behaviors related to physical activity and inactivity among caregivers of 6-10 year old children. Additionally, different ethnic groups based on their personal experience gave different meaning to weight normalcy, physical activity and inactivity. Across different cultures, familial differences were found with regards to specific views on preventive strategies related to childhood obesity and factors that influence their understanding of weight status. Other findings included (a) gender differences with relation to caregivers' perception of physical activity, (b) safety of children as a perceived benefit of television viewing, (c) caregivers' perception of children needing other children to stay physically active, (d) caregivers' role in increasing physical activity and limiting physical inactivity, and (e) perceived role of physical activity and inactivity in overweight and obesity were important findings that emerged from the data. Additionally, caregivers' perception of community support for the prevention of childhood obesity included changes in the environment to increase physical activity among families and increased nutrition education programs to support food-related behavior change.

Implications for Praxis

Physical Activity

Findings from this study suggest that caregivers see illness as the only obstacle to movement, otherwise children are naturally seen as active. With regards to physical activity, male participants emphasized the difference in physical fitness achieved from sports programs as compared to outdoor play, while female participants' perception of this age group focused on children's preference for play over other activities. Recognizing gender differences among caregivers in their perception of children's activity is important when designing intervention programs.

Physical activity for children is perceived as a positive element of their upbringing, although familial differences were observed in regard to appropriate levels of physical activity for children. Some participants perceived appropriate levels of physical activity as child-dependent, while others had specific time limits for the different types of activities. These included thirty minutes to one hour of physical activity for activities such as running, playing basketball and bike riding. In the case of very active children, caregivers suggested that appropriate levels might be defined by the child's tolerance, although there is a need to prevent children from being worn out or overly tired.

Gender differences were reported as it relates to patterns of physical activity among children. Specifically, girls that enter puberty were observed to present a tendency to be less active, while team sports for females in this age group might be more limited. This study supports previous findings that girls are less active than boys (Ernst, & Pangrazi, 1999; Hovell, Sallis, Kolody, & McKenzie, 1999; Lindquist et al., 1999; Mota, & Queiros, 1996;

National Center for Chronic Disease Prevention and Health Promotion, 1999). These studies indicate the need for special attention to females especially in pre-puberty and puberty stages of development. Such considerations may require the need for intervention programs that can increase physical activity among girls. An intervention study examined the impact of a school-based program on physical activity levels and body mass index (BMI) of 606 fourth-grade students. Results showed no difference in BMI between the groups; however, researchers found that the treatment was effective at increasing the physical activity level of children, especially among the girls (Pangrazi, Beighle, Vehige, & Vack, 2003).

An important finding in this study was that across all the cultures caregivers identified the need for children to have other children to stay physically active and to reduce television viewing. Caregivers perceived the benefit of having siblings and relatives to engage children in play and the difficulty that single children have with no one to play with, which can impact their overall activity levels. These findings suggest the need to consider caregivers' perception of factors that impact children's physical activity level in one- child family homes when designing childhood obesity intervention programs. A study by Lindquist et al. (1999) found that one child-families in the US had higher levels of physical fitness. The potential difference between these two study populations suggests the need to further examine scientific and lay definition of physical activity terminology when comparing qualitative and quantitative data across studies in different cultures and societies.

Caregivers' perception of current practice of physical activity included children's involvement in outdoor play and sports programs. Children's outdoor play takes place in school playgrounds and away from the school. Caregivers were varied on their perception of children's physical activity. Fathers reported that children are more active during the weekends with their relatives and when involved in organized sports. However, mothers reported on children's neighborhood outdoor play and indicated that children's physical activity was more likely to take place on school playgrounds. A study by Gavarry (2003) in a sample of one-hundred and eighty-two 6-20 year old children and youth found that elementary school subjects irrespective of their gender were more inactive during their free days than during school days. In line with these findings, caregivers in this study emphasized the importance of school physical education programs for children. This recognition of the value of physical education programs supports findings of Tsgadi et al. (2002), who found that participation in physical activity was highest in school than before or after school.

With regards to assessing children's activity, caregivers reported that they monitor their activity by questioning the children or by observing them. Additionally, caregivers reported children's activity by day of week and time of day. Gavarry (2003) supports these findings, specifically with regards to using type of day, i.e., school day versus weekend to obtain information on children's activity. This important finding has implications for design of research in obtaining activity data from caregivers of young children.

According to Arluk et al. (2003) fathers' participation in children's physical activity and the presence of parents at home when the child arrives from school were found to be related to children's weight status. In accord with this finding, this study found that caregivers in all groups delineated the role of parents in promoting physical activity and limiting physical inactivity. Participants from among the fathers group reported that parent involvement in physical activity is likely to occur on the weekends. Additionally, participants in this group reported an observed increase in physical activity opportunities for children in the CNMI over the past two decades and suggested that children's lack of involvement in such activities may be due to parents' lack of support. One suggested reason for this lack of support was the family's socioeconomic status. Because, caregivers perceived children to be inherently active, they indicated that children require active parental involvement mainly to keep them occupied and to organize structured and unstructured activities for them. This finding suggests that caregivers may have culturally-based views with regards to their role in promoting physical activity, which may have implications for social marketing messages.

Physical Inactivity

Although caregivers' definition of physical activity included types and nature of physical activity along with its perceived benefits, the definition of physical inactivity focused more on types of physical inactivity and perception of physically inactive individuals. Terms such as "couch potato" and "lazy" were used to define physical inactivity. Although, these terms have negative connotation, in contemporary society, they may be associated with individuals who follow a more sedentary lifestyle. According to the US Department of Health and Human Services (1996) a sedentary lifestyle involves little or no physical activity.

Because of the increasing hours of television use among children (Stephens, 2002), this study explored caregivers' perception and attitude toward children's television use, and found ethnic differences in the value placed on television viewing. For instance Filipino participants focused on advantages of television viewing, while Chamorro participants focused on the negative aspects of television viewing. Sociocultural differences among the caregivers with regards to television viewing were also observed with computer use. The study found that fathers and Filipino participants did not relay a negative attitude toward computer use; however, among the Chamorro participants caregivers indicated a more negative attitude. Content analysis of the writing samples suggests that Carolinian participants share both negative and positive views about television use. This finding was further validated by the focus group results, which suggest that from among all the groups, Carolinian participants seemed to focus more on the advantages and disadvantages of television viewing than any other group. Caregivers seemed concerned with excessive periods of time spent watching television, suggesting that this practice may not be healthy for children. In regards to the disadvantages of television viewing, caregivers in this group also felt that television may affect their child's attention span, decrease their appetite, expose them to violence, and teach them inappropriate words. According to Bruss et al. (2003) children's dietary intake is highly valued in this society, therefore decrease in appetite may be perceived as a disadvantage of television viewing.

Across all the groups, the one advantage of television viewing was safety and supervision. Caregivers, who expressed concern with safety and supervision, believed that it is easier to have the children at home watching television so they can keep track of them and offer parents peace of mind. Childhood obesity intervention programs should consider this finding as it might interfere with limiting television viewing of children.

As for appropriate limits of television viewing and computer use, majority of the participants did not seem to have formulated restrictive views on this matter, although some suggested one or two hours per day. Reported television and computer use was varied among the different groups. In general, participants reported one to two hours of television and computer use during the week and as much as four hours during the weekend. This practice is in line with CDC's recommendation that suggests that children's television viewing be limited to two hours per day during school days (http://www.cdc.gov/nccdphp/dnpa/physical/recommendations/young.htm). Additionally, participants in the different groups reported different practices. This finding suggests the need for investigating culture-specific practices within communities prior to the design of population-based intervention programs. For instance, among the Filipino group, although children's TV use is seen within the purview of each family dynamic, caregivers reported one to two hours of television use daily during the week, with higher weekend and holiday usage. Caregivers in the Chamorro group reported two or more hours of television and computer use daily during the week.

With regards to pattern of television and computer use, caregivers noted that during weekdays children are governed by different limits with regards to computer use than during the weekends. Among the Carolinian group TV and computer use was reported as one hour during the week, with more time on the weekends. Fathers reported that during weekdays, children typically watch about one hour of television. Caregivers reported that they find it difficult to limit their children's television viewing when away from home. Additionally, it was noted that because of the recent increased access to television and computer games there may be an increase in physical inactivity among children. This finding suggests the need for establishing a monitoring system that can collect longitudinal data of the patterns of physical inactivity in this population for the purpose of tracking community-based intervention programs. Such a system may employ parental reporting of children's television viewing, which has been shown to have high reliability (Andersen et al., 1985).

Results of this study also showed that patterns of physical inactivity might depend on the child's preference and culture of the household, which uses discipline and structure to discourage television viewing. Caregivers either reported that their children are intensely interested in television and computer use or that they prefer to be physically active or engaged in outdoor play. Although, among those typically disinterested in television, higher TV use may be observed when they don't have any playmates. In general, children seem to set their own limit for television viewing. The participants identified factors that influence children's television viewing and outdoor play. These included (a) personal preference for outdoor play, (b) personal preference for other activities such as reading or math work, (c) playmates, and (d) weather conditions. However, for some school aged children weekends seemed to be a challenge with regards to television viewing and computer use. This finding was also observed by Tsgadi, Taxildaris, Laparidis, and Michalopoulou (2002) who found that during the weekend ten-year old Greek children's physical activity and inactivity was varied among the study participants. Some children were found to be more physically inactive, while others were more physically active on the weekends.

Intervention Strategies to Promote Physical Activity and Limit Physical Inactivity

This study found that although across all groups caregivers valued physical activity, intervention strategies to increase children's physical activity was employed by only a sample of caregivers. For instance, among the Chamorro group, caregivers who were following medical recommendations for overweight children indicated racing outdoors with their children. Other strategies reported by caregivers in this group included (a) having children go out biking, (b) walking in the park, and (c) playing catch with the children. According to Mandigo and Thompson (1998), six strategies may be used to increase children's physical activity. These include (a) recognizing developmentally appropriate activity for children, (b) creating fun-filled activity, defined as balance between individual skill and challenge of activity, (c) giving children a sense of control, by permitting them to change the activity, (d) setting clear goals and objectives that can be evaluated through feedback from the children, (e) avoiding giving negative feedback to the children or putting pressure to achieve tasks, and finally, (f) promoting intrinsic versus extrinsic motivation. Intervention programs should consider that valuing physical activity might not necessarily mean strategies are being employed in increasing children's physical activity. Also, differences among caregivers may exist in the use of strategies to promote physical activity. In an effort to sustain regular physical activity in children, caregivers may use strategies proposed by Mandingo and Thompson (1998) to develop culture-specific approaches that are acceptable to the family.

With regards to strategies used by caregivers to reduce activities that are physically inactive such as television viewing and computer use, Carolinian participants along with the fathers reported that they try to maintain a schedule during weekdays to control these activities. Additionally, they indicated that they maintain different rules and limits for weekdays than weekends. Because children may have the tendency to watch television during their get-togethers, there is a perceived need for parental intervention in limiting children's viewing and encouraging outdoor play. Among the Carolinian participants, it was noted that working parents may have difficulty in supervising their children's television viewing.

With regards to parental involvement in reducing physical inactivity, caregivers also reported that either their children are disinterested in television, which does not require any action from them, or that they are intensely interested in television and will need very restrictive limits. Although caregivers recognize their role in limiting television viewing, they reported their challenges with this task. Issues raised were: children not following parent's directions, caregivers having to take care of more than one child at a time, or children in the same household having different preferences and tendency for physical inactivity. Overall caregivers reported that they use different strategies to get compliance from their children with regards to television viewing. These include encouraging children to engage in other activities such as reading books, or playing board games with siblings; raising one's voice; setting limits with monitoring to ensure compliance; using rewards; or spending time with the children.

Physical Activity and Inactivity in Prevention of Childhood Obesity

Caregivers recognized the psychological and physiological consequences of childhood obesity and the need for medical referral and weight control measures. Participants identified different environmental and societal factors related to overweight status among children. Frequent social gatherings, time spent at school, food availability and accessibility, media, cultural beliefs and practices, and physical activity are factors that are perceived to interact with childhood obesity. Participants in all the groups identified the importance of physical activity in preventing childhood obesity and reducing mortality.

Filipino participants identified the following factors related to children not being overweight (a) genetics, (b) fondness for activities, (c) ability to burn body fat, (d) higher activity level, (e) parental involvement in ensuring that children play for at least 2 hours per day, (f) child's preference for swimming, (g) food choices, and (h) eating the right amount and type of food. With regards to slim children, Carolinian participants suggested that caregivers should seek medical assistance in diagnosing the problem. Specifically, it was suggested that the following issues be carefully examined (a) quantity of food consumed, (b) genetic make-up, and/or (c) potential health problems. With regards to obese children, caregivers suggested that they might need more attention and active parental involvement.

Caregivers also recognized the role of diet and physical activity and inactivity in overweight and obesity. With regards to physical activity and inactivity, Trembley and William (2003) found that children's BMI was negatively associated with organized and unorganized Strategies identified by the Filipino participants emphasized the role of caregivers in controlling the child's food. Among the Chamorro group, caregivers who had sought medical assistance for overweight children indicated that they manage overweight children by limiting certain foods, while increasing physical activity. All the focus group participants, indicating that more active children are less overweight, emphatically reported the relationship of weight and activity. Fathers also noted the importance of children's activity in maintaining their weight, especially with the changing time.

In general the extended family, health care providers, community members, and personal experience all seemed to influence caregivers' awareness and understanding of children's weight status. There is a common belief that children's individual characteristic determines their weight status. Although parents believe that individual characteristics determine their child's weight status, most recognize specific factors that interact with these characteristics. These include genetic makeup, physiology and metabolism, activity level, and dietary intake. The caregivers reported individual weight differences were influenced by activity level. These included children who are predisposed to being active or inactive, those who are generally interested in activities, and those whose parents ensure daily play.

Physical activity as an intervention in helping children normalize their weight status was indicated by caregivers. Additionally, participants in the Chamorro and Carolinian group emphasized the role of parents in increasing children's physical activity. According to Kimm et al. (2002), physical activity levels among children declines with increasing age mainly due to changes in children's preference for physical activity and frequency of parents transporting children to activity locations. Therefore, the need for reinforcers (incentives) that encourages children to engage in physical activity, especially vigorous or high-intensity activities are indicated (Sallis et al., 1999). Among the participants in the father's group, the need to tell children to participate in physical activity, enrolling them in gyms so they can be encouraged to be active, and promising them a reward for engaging in physical activity were reported.

Arline, Salbe, Weyer, Lindsay, Ravussin, and Tataranni (2002) found that among Pima Indians early childhood obesity at age five was the foremost predictor of childhood obesity at age ten. Based on these findings, the researchers emphasized the importance of initiating childhood obesity prevention strategies in early childhood. Sociocultural and familial differences were observed in strategies used for the prevention and control of underweight and overweight children among the caregivers in this study. Most strategies focused on overweight status, even though caregivers seemed concerned with underweight status as well.

With regards to preventing overweight status, participants in the father's group suggested monitoring and telling children to control their intake, while subjects in the Chamorro group suggested engaging children in sports. The participants in the Filipino group emphasized the role of diet and exercise in the prevention of overweight status in children. This knowledge of the main theory of the law of thermodynamics that indicates energy intake should balance with energy expenditure can help in understanding the role of physical activity and exercise interventions in the prevention of childhood obesity (Roberts, 2000).

Caregivers had similar strategies for controlling overweight status in children. Among the Chamorro group, strategies included (a) encouraging overweight children to go to the gym to work out, (b) telling children to do more activities like jogging, running and walking, (c) encouraging slightly overweight children to get involved in sports and fitness programs, (d) encouraging children to go out biking, and (e) limiting their intake and offering them dinner far in advance of bedtime. Additionally, caregivers noted that when using medical recommendations to help overweight children, adjustments might have to be made to meet individual family needs.

The emphasis on physical activity in the prevention and control of childhood obesity among the study participants is supported by scientific research. Roberts (2000) suggests that general endurance training and sustained activities that use large muscles are among strategies that are recommended in the prevention and control of obesity. In a study of thirty-five children, increases in maximal oxygen uptake (and indicator of aerobic fitness) was observed as a result of a general endurance training program which included three, ninety-minute weekly sessions at an intensity of more than 80% of the maximum heart rate (Obert, Mandigouts, Nottin, Vinet, N'Guyen, & Lecoq, 2003). Furthermore, the effectiveness of scheduled endurance training programs focuses on type, intensity, frequency, and duration of the exercise (Roberts, 2000). With regard to type, sustained activities such as swimming, jogging, aerobic dance, and other similar activities that use large muscle groups are indicated. Because measuring children's heart rate may not be feasible, there may be other ways of measuring the intensity of exercise, such as the Borg Scale adapted to children. Borg Scale is a rating system that the individual uses to indicate their perceived level of exertion. The scale is from six to twenty with seven indicating very, very light exertion, and nineteen indicating very, very hard exertion. However, a newer scale has been devised referred to as the Children's OMNI Scale that utilizes pictures, numbers (0-10) and different verbal descriptors (not tired at all - very, very tired) of exertion. The use of this perceived exertion scale might be more appropriate than using of the Borg scale that was developed to be used with adults (Robertson, 2004). As for frequency and duration, Roberts (2000) recommends two to three days of thirty to forty minute sessions per week. Additionally, as with other activities, children's physiological conditions, previous experience and ability to perform certain activities should be taken into consideration prior to engaging in endurance training programs.

With regards to chronic disease prevention, physical activity and dietary intervention were noted. The participants in all the groups emphasized the importance of exercise, especially because physical activity was seen as a more culturally acceptable behavior to adopt than restricting foods through dietary changes. According to Bruss et al. (2003), dietary intake of children elicits a strong emotional response among caregivers in this population. Because of the perceived seriousness of the magnitude of chronic diseases, strategies identified by fathers, in the prevention of chronic diseases focused on less culturally acceptable behavior such as restricting and monitoring the diet of overweight children in families with a history of diabetes. Participants in this group also indicated that everyone should take responsibility for this matter and work together to support and role model the child.

Differences among male and female participants were observed in the instruction of children and assistance provided in adopting behaviors related to the prevention of childhood obesity and chronic diseases. Male participants reported to use social control through verbal messages and injunctions, while females reported to obtain compliance by active parental involvement through control and training. Although verbal messages were the primary manner in instructing children, fathers also saw a role for older children in setting examples for their younger siblings and engaging overweight children in more activities around the house. Fathers also reported that parents needed to inform their overweight children about their weight and teach them about the consequences of being overweight. Female participants believed that overweight children would benefit from parental involvement especially with regards to reducing the purchase of fatty foods. In addition to diet, mothers also identified the role of exercise and physical activity in preventing childhood overweight and obesity

Among participants sociocultural beliefs related to weight normalcy were observed. This is an important finding in the design of nutrition education intervention programs. For instance, female participants in the Chamorro group indicated that fat is perceived as wealth and being fat and large is a representation of it. Both Chamorro and Carolinian participants indicated that culturally people prefer to see children as being fat. Underweight status among children seems to be a more sensitive issue than obesity. According to Bruss et al. (2003), these attitudes may positively or negatively influence caregivers' behavior toward children's weight status.

Analysis of data also suggests that different groups within the community reinforce caregivers' perception of weight normalcy. Differences were seen among the different ethnic groups in communicating acceptable weight status. Informal network which involves the immediate and extended family through a socially constructed conception of weight communicate weight normalcy messages to caregivers. Additionally, certain ethnic groups rely on the formal network which involves the doctors and nutritionists for weight status information. Filipino participants recognized the doctor as a more accurate source of information on appropriate weight status and advice than another parent. In addition to doctors, Filipino participants also rely on nutritionists and regular annual medical check up to learn about the child's weight status. Grandmothers, aunts/uncles, and wives were reported as those that influence fathers' perception of their child's weight status. Additionally, fathers reported that within the Chamorro culture there is a familial hierarchy that allows them to feel comfortable in advising their nieces and nephews in regards to weight control measures. However, advising their friends was seen as an intrusion. Carolinian participants identified both the family and doctors in influencing their perception of their child's weight status. Among the Carolinians, husbands were also seen as influencing primary caregivers' perception of child's weight status. Chamorro female participants reported that their mother-in-law and their husbands also influence their perception of their child's weight status. Carolinian and Filipino participants reported to rely on medical sources of weight assessment information in addition to using their own personal judgment. Visual assessment of child's weight, height and weight charts, personal feeling, and child fitting into clothes were used by caregivers to formulate personal judgment on child's weight status. With regards to caregivers' source of information on children's weight normalcy, Anjali et al. (2001) found that WIC mothers used their own perception to establish weight normalcy with disregard to weight status information offered by health professionals.

The potential for developing "health promoting" communities exists in most communities as long as there is a process to develop and apply strategies suitable to that community (Kickbusch & O'Byrne, 1997). Towards this process, previous research has shown the importance of engaging community members in identifying their own needs and finding solutions to their own problems (Matomora, 1989). Caregivers identified ways that the community might support them in preventing childhood obesity. Specifically, the focus of these strategies was on education and environment. With regards to environment, caregivers mainly focused on strategies to increase physical activity opportunities for families, which is in accord with recommendations from CDC (2003) and PAHO (2002). These included more public exercise places, such as gyms and outdoor places that promote family activity; government's assistance with village-based community centers specifically with obtaining donated exercise equipments from local gyms; making physical activity programs accessible and free to the public; and ensuring adequate advertisement of such activities for the public. Additionally, caregivers focused on challenges faced with food related issues. One such issue was the perceived higher cost of purchasing healthier foods, while another issue was the sociocultural characteristic of the community which offers frequently held social gatherings (parties) that involve generous food offerings and hospitality. In addition to making physical activity more accessible to the families, caregivers identified the need for nutrition education topics related to children. These include (a) food substitution, (b) amount of food needed by children, (c) additional knowledge of foods, (d) nutrients, (e) strength building foods, and (f) food preparation.

Caregivers identified four potential sources of information in the education of families. These include (a) community-based education sessions, (b) media, (c) published literature, and (d) health care professionals. The participants discussed the venue and format of the community-based sessions. The village-based community centers were identified as a place where classes could be offered to families. Caregivers found the focus group format effective and suggested using it in conducting nightly classes for the families in the village. For those unable to leave their home, it was suggested that educational programs be offered on cable station. Participants in the Chamorro group also reported accessing nutrition education information through US broadcast radio programs, while learning about community-based workshops through the local radio stations. Among the Filipino participants nutrition information was accessed through newspapers, books, and government programs.

Caregivers suggested offering free magazines with practical useful information for parents such as recommended vegetables and other nutritious foods. The need to make published health information accessible to the community outside of health care clinics was also identified by the participants. Caregivers suggested churches, grocery stores and office waiting areas as places were such information can be made accessible to families. Also, the schools were identified as a place where information can be sent home to the children. Filipino participants emphasized the importance of the health care professionals as a reliable source of information for the families. Because doctors are perceived as more accurate on diagnosing appropriate weight status and providing medical advice, physicians were identified as sources of information for families who have concerns with their children's weight status. Additionally, participants stated that one way families might access health care professionals is through community-based workshops that are offered by the public health agency. Caregivers indicated that they find the information from the public health sector helpful and accessible.

Finally, because of the devastating consequences of chronic diseases such as Type II diabetes, families in the CNMI are facing major lifestyle choices (CNMI National Food and Nutrition Policy and Ten-Year Plan of Action, 1996). Over the past two decades the CNMI community has become more aware of these issues. Today, there is a general concern in the community regarding the effect of these nutrition problems on individuals and families. Results of this study suggest that families may be aware of the role of diet and activity in chronic diseases. However, they may need other interventions, such as home visits made by health professionals. Caregivers expressed that information and awareness may not be adequate for bringing about lifestyle changes and suggested the need for skill building and repeated follow-up activities. This finding supports the intended purpose of public health nutrition programs, which are designed to bring about a specific health outcome and/or behavior change. Achieving such outcomes in most instances require long-term endeavors with multiple influences. According to Center for Disease Control (CDC) guidelines, intervention programs that work are not just a single episode such as a video or guest speakers, rather they are complete programs (Collins, Robin, Wooley, Fenley, Hunt, Taylor, Haber, & Kolbe, 2002). Also, intervention studies suggest that although knowledge acquisition is necessary, it is not sufficient to promote behavior change. The literature further suggests that effective interventions resulting in behavior change require a series of sessions that include awareness, skill building and problem solving activities (Boyle, 2003). Therefore, it can be concluded that behavior change in the context of public health programs require knowledge along with adequate skill building activities in making informed decision and bringing about the needed change (Miller, Edwards, Kissling, & Sanville, 2002). Other education considerations identified by caregivers were to offer information in the vernacular as indicated by the participants in the Filipino group. Additionally, caregivers also identified the need for visiting schools and training the school community.

Conclusion

Childhood obesity is a growing epidemic and its prevention is beneficial to the individual, family, and society (Dwyer, Stone, Yang, Webber, Must, Feldman, Nader, Perry, Parcel, 2000). The financial cost of overweight and obesity is a burden carried by the individual and society (Wolf & Colditz, 1998). This growing global epidemic, poses a future challenge for developing nations that do not have the economic resources to carry the burden of the health complications from this preventable condition (World Development Indicators, 2001). Identifying effective intervention strategies in the prevention of childhood obesity is a necessary component of public health nutrition and health education program planning and implementation. It requires investigation of the problems of obesity using different disciplines to study the characteristics of the populations most affected by obesity. Collaborative interdisciplinary approaches to the study of childhood obesity are more relevant today than ever before. Gaining a deeper understanding of the sociocultural factors in influencing primary care giver practices associated with childhood obesity is needed in developing target nutrition intervention strategies in the prevention of this condition. The literature lacks information with regards to the sociocultural influences of the primary care giver on childhood obesity. Understanding the relationship of the primary care giver's level of cultural identity or connectedness to a cultural set of norms, values and beliefs related to childhood obesity and its different factors is necessary.

Over the past two decades, although, there has not been sufficient time for a major genetic shift in the general population, there are dramatic increases in childhood and adult obesity (Troiano et al, 1995), suggesting a more prominent role due to environmental factors. However, it is not clear why some communities have seen a more intense increase than others have. Of increasing concern is the marked presence of childhood obesity among African Americans, Native Americans and Hispanics in the US (Jackson, 1993; Troiano et al., 1995; Goran, 2001; Dwyer et al., 2000). Information on Pacific Islanders in the US is limited. However, in general, more economically developed Pacific Island nations have experienced an increase in overweight and obesity in their communities with rates similar to those in US Native American populations (Popkin & Doak, 1998). Native American of North America may have some of the highest rates of overweight and obesity (Potvin, Desrosiers, Trifonopoulos, Leduc, Rivard, Macaulay, & Paradis, G., 1999). The increasing rates of childhood obesity among ethnic minority populations in the US suggest the potential influence of culture/ethnicity and family on childhood obesity.

This study used qualitative methods to present a fresh perspective on factors related to childhood obesity. It examined value and belief systems of people with regards to physical activity and inactivity and how they are revealed in sociocultural and familial factors related to childhood obesity. Moreover, it offers an insight into caregivers' perception, attitude and knowledge of physical activity and inactivity, which are associated with childhood obesity. Caregivers have an important role in promoting physical activity and limiting physical inactivity in 6-10 year old children. In under-studied communities that have experienced increasing rates of childhood obesity, it is necessary to obtain baseline information with regards to sociocultural and familial factors in order to design more effective and targeted programs.

Findings from this study offer practical theories for use by educators in designing effective education programs for use in multiethnic settings. Despite an increasing number of education intervention programs, epidemiological studies suggest a rapid increase in childhood obesity. Historically, strategies have focused on treating obesity as a medical disorder through prescriptions for less television viewing, more exercise, reduced fat intake, and fewer high calorie snack foods. These findings have important implications for health care professionals in the US and globally specifically in the prevention of childhood obesity.

In summary, findings from this study provides a rich point of analysis for scholars interested in exploring issues central to health promotion, family dynamics, physical fitness, and cultural studies. Major issues were identified that call for additional investigation. For instance, the impact of the health care provider and the community in promoting and supporting an environment that promotes physical activity in ethnically diverse populations need further investigation. Also, because the goal of health promotion is behavior modification, the level of cultural competence (sensitivity to sociocultural and familial factors related to childhood obesity) among health care professionals in community-based intervention programs needs further examination. It is important that communities begin to follow physical activity recommendations (Strong et. al, 2005) made based upon the best evidence currently available. However, in implementing these recommendations public health officials need to recognize the inherent and unique cultural influences that each community may impose that might offer additional barriers to behavior change.

References

Aboud, F.E., Christina, J. (1970). Development of ethnic identity. In Eckensberger, L., Poortinga, Y., Lonner, W.J. (Eds.), *Cross-cultural contributions to Psychology*, Swets and Zeitlinger, Lisse.

Andersen, R. E., Crespo, C. J., Bartlett, S. J., Cheskin L. J., Pratt, M. (1998). Relationship of physical activity and television watching with body weight and level of fatness among children. *Journal of American Medical Association,* **279**, 12, 1561-1567.

Andersen, D. R., Field, D. E., Collins, P.A., Lorch, P. & Nathan, J.G. (1985). Estimates of young children's time with television: a methodological comparison of parent reports with time-lapse video home observation. *Child Development,* **56**, 1345-1357.

Anjali, J., Sherman, S.N., Chamberlin, L.A., Carter, Y., Powers, S.W., Whitaker, R.C. (2001). Why don't low-income mothers worry about their preschoolers being overweight? *Pediatrics*, **107**, 5, 1138-1146.

Arline, D., Salbe, A. D., Weyer, C., Lindsay, R. S., Ravussin, E., & Tataranni, P. A. (2002). Assessing risk factors for obesity between childhood and adolescence: I. Birth weight, childhood adiposity, parental obesity, insulin, and leptin. *Pediatrics,* **110**, 299-306.

Arluk, S.L., Branch, J.D., Swain, D.P. & Dowling, E.A. (2003). Childhood obesity's relationship to time spent in sedentary behavior. *Military Medicine,* **168**, 7, 583-586.

Bailey, R. C., Olson, J., Pepper, S. L., Porszaz, J., Barstow, T. J., & Cooper, D. M. (1995). The level and tempo of children's physical activities: An observational study. *Medicine and Science in Sport and Exercise*. **27**, 1033-1041.

Baranowski, T., Nader, P. R., Dunn, K., & Vanderpool, N. A. (1982). Family self-help: Promoting changes in health behavior. *Journal of Communication,* **32**(3), 161-172.

Baughcum, A.E., Burklow, K.A., Deeks, C.M., Powers, S.W., Whitaker, R.C. (1998). Maternal feeding practices and childhood obesity: a focus group study of low-income mothers. *Archives of Pediatrics and Adolescent Medicine*, **152**(10): 1010-1014.

Baughcum, A.E., Chamberlin, L.A., Deeks, C.M., Powers, S.W., Whitaker, RC. (2000). Maternal perceptions of overweight preschool children. *Pediatrics,* **106**, 1380-1386.

Bogden, R. C., & Biklen, S. K. (1998). *Qualitative Research for Education: An Introduction to Theory and Methods*. Allyn and Bacon, MA: A Viacom Company.

Bouchard, C. (1997). Obesity in adulthood - The importance of childhood and parental obesity. *New England Journal of Medicine,* **337**, 926-927.

Boyle, M. (2003). Community Nutrition in Action: an entrepreneurial approach. Belmont, CA: Wadsworth.

Bruss, M. B., Morris, J. R., & Dannison, L. (2003). Prevention of childhood obesity: Sociocultural and familial factors. *Journal of American Dietetic Association,* **103**, 1042-1045.

Center for Disease Control (CDC). National Center for Chronic Disease Prevention and Health Promotion, *Nutrition and Physical Activity*. http://www.cdc.gov/nccdphp/dnpa/obesity/faq.htm#adults. Page last updated December 8, 2003.

Clarke, W.R., Lauer, R.M. Does childhood obesity track into adulthood? (1993). *Critical Reviews in Food Science and Nutrition*, **33**(4-5): 423-430.

Collins, J., Robin, L., Wooley, S., Fenley, D., Hunt, P., Taylor, J., Haber, D., & Kolbe, L. (2002). Programs-that-work: CDC's guide to effective programs that reduce health-risk behavior of youth. *Journal of School Health,* **72** (3), 93-99.

CNMI Census, 2000.

CNMI National Food and Nutrition Policy and Ten-Year Plan of Action. (1996). Prepared and submitted by the CNMI National Food and Nutrition Advisory

Council in collaboration with the World Health Organization.

CNMI Statistical Yearbook (1999).

Crespo, C. J., Smit, E., Troiano, R. P., Bartlett, S. J., Macera, C. A., & Andersen, R. E. (2001). Television watching, energy intake, and obesity in US children: results from the third National Health and Nutrition Examination Survey, 1988-1994. *Archives of Pediatrics & Adolescent Medicine,* **155**(3), 360-365.

Creswell, J. W. (1998). *Qualitative Inquiry and Research Design: Choosing Among Five Traditions.* CA: Sage Publications.

Cutting, T.M., Fisher, J.O., Grimm-Thomas, K., Birch, L.L. (1999). Like mother, like daughter: familial patterns of overweight are mediated by mother's dietary disinhibition. *American Journal of Clinical Nutrition,* **69**, 608-613.

Drewnowski, A. Popkin, B.M. (1997). The Nutrition Transition: New Trends in the Global Diet. *Nutrition Reviews,* **55** (2), 31-43.

Dwyer, J.T., Stone, E.J., Yang, M., Webber L.S., Must, A., Feldman, H.A., Nader, P.R., Perry, C.L., Parcel, G.S. (2000). Prevalence of marked overweight and obesity in a multiethnic pediatric population: findings from the Child and Adolescent Trial for Cardiovascular Health (CATCH) study. *Journal of the American Dietetic Association,* **100** (10), 1149-1154.

Ernst, M. P., & Pangrazi, R. P. (1999). Effects of a physical activity program on children's activity levels and attraction to physical activity. *Pediatric Exercise Science*, **11**, 393-405.

Frideres, J., Goldenberg, S. (1982). Ethnic identity: myth and reality in Western Canada. *International Journal of Intercultural Relations*, **6**, 137-151.

Gabel, S., Lutz, S. (2000). Household, parent, and child contributions to childhood obesity. *Family Relations,* **49**(3), 293-300.

Garn, S.M., Clark, D.C. (1976). Trends in fatness and the origins of obesity. *Pediatrics,* **57**(4), 443-456.

Gavarry, O. (2003). Habitual Physical Activity in Children and Adolescents during School and Free Days. *Medicine and Science in Sports and Exercise,* **35** (3), 525-531.

Goran, M.I. (2001). Metabolic precursors and effects of obesity in children: a decade of progress, 1990-1999. *American Journal of Clinical Nutrition,* **73**(2), 158-171.

Gortmaker, S. L., Cheung, L. W., Peterson, K., E., Chomitz, G., Cradle, J. H., Dart, H.,

Fox, M. K., Bullock, R. B., Sobol, A. M., Colditz, G., Field, A. E. & Laird, N. (1999). Impact of a school-based interdisciplinary intervention on diet and physical activity among urban primary school children. *Archives of Pediatrics and Adolescent Medicine*, **153** (9), 975- 983.

Hovell, M. F., Sallis, J. F., Kolody, B., & Mckenzie, T. L. (1999). Children's physical activity choices: a developmental analysis of gender, intensity levels, and time. *Pediatric Exercise Science*, **11**, 158-168.

International Obesity Task Force. Managing the global epidemic of obesity. Report of WHO Consultation on Obesity. Geneva, June 5-7, 1997. Geneva: World Health Organization.

Kickbusch, I., & O'Byrne, D. (1997). Promoting health where the people are. *World Health,* May/June, 4-5.

Jackson, M. Y. (1993). Height, weight, and body mass index of American Indian schoolchildren, 1990-1991. *Journal of the American Dietetic Association,* **93**(10), 1136-1140.

Janz, K. F., Levy, S. M., Burns, T. L., Torner, J. C., Willing, M. C. & Warren, J. J. (2002). Fatness, physical activity, and television viewing in children during the adiposity rebound period: The Iowa Bone Development Study. *Preventive Medicine,* **35**, 563-571.

Kimm, S.Y., Glynn, N.W., Kriska, A.M., Barton, B.A., Kronsberg, S.S., Daniels, S.R., Crawford, P.B., Sabry, Z. I., Liu, K. (2002). Decline in physical activity in black girls and white girls during adolescence. *New England Journal of Medicine,* **347** (10), 709-715.

Klesges, R.C., Klesges, L.M., Eck, L.H., Shelton, M. (1995). A longitudinal analysis of accelerated weight gain in preschool children. *Pediatrics,* **95** (1), 126-130.

Krathwohl, D. R. (1998). *Methods of Educational and Social Science Research: An Integrated Approach* (2nd ed.). New York: Longman.

Kumanyika, S. (1993). Ethnicity and obesity development in children. *Annals of the New York Academy of Sciences,* **699**, 81-90.

Lewis, B.A., Marcus, B.H., Pate, R.R. & Dunn, A.L. (2002). Psychological mediators of physical activity behavior among adult and children. *American Journal of Preventive Medicine,* **23** (2S), 26-35.

Mandigo, J.L. & Thompson, L.P. (1998). Go with their flow: How flow theory can help practitioners to intrinsically motivate children to be physically active. *The Physical Educator,* **55** (3), 145-159.

Maslow, A.H. (1954). *Motivation and personality.* New York: Harper & Row.

Matomora, M. K. S. (1989). A people-centered approach to primary health care Implementation in Mvumi, Tanzania. *Social Science & Medicine,* **28** (10), 1031-1038.

Miller, C. K., Edwards, L., Kissling, G., Sanville, L. (2002). Evaluation of a theory-based nutrition intervention for older adults with diabetes mellitus. *Journal of the American Dietetic Association,* **102**, 1069-1074, 1079-1081.

Moore, L.L., Gao, D., Bradlee, L., Cupples, L.A., Sundarajan-Ramamurti, A., Proctor, M.H., Hood, M.Y., Singer, M.R. & Ellison, R.C. (2003). Does early physical activity predict body fat change throughout life? *Preventive Medicine,* **37**, 10-17.

Mota, J., & Queiros, P. (1996). Children's behavior: physical activity regarding parents' perception vs. children's activity. *International Review for the Sociology of Sport,* **31**, 173-178.

Myers, S. & Vargas, Z. (2000). Parental perceptions of the preschool obese child. *Pediatric Nursing,* **26**, i1, 23.

National Center for Chronic Disease Prevention and Health Promotion. (1999). Patterns and trends in physical activity, 200-201.

National Institute of Health. (1998). Clinical Guidelines on the identification, evaluation, and treatment of overweight and obesity in adults -- the evidence report. *Obesity Research,* 6(supplemental 2), 51S-209S.

Obert, P., Mandigouts, S., Nottin, S., Vinet, A., N'Guyen, L. D., & Lecoq, A. M. (2003). Cardiovascular responses to endurance training in children: effect of gender. *European Journal of Clinical Investigation*, **33** (3), 199-208.

O'Loughlin, J.O., Paradis, G., Meshefedjian, G., Gray-Donald, K. (2000). A five-year trend of increasing obesity among elementary schoolchildren in multiethnic, low-income, inner city neighborhoods in Montreal, Canada. *International Journal of Obesity,* **24**, 1176-1182.

Pan American Health Organization (PAHO), Physical Activity Fact Sheet Series 4 of 5Page 2 of 2 PAHO, January 2002, http://www.paho.org/English/HPP/HPN/whd2002factsheet4.pdf.

Pangrazi, R. P., Beighle, A., Vehige, T., & Vack, C. (2003). Impact of Promoting Lifestyle Activity for Youth (PLAY) on children's physical activity. *Journal of School Health,* **73**(8), 317-321

Patton, M. Q. (1990). *Qualitative evaluation and research methods*, 2nd. ed. Newbury Park, CA: Sage Publications.

Phinney, J. S. (1990). Ethnic identity in adolescents and adults: Review of research. *Psychological Bulletin,* **108**, 499-514.

Pinhey, T.K., Rubenstein, D.H., Colfax, R.S. (1997). Overweight and happiness: the reflected self-appraisal hypothesis reconsidered. *Social Science Quarterly*, **78**(3), 747-755.

Popkin, B.M., Doak, C.M. (1998). The obesity epidemic is a worldwide phenomenon. *Nutrition Reviews,* **56** (4), 106-114.

Potvin, L., Desrosiers, S., Trifonopoulos, M., Leduc, N., Rivard, M., Macaulay, A. C., & Paradis, G. (1999). Anthropometric characteristics of Mohawk children aged 6 to 11 years: a population perspective. *Journal of the American Dietetic Association,* **99**(8), 955-961.

Powdermaker, H. (1997). An anthropological approach to the problem of obesity. In C. Counihan & P. Van Esterik (Eds.), *Food and culture: A reader* (pp. 203-210). New York: Routledge.

Rimal, R. N., & Flora, J. A. (1998). Bidirectional familial influences in dietary behavior: Test of a model of campaign influences. *Human Communication Research,* **24**(4), 610-637.

Roberts, S.O. (2000). The role of physical activity in the prevention and treatment of childhood obesity. *Pediatric Nursing*, (**26**), 33–43.

Robertson, R. J. (2004). Perceived exertion for practitioners. Human Kinetics, IL: Champaign.

Rosenthal, D.A., Feldman, S.S. (1992). The nature and stability of ethnic identity in Chinese youth: effects of length of residence in two cultural contexts. *Journal of Cross-cultural Psychology*, **23**(2), 214-227.

Ross, C.E., Mirowsky, J. (1983). Social epidemiology of overweight: a substantive and methodological investigation. *Journal of Health and Social Behavior,* **24** (3), 288-298.

Rush, E. C. (2003). Body composition and physical activity in New Zealand Maori, Pacific and European children aged 5-14 years. *The British Journal of Nutrition,* **90** (6), 1133-1139.

Sallis, J.F. & Owen, N. (1999). Physical activity and behavioral medicine. Thousand Oakes, CA: Sage, pp. 8-9:128-133, 167-171.

Sallis, J.F., Alcaraz, J.E., McKenzie, T.L. & Hovell, M.F. (1999). Predictors of change in children's physical activity over 20 months: Variations by gender and level of adiposity. *American Journal of Preventive Medicine,* **16** (3), 222-229.

Sallis, J.F., Prochaska, J. & Taylor, W.C. (2000). A review of correlates of physical activity for children and adolescents. *Medicine and Science in Sports and Exercise,* **32** (5), 963-975.

Sallis, J.F. & Saelens, B.E. (2000). Assessment of physical activity by self-report: status, limitations, and future directions. *Research Quarterly for Exercise and Sport,* **71** (2 suppl), 1-14.

Serdula, M.K., Ivery, D., Coates, R.J., Freedman, D.S., Williamson, D.F., Byers, T. (1993) Do obese children become obese adults? A review of the literature. *Preventive Medicine,* **22**, 167-177.

Stephens, M. (2002). Children, physical activity and public health: another call to action. *American family physicians*, **65**, 6, 1033-1034.

Strauss, R. S., & Pollack, H. A. (2001). Epidemic increase in childhood overweight, 1986-1998. The *journal of the American Medical Association,* **286** (22), 2845-2848.

Strong, W.B., Malina, R.M., Blimkie C.J.R., Daniels, S.R., et al. (2005). Evidence based physical activity for school-age youth. *The Journal of Pediatrics,* **146**(6):732-737.

Tardy, R. W., & Hale, C. L. (1998b). Getting "plugged in": A network analysis of health-information seeking among "stay-at-home moms." *Communication Monographs,* **65**(4), 336-357.

Tremblay, M.S. & Williams, J.D. (2003). Is the Canadian childhood obesity epidemic related to physical inactivity? *International Journal of Obesity and Related Metabolic Disorders,* **27** (9), 1100-1105.

Troiano, R.P., Flegal, K.M., Kuczmarski, R.J., Campbell, S.M., Johnson, C.L. (1995). Overweight prevalence and trends for children and adolescents. The National Health and nutrition Examination Surveys, 1963 to 1991. *Archives of Pediatrics and Adolescent Medicine,* **149**(10): 1085-1091.

Trost, S.G., Sirard, J.R., Dowda, M., Pfeiffer, K.A. & Pate, R.R. (2003). Physical activity in overweight and nonoverweight preschool children. *International Journal of Obesity and Related Metabolic Disorders,* **27** (7), 834-839.

Tsgadi, C., Taxildaris, K., Laparidis, K., & Michalopoulou, M. (2002). Assessing physical activity and physical characteristics of prepubescent children in Greece. *The Physical Educator,* **59** (2), 75-82.

US Census Bureau, 2000.

U.S. Department of Health and Human Services. (1996). Physical *activity and health: a report of the Surgeon General.* Atlanta: U.S. Department of Health and Human Services, Centers for Disease Control and Prevention National Center for Chronic Disease Prevention and Health Promotion.

Utter, J., Neumark-Sztainer, D., Jeffery, R. & Story, M. (2003). Couch potatoes or French fries: Are sedentary behaviors associated with body mass index, physical activity, and dietary behaviors among adolescents? *Journal of American Dietetic Association,* **103** (10), 1298-1305.

Welk, G. J. (2000). Physical activity protects against the health risks of obesity. President's Council on Physical Fitness and Sports. *Research Digest,* **3**(12), 1-6.

Wertsch, J. V. (1991). *Voices of the mind: A sociocultural approach to mediate action.* Cambridge, MA: Harvard University Press.

Whitaker, R.C., Pepe, M.S., Wright, J.A., Seidel, K.D., Dietz, W.H. (1998). Early Adiposity rebound and the risk of adult obesity. *Pediatrics,* **101** (3), 1-6.

Whitaker, R.C., Wright, J.A., Pepe, M.S., Seidel, K.D., Dietz, W.H. (1997). Predicting obesity in young adulthood from childhood and parental obesity. *New England Journal of Medicine,* **337**, 869-873.

Wilkinson, W. K. & Migotsky, C. P. (1994). A factor analytic study of epistemic style inventories. *Journal of Psychology,* **128**, 499 - 516.

Wolf, A.M., Colditz, G.A. (1998). Current estimates of the economic cost of obesity in The United States. *Obesity Research,* **6**(2), 97-106

World Development Indicators. (2001). World Bank Organization.

INDEX

A

academic performance, 28
academics, 10
acceptance, 30, 140, 156, 157, 158, 159, 160, 162, 163, 165, 166, 167, 205
access, 2, 19, 95, 106, 113, 162, 168, 204, 206, 228, 235, 241, 246
accounting, 72
acculturation, 7, 202
accumulation, 6, 7, 12
accuracy, 17, 54, 214
achievement, 118
acid, 129, 158, 165, 177
activity level, 11, 32, 186, 206, 219, 230, 231, 239, 243, 250
adaptation, 19, 133, 176
addiction, 227
adipocyte, 132, 133, 177
adipose, 6, 7, 24, 72, 73, 110, 128, 129, 133, 170, 177
adipose tissue, 6, 7, 24, 72, 73, 110, 128, 129, 133, 170, 177
adiposity, vii, 1, 8, 15, 16, 17, 19, 27, 35, 40, 72, 73, 84, 85, 94, 96, 123, 135, 136, 137, 171, 182, 205, 209, 210, 249, 251, 253
adjustment, 24, 72, 174
adolescence, ix, x, 8, 9, 11, 17, 20, 22, 23, 29, 33, 35, 40, 48, 49, 78, 89, 90, 93, 96, 99, 121, 135, 136, 137, 179, 184, 192, 196, 197, 210, 249, 251
adolescent boys, ix, 74, 89, 92, 93, 94, 95
adolescent female, 3, 25
adolescents, viii, ix, x, 7, 9, 17, 20, 28, 30, 36, 37, 39, 43, 44, 48, 49, 67, 69, 71, 74, 75, 77, 78, 79, 80, 81, 82, 83, 84, 85, 86, 87, 89, 90, 91, 92, 93, 94, 95, 96, 97, 99, 100, 101, 103, 104, 106, 107, 108, 111, 113, 114, 115, 116, 117, 118, 119, 120, 121, 122, 123, 124, 125, 135, 136, 137, 174, 182, 183, 184, 192, 193, 194, 196, 197, 198, 252, 253
adrenal insufficiency, 132
adult obesity, 6, 10, 23, 31, 52, 53, 54, 70, 72, 85, 141, 183, 197, 200, 201, 204, 254
adult population, 67, 75, 124, 135
adulthood, vii, ix, 2, 6, 8, 9, 13, 17, 22, 27, 29, 40, 49, 70, 71, 72, 74, 82, 89, 90, 93, 111, 112, 125, 126, 131, 132, 155, 182, 197, 205, 249, 250, 254
adults, 2, 6, 7, 8, 9, 10, 16, 17, 18, 19, 20, 27, 28, 31, 32, 35, 38, 41, 42, 44, 46, 47, 53, 67, 71, 82, 83, 85, 90, 97, 101, 109, 116, 126, 140, 170, 175, 176, 182, 184, 192, 194, 200, 210, 223, 233, 244, 249, 251, 252, 253
advertisements, 115, 119, 121, 125, 161, 162, 167, 181
advertising, 119, 181, 193, 196
advocacy, 118
aetiology, 141, 148, 178
affect, 8, 10, 17, 24, 26, 43, 54, 71, 73, 120, 132, 162, 163, 204, 226, 240
Africa, vii, viii, 1, 2, 3, 4, 5, 7, 8, 10, 11, 13, 14, 15, 16, 17, 18, 20, 21, 22, 23, 25, 27, 28, 29, 30, 31, 32, 36, 41, 42, 43, 46, 47, 48, 50, 51, 54, 56, 57, 58, 59, 60, 61, 62, 63, 64, 65, 66, 67, 87, 102, 119, 122, 173
African Americans, 122, 205
Afrikaans, 30
afternoon, 220, 225
age, viii, ix, 2, 3, 6, 7, 8, 9, 11, 13, 15, 16, 17, 18, 19, 20, 21, 22, 23, 24, 25, 26, 27, 28, 30, 31, 32, 36, 37, 42, 44, 47, 49, 52, 58, 69, 70, 71, 73, 75, 76, 77, 78, 79, 89, 91, 93, 97, 100, 102, 103, 110, 118, 120, 123, 126, 131, 137, 141, 143, 156, 157, 158, 160, 163, 165, 170, 173, 174, 175, 182, 183, 184, 185, 187, 188, 190, 197, 202, 203, 204, 208, 209, 210, 213, 215, 217, 218, 219, 231, 238, 243, 253
agent, 128

agricultural sector, 57
agriculture, 29
alcohol, 109
alertness, 221
alternative, 150, 165
alternatives, 193
alters, 149, 166
amino acids, 167
amniotic fluid, 133, 136, 166
amphetamines, 192
amputation, 71
anemia, 13, 48
animals, 14, 73, 178
anorexia, 5, 123, 129, 178, 195
anorexia nervosa, 178, 195
anxiety, ix, 89, 110, 170, 202
appendix, 3, 33
appetite, xi, 14, 42, 73, 110, 129, 132, 133, 138, 169, 177, 178, 179, 180, 195, 205, 226, 240
Arab countries, viii, 70, 79, 102
Argentina, 173
argument, 140, 141, 182
Armenia, 102
artery, 42, 183
arthritis, 17, 90
Asia, vii, 1, 4, 46, 47, 86, 87, 90, 93, 94, 102, 122, 125, 173
Asian countries, 102
assessment, 18, 29, 34, 41, 79, 120, 123, 159, 163, 165, 170, 171, 175, 184, 185, 187, 216, 232, 245
assets, 52, 54, 56
assignment, 228
association, vii, 1, 6, 12, 18, 19, 20, 21, 22, 25, 43, 49, 53, 72, 73, 113, 114, 129, 132, 137, 148, 159, 163, 171, 180, 184, 203, 204, 205, 206, 207
assumptions, 15, 38
asthma, 71, 83, 92, 100, 126
asymptomatic, 71
atherosclerosis, 6, 17, 35, 71, 82, 87, 182, 183
athletes, 10, 72, 112
attention, 29, 52, 71, 82, 141, 147, 160, 179, 226, 230, 239, 240, 243
attitudes, xi, 10, 118, 141, 158, 160, 199, 201, 202, 204, 205, 214, 216, 227, 236, 237, 238, 245
attractiveness, 203
Australia, 36, 46, 53, 67, 101, 119, 153, 173
Austria, 94
authenticity, 214
autoimmune disease, 182
availability, 2, 10, 24, 28, 53, 58, 90, 106, 129, 130, 133, 173, 176, 202, 229, 242
avoidance, 163, 190
awareness, xii, 29, 30, 186, 200, 216, 230, 235, 243, 247

B

back pain, 183
Bahrain, viii, 43, 69, 75, 77, 102, 103
Bangladesh, 54, 125
barriers, 143, 188, 206, 249
basic services, 56
behavior, xii, 31, 73, 85, 87, 161, 162, 163, 166, 200, 201, 202, 203, 205, 207, 208, 210, 212, 216, 233, 238, 244, 245, 247, 248, 249, 250, 251, 252
behavior modification, xii, 200
behavioral change, 201, 210
Beijing, 102, 173
Belgium, 93, 175
belief systems, 201, 248
beverages, 111, 156, 162
bias, 83, 215
binding, 129, 132
biological processes, 110
birth, 8, 9, 13, 17, 18, 19, 21, 22, 23, 36, 42, 48, 49, 58, 73, 77, 97, 111, 115, 125, 134, 156, 184, 197, 205
birth weight, 13, 18, 19, 23, 49, 58, 73, 111, 184, 205
birthweight, 22, 23, 26
black women, 13
bladder, 17
blindness, 71
blocks, 31
blood, 5, 7, 42, 43, 49, 71, 72, 90, 110, 128, 129, 134, 179, 182, 192, 198
blood pressure, 49, 192
BMI, ix, 6, 12, 13, 14, 15, 16, 17, 18, 19, 20, 23, 27, 28, 33, 41, 57, 73, 74, 75, 76, 77, 78, 79, 80, 85, 89, 90, 91, 94, 101, 102, 103, 110, 113, 114, 115, 116, 117, 120, 123, 170, 171, 173, 174, 175, 180, 181, 183, 185, 186, 187, 188, 190, 192, 194, 200, 201, 204, 205, 206, 207, 210, 237, 239, 243
body, ix, 4, 6, 9, 10, 12, 13, 14, 15, 16, 17, 20, 23, 24, 25, 26, 28, 30, 32, 33, 35, 36, 37, 38, 39, 40, 41, 42, 43, 44, 46, 48, 54, 57, 72, 73, 75, 76, 78, 82, 83, 84, 85, 87, 89, 91, 94, 95, 97, 98, 110, 111, 114, 120, 122, 126, 128, 130, 131, 133, 134, 136, 137, 138, 141, 157, 170, 173, 177, 182, 184, 191, 193, 195, 196, 197, 198, 200, 201, 205, 209, 210, 217, 221, 230, 231, 237, 239, 243, 249, 251, 253
body composition, 4, 10, 15, 17, 23, 26, 33, 43, 44, 83, 122, 136, 209
body density, 16
body dissatisfaction, 184

body fat, 9, 10, 12, 13, 15, 16, 17, 20, 23, 24, 25, 35, 36, 38, 39, 41, 42, 46, 48, 73, 76, 84, 94, 95, 126, 131, 141, 170, 205, 209, 210, 230, 237, 243, 251
body image, 87
body mass index, 6, 37, 38, 39, 40, 42, 43, 44, 46, 57, 72, 75, 76, 78, 82, 85, 97, 98, 120, 126, 193, 197, 198, 201, 209, 239, 251, 253
body shape, 30, 83
body size, 205
body weight, ix, 6, 10, 23, 24, 32, 83, 85, 89, 91, 110, 111, 114, 133, 138, 177, 195, 196, 200, 249
Bolivia, 55
bone mass, 36
bowel, 178
boys, viii, ix, 2, 3, 6, 9, 10, 14, 15, 22, 25, 27, 34, 40, 43, 46, 69, 74, 75, 76, 77, 78, 79, 80, 81, 83, 89, 90, 91, 92, 93, 94, 100, 102, 107, 108, 113, 114, 116, 143, 173, 176, 181, 184, 190, 197, 204, 206, 210, 218, 222, 238
brain, xi, 42, 129, 169, 177, 178, 179, 180, 196
Brazil, vii, 1, 3, 5, 7, 10, 12, 19, 20, 21, 25, 38, 39, 40, 43, 47, 49, 68, 85, 94, 112, 127, 135, 136
breakdown, 12
breakfast, 111, 161, 162, 181, 189, 190
breast milk, 137, 182
breastfeeding, 26, 48, 53, 58, 59, 64, 65, 137, 182
breathing, 71, 83, 96
Britain, 46, 53, 176, 196
Bulgaria, 90, 175
bulimia, 5, 123, 184
bullying, 197
Burkina Faso, 55
burn, 230, 243
burning, 231

C

calcification, 42
calcium, 5, 25
calorie, 32, 35, 114, 120, 177, 188, 189, 191, 197, 248
campaigns, 116, 141
Canada, 10, 250, 252
cancer, 4, 49, 90, 111, 117, 182
car accidents, 115
carbohydrate, ix, 14, 24, 78, 90, 93, 182, 189
cardiovascular disease, ix, 13, 17, 30, 43, 44, 83, 89, 119, 132, 182, 191
cardiovascular risk, 9, 35, 36, 86, 194
caregivers, xi, xii, 30, 119, 199, 200, 201, 205, 208, 213, 214, 216, 217, 218, 219, 220, 222, 223, 224, 225, 226, 227, 228, 229, 230, 231, 232, 233, 234, 236, 237, 238, 239, 240, 241, 242, 243, 244, 245, 246, 247, 248
categorization, 56
Caucasians, 184, 207
cell, 25, 110, 196
cell cycle, 196
Census, 96, 211, 212, 250, 253
centigrade, 115
central nervous system, 128
centriole, 179
channels, 223, 225
child development, 19
childcare, 201
childhood, vii, viii, ix, x, xi, xii, 1, 2, 3, 6, 8, 9, 11, 13, 17, 18, 21, 22, 25, 27, 28, 29, 30, 31, 32, 33, 36, 37, 39, 40, 41, 42, 43, 44, 46, 49, 51, 52, 53, 54, 59, 64, 66, 67, 68, 69, 70, 71, 72, 73, 74, 75, 76, 78, 79, 81, 82, 83, 84, 85, 89, 90, 95, 96, 97, 99, 101, 102, 109, 112, 114, 116, 118, 119, 120, 121, 123, 125, 126, 131, 132, 134, 135, 136, 137, 138, 139, 140, 141, 142, 143, 145, 147, 148, 149, 150, 157, 158, 166, 167, 169, 170, 171, 173, 175, 179, 180, 181, 182, 183, 184, 185, 186, 190, 192, 194, 197, 199, 200, 201, 202, 203, 204, 207, 208, 210, 211, 212, 214, 216, 229, 230, 233, 234, 237, 238, 239, 242, 243, 244, 245, 246, 247, 248, 249, 250, 252, 253, 254
childrcn, vii, viii, ix, x, xi, 1, 2, 3, 4, 5, 6, 7, 8, 9, 10, 11, 12, 13, 14, 16, 17, 18, 19, 20, 21, 22, 23, 24, 25, 26, 27, 28, 29, 30, 31, 32, 33, 34, 35, 36, 37, 38, 39, 40, 41, 42, 43, 44, 45, 46, 47, 48, 49, 50, 51, 52, 53, 54, 55, 56, 58, 59, 64, 65, 66, 67, 68, 69, 70, 71, 72, 73, 74, 75, 76, 77, 78, 79, 80, 81, 82, 83, 84, 85, 86, 87, 90, 93, 94, 96, 97, 98, 99, 100, 101, 102, 103, 104, 105, 106, 107, 108, 109, 110, 111, 112, 114, 115, 116, 117, 118, 119, 120, 121, 122, 123, 124, 125, 126, 130, 131, 132, 135, 136, 137, 139, 140, 141, 142, 143, 144, 145, 147, 148, 150, 151, 155, 156, 157, 158, 159, 160, 161, 162, 163, 165, 166, 167, 168, 169, 170, 171, 173, 174, 175, 176, 177, 178, 179, 180, 181, 182, 183, 184, 185, 186, 187, 188, 189, 190, 191, 192, 193, 194, 195, 196, 197, 199, 200, 201, 202, 203, 204, 205, 206, 207, 208, 209, 210, 211, 212, 213, 214, 215, 216, 217, 218, 219, 220, 221, 222, 223, 224, 225, 226, 227, 228, 229, 230, 231, 232, 233, 234, 235, 236, 237, 238, 239, 240, 241, 242, 243, 244, 245, 246, 248, 249, 250, 251, 252, 253
Chile, 102
China, vii, 1, 3, 5, 7, 10, 11, 12, 16, 21, 35, 38, 46, 49, 102, 126, 173
cholesterol, 78, 131, 137, 179
chromosome, 131, 179

cigarette smoking, 184
circulation, 178
classes, 76, 114, 157, 176, 234, 246
classification, x, 21, 76, 127, 131, 134, 176, 204
classroom, 91, 160, 210, 237
classrooms, 91
clinical syndrome, 30
cloning, 84
clustering, 74
clusters, 5
cocaine, 129
coding, 132, 214
cognition, 36, 150
cognitive function, 27
cohort, 42, 44, 71, 82, 83, 107, 125, 137, 182, 197, 205
collaboration, 30, 250
Colombia, 55, 58
colon, 183
commercials, 161, 162, 181
commitment, 29
communication, 109, 123
communication systems, 109
community, xii, 3, 12, 21, 30, 31, 32, 43, 50, 67, 72, 73, 79, 94, 116, 117, 118, 125, 170, 186, 187, 192, 200, 201, 202, 203, 204, 213, 214, 215, 216, 230, 232, 234, 235, 237, 238, 241, 243, 245, 246, 247, 248, 249
community support, xii, 200, 214, 216, 238
compassion, 187
competence, 248
competition, 160
complement, vii, 1
complex carbohydrates, 12
complexity, 13, 133, 145, 149, 150
compliance, 229, 233, 242, 245
complications, 8, 13, 26, 28, 35, 40, 71, 90, 100, 111, 147, 183, 192, 247
components, 13, 15, 24, 72, 113, 129, 131, 132, 133, 202, 220
composition, 19, 20, 26, 35, 38, 48, 112, 113, 130, 133, 136, 137, 252
computer use, 206, 207, 224, 225, 227, 228, 236, 240, 241, 242
concentration, 72, 131, 162
conception, 232, 245
concordance, 131, 158
conduct, x, 52, 99
confidence, 22, 77
confidence interval, 22, 77
confidentiality, 213
conflict, 163, 205, 236, 237
consensus, 185, 202, 209
consent, 213, 214
conservation, 10
consumers, 29, 114
consumption, 4, 12, 41, 77, 79, 111, 112, 113, 114, 115, 117, 118, 119, 120, 122, 126, 133, 156, 158, 160, 161, 162, 163, 165, 167, 168, 177, 181, 182, 187, 189
consumption frequency, 158
consumption patterns, 119
content analysis, 115, 119, 167, 196, 217, 218, 223, 226
context, 2, 3, 4, 10, 11, 18, 24, 29, 31, 32, 65, 149, 150, 157, 160, 167, 201, 202, 203, 206, 247
continuity, 132, 133
control, vii, xi, 2, 20, 22, 24, 29, 30, 32, 36, 53, 66, 81, 82, 110, 120, 125, 134, 138, 156, 160, 162, 163, 169, 177, 178, 179, 182, 185, 187, 188, 194, 195, 198, 202, 205, 208, 210, 212, 224, 226, 227, 228, 233, 242, 243, 244, 245
control condition, 160
control group, 110, 162
conversion, 132
conviction, 148, 187
cooking, 142, 237
corn, 159
coronary artery disease, 121, 182
coronary heart disease, 82, 86, 90
correlation, 15, 16, 18, 26, 115, 159, 160, 163
cortisol, 128, 179
costs, 32, 112, 121, 195
coverage, 103, 176
critical period, 8, 9, 19, 22, 132, 163
Croatia, 175
cross-sectional study, ix, 24, 27, 77, 85, 89
Cuba, 102
cultural differences, 205
cultural values, 203
culture, vii, 1, 29, 32, 87, 202, 203, 224, 225, 226, 232, 241, 242, 245, 248, 252
curriculum, 117, 118, 210
CVD, 100, 122
cycling, 181, 190
Czech Republic, 175

D

danger, 192
data analysis, 8, 13, 48
data collection, 54, 56, 95, 173, 214
database, 142
dating, 78
DBP, 78
death, 4, 70, 71, 140, 234

death rate, 4
defects, 73
deficiency, 7, 25, 44, 46, 84, 130, 132, 133, 138, 176, 177, 178, 179, 180, 195
deficit, 131, 189
definition, viii, 6, 18, 37, 69, 94, 95, 96, 170, 193, 204, 205, 212, 214, 216, 239, 240
demand, x, 115, 127, 134
demographic change, 113, 125
demographic characteristics, 75
demographic data, 92
demographic factors, 5, 112
demographic transition, 3
demographics, 3, 200
Denmark, 139, 141, 142, 143, 144, 175
density, 22, 78, 79, 83, 125
Department of Health and Human Services, 37, 95, 253
dependent variable, 56
deposition, 14, 15, 23, 24, 32, 41, 138, 177
deposits, 14
depression, 100, 110, 125, 184
deprivation, 19, 25, 132, 184
desire, 178, 219
detection, 14
developed countries, vii, 1, 7, 18, 26, 51, 53, 76, 108, 109, 117, 173
developing nations, 74, 102, 247
developmental change, 166
deviation, 18
diabetes, 18, 71, 83, 90, 92, 97, 100, 132, 183, 184, 192, 197, 198, 251
diagnostic criteria, 71
diastolic blood pressure, 78
diet, ix, x, xi, 4, 5, 12, 13, 19, 20, 22, 23, 24, 26, 29, 30, 32, 85, 90, 93, 96, 109, 110, 112, 113, 123, 125, 130, 131, 133, 135, 138, 139, 140, 141, 142, 143, 144, 145, 147, 148, 149, 150, 151, 155, 156, 163, 169, 173, 177, 181, 182, 186, 187, 188, 189, 190, 191, 192, 193, 197, 201, 203, 205, 206, 208, 210, 211, 230, 231, 233, 234, 235, 237, 243, 244, 245, 247, 250
dietary fat, 22, 112, 113, 117, 126, 182
dietary habits, 95, 202, 203
dietary intake, 13, 180, 210, 233, 234, 240, 243
dieting, xi, 87, 149, 169, 188
differentiation, 132, 133
direct measure, 17
disaster, 68
discipline, 225, 241
discrimination, 100
disorder, vii, ix, 1, 5, 20, 31, 71, 84, 89, 120, 248
disposition, 8
distress, 163, 184
distribution, 5, 9, 10, 15, 16, 17, 22, 35, 36, 46, 47, 48, 49, 76, 84, 120, 132, 173
diversity, 2, 13
division, 25
DNA, 25
doctors, 148, 232, 235, 245, 246
dopamine, 192
Down syndrome, 131
drug treatment, 191
drugs, 30, 133, 192
duration, 22, 55, 65, 116, 128, 142, 150, 244
dyslipidemia, 71, 90

E

earnings, 197
East Asia, 4
Eastern Europe, 93
eating, vii, xi, 1, 2, 5, 31, 70, 73, 77, 85, 110, 114, 116, 117, 118, 120, 123, 139, 140, 141, 146, 147, 148, 151, 155, 160, 161, 162, 163, 166, 173, 176, 177, 178, 179, 181, 184, 185, 186, 187, 188, 189, 190, 191, 193, 202, 203, 204, 207, 223, 230, 234, 243
eating disorders, 123, 188
economic development, 27, 30, 42, 52, 66, 112
economic growth, viii, 4, 39, 51, 66
economic policy, 39
economic resources, 247
economic status, viii, 32, 51, 52, 53, 54, 79, 107, 114, 194
economics, 53, 66
educational attainment, 184
educational background, 150
educational programs, 235, 246
Egypt, viii, 7, 52, 55, 57, 69, 79, 102, 103, 125, 173
electricity, 54, 56
elementary school, 35, 210, 213, 239, 252
emergence, 26, 30, 71, 238
employment, 57, 73
endocrine, vii, x, 24, 110, 127, 128, 133, 138
endocrine system, 110
endurance, 244, 252
energy, viii, ix, x, xi, 3, 5, 6, 7, 10, 11, 13, 14, 19, 20, 21, 23, 24, 28, 32, 38, 40, 53, 69, 70, 72, 73, 75, 83, 84, 103, 109, 110, 111, 112, 113, 114, 116, 117, 121, 122, 125, 127, 128, 129, 131, 132, 133, 134, 136, 141, 156, 169, 176, 177, 178, 179, 180, 181, 182, 188, 189, 193, 195, 221, 223, 244, 250
energy density, 28, 32, 112, 121, 181, 195
England, 35, 40, 43, 49, 67, 117, 152, 170, 173, 176, 194, 249, 251, 254

enthusiasm, 160
environment, x, 11, 20, 25, 29, 30, 73, 84, 100, 111, 114, 118, 126, 127, 130, 131, 134, 140, 142, 147, 159, 166, 176, 200, 202, 234, 236, 238, 246, 248
environmental change, xii, 130, 131, 200, 216
environmental conditions, 131
environmental factors, 2, 7, 11, 24, 42, 70, 73, 75, 96, 111, 117, 123, 126, 128, 130, 131, 200, 201, 248
environmental influences, ix, 70, 204
enzymes, 132, 134, 177
epidemic, xi, 2, 32, 38, 40, 45, 47, 50, 67, 68, 70, 71, 72, 73, 82, 85, 87, 100, 102, 110, 111, 120, 121, 124, 126, 140, 152, 169, 176, 193, 247, 251, 252, 253
epidemiology, 44, 46, 47, 68, 83, 124, 126, 196, 252
epilepsy, 179
epithelial cells, 178
essential fatty acids, 196
estimating, 17
ethnic background, 212
ethnic groups, xi, xii, 2, 13, 14, 15, 16, 17, 38, 72, 171, 174, 200, 201, 202, 203, 211, 213, 216, 232, 238, 245
ethnic minority, 200, 248
ethnicity, 53, 203, 204, 206, 248
etiology, x, 6, 14, 18, 39, 72, 74, 127, 128, 130, 131, 134, 135, 200
EU, 101
Europe, ix, 10, 53, 67, 72, 74, 89, 90, 93, 94, 97, 101, 123, 175, 194
evening, 218, 226, 229
everyday life, 181
evidence, ix, x, 2, 8, 11, 21, 22, 25, 27, 38, 70, 74, 82, 96, 99, 100, 102, 103, 109, 113, 117, 118, 119, 126, 130, 162, 163, 170, 179, 180, 182, 184, 185, 187, 190, 191, 193, 196, 209, 248, 251
evolution, 121
excuse, 148
exercise, x, xi, 11, 24, 30, 48, 70, 71, 76, 83, 97, 110, 112, 116, 122, 131, 139, 140, 142, 143, 144, 145, 146, 147, 148, 149, 150, 151, 169, 175, 176, 177, 179, 180, 185, 187, 190, 191, 193, 200, 202, 207, 217, 220, 221, 227, 230, 233, 234, 244, 245, 246, 248
exertion, 244, 252
expenditures, 10, 100, 112, 126, 141
expertise, 71, 151
experts, 120, 151, 209
exposure, xi, 19, 84, 115, 120, 135, 155, 156, 157, 158, 159, 162, 163, 165, 166, 167, 181
expression, 129, 131, 132, 177, 178
extrapolation, 81
extreme poverty, 58
extrinsic motivation, 208, 242

F

facial expression, 157, 164, 165
facial responses, 168
factor analysis, 56, 57
failure, 71, 205
family, viii, x, xi, 11, 12, 30, 39, 51, 59, 65, 73, 76, 114, 115, 117, 118, 124, 139, 140, 141, 142, 143, 144, 145, 146, 147, 149, 150, 151, 159, 167, 169, 175, 180, 185, 186, 187, 188, 189, 191, 192, 198, 202, 203, 207, 216, 218, 222, 227, 229, 230, 231, 232, 233, 234, 239, 240, 241, 242, 243, 244, 245, 246, 247, 248, 253
family history, 175, 198
family income, 175
family members, 11, 39, 159, 167, 202
famine, 3, 8, 67, 84, 109, 135, 176
farms, 3, 21
fast food, 95, 114, 161, 166, 173, 181, 182
fasting, 20, 71, 91, 129, 133, 178, 198
fat, 5, 6, 7, 8, 9, 11, 12, 13, 14, 15, 16, 17, 18, 19, 20, 21, 22, 23, 24, 25, 27, 28, 32, 35, 40, 41, 46, 47, 48, 49, 73, 78, 83, 94, 109, 110, 112, 113, 114, 120, 131, 133, 136, 138, 140, 141, 147, 149, 162, 163, 166, 168, 170, 177, 181, 182, 189, 196, 200, 204, 206, 207, 209, 210, 223, 231, 232, 245, 248
fatty acids, 167, 182, 191
feedback, 208, 242
females, 12, 14, 15, 16, 74, 77, 86, 93, 119, 160, 184, 206, 218, 238, 239, 245
fetal growth, 184, 185
fetal nutrition, 123
fetus, 22
Filipino, 204, 211, 213, 216, 217, 221, 222, 223, 224, 225, 226, 227, 230, 232, 235, 237, 240, 241, 243, 244, 245, 246, 247
Finland, 94, 175
First World, 136
fish, 189
fitness, 10, 84, 142, 207, 244
flavor, xi, 155, 157, 158, 159, 166, 168
fluid, 136
focus groups, 202, 212, 213, 214, 215
focusing, 73, 141, 144, 214
folic acid, 5
food, xi, xii, 2, 5, 10, 12, 19, 22, 28, 29, 30, 31, 32, 41, 47, 53, 58, 72, 73, 77, 79, 95, 106, 108, 109, 112, 114, 115, 119, 120, 122, 124, 125, 129, 130, 131, 132, 134, 137, 138, 140, 141, 142, 144, 145, 146, 147, 149, 151, 155, 156, 157, 158, 159, 160,

161, 162, 163, 165, 166, 167, 168, 169, 173, 176, 177, 178, 180, 181, 187, 188, 189, 191, 192, 193, 195, 200, 201, 202, 203, 204, 216, 221, 226, 229, 230, 231, 234, 235, 236, 238, 242, 243, 246
food industry, 30, 47, 193
food intake, 19, 32, 112, 125, 129, 131, 132, 134, 137, 138, 162, 163, 177, 178, 180, 191, 192, 195
Ford, 82
formal education, 114
France, 84, 175
friends, 145, 216, 219, 220, 222, 232, 233, 245
fruits, 109, 114, 158, 160, 163, 210

G

gallbladder, 90
gastrointestinal tract, 110
gender, ix, 2, 8, 16, 27, 29, 30, 53, 58, 76, 77, 89, 92, 94, 105, 106, 107, 110, 163, 170, 204, 205, 206, 207, 210, 219, 238, 239, 250, 252, 253
gender differences, 2, 8, 27, 94, 105, 206, 210, 219, 238
gene, x, 11, 13, 25, 44, 73, 84, 110, 127, 128, 129, 131, 132, 133, 134, 135, 138, 177, 179, 195
gene expression, 25, 128
gene therapy, 133
general practitioner, 192
generation, 70, 101, 176
genes, 11, 12, 73, 110, 121, 131, 132, 134, 179, 231
genetic disorders, 111
genetic factors, vii, 24, 44, 93, 110, 130, 131, 180, 205
genetic mutations, 73
genetic syndromes, x, 127, 128, 131
genetics, x, 84, 110, 111, 127, 128, 130, 131, 134, 200, 230, 243
geography, 32
Georgia, 51
Germany, 91, 118, 137, 175, 203
gestation, 8
gestational age, 8, 9, 185, 197, 205
girls, viii, ix, 2, 3, 6, 8, 9, 10, 11, 13, 14, 15, 21, 22, 23, 24, 25, 26, 27, 28, 34, 35, 36, 40, 41, 44, 69, 70, 72, 74, 75, 76, 77, 78, 79, 80, 81, 83, 84, 87, 89, 91, 92, 93, 94, 100, 102, 107, 108, 114, 116, 119, 120, 122, 143, 168, 173, 174, 176, 181, 184, 190, 197, 204, 206, 210, 218, 219, 238, 239, 251
gland, 180
gluconeogenesis, 192
glucose, 17, 18, 37, 71, 83, 87, 110, 111, 128, 185, 192, 198
glucose tolerance, 17, 18, 83
GNP, 4, 54, 112
goals, 187, 202, 208, 242
gold, 170
good behavior, 160
gout, 17, 90, 183
government, 29, 235, 246
grades, 117, 210
grains, 109
graph, 105
Great Britain, 67
Greece, 74, 85, 90, 94, 97, 101, 175, 253
group identity, 203
group membership, 202
groups, viii, ix, xi, 2, 7, 9, 16, 19, 21, 24, 53, 54, 65, 69, 70, 75, 76, 79, 85, 91, 109, 112, 118, 123, 133, 141, 144, 145, 146, 147, 156, 157, 159, 162, 169, 173, 176, 190, 199, 200, 201, 204, 206, 210, 213, 214, 215, 216, 217, 222, 223, 225, 226, 228, 230, 231, 232, 233, 237, 239, 240, 241, 242, 244, 245
growth, vii, viii, 1, 2, 5, 6, 8, 9, 17, 18, 19, 20, 21, 22, 23, 24, 25, 26, 27, 28, 31, 32, 33, 34, 35, 36, 37, 38, 39, 42, 43, 44, 45, 46, 48, 49, 51, 53, 56, 67, 75, 84, 86, 92, 94, 97, 101, 111, 122, 128, 133, 134, 135, 136, 137, 170, 174, 176, 178, 179, 181, 183, 185, 193, 204, 205
growth factor, 24, 133, 136
growth hormone, 19, 128, 134, 178
growth rate, 19, 24, 25, 44, 84
growth spurt, 9, 22, 46, 94, 170
Guatemala, 55, 58
guidance, 186
guidelines, 5, 29, 39, 116, 117, 185, 186, 187, 190, 191, 247
Guinea, 44
gut, xi, 128, 169
gymnastics, 142

H

happiness, 204, 252
HE, 42
health, vii, viii, ix, 1, 2, 3, 5, 6, 17, 18, 20, 22, 26, 29, 30, 31, 32, 40, 41, 44, 45, 46, 47, 56, 67, 68, 69, 70, 72, 74, 75, 81, 82, 83, 84, 85, 86, 87, 93, 97, 99, 100, 105, 111, 112, 115, 117, 118, 119, 121, 122, 124, 125, 136, 140, 141, 148, 149, 151, 176, 188, 193, 194, 201, 205, 208, 209, 210, 217, 221, 223, 230, 233, 234, 235, 243, 246, 247, 248, 249, 250, 251, 253
health care, vii, 1, 119, 125, 141, 230, 234, 235, 243, 246, 248, 251
health care costs, 119, 125
health care professionals, 235, 246, 248
health education, 117, 201, 247

health information, 246
health problems, 17, 93, 136, 230, 243
health psychology, 121
health status, 6, 40
heart disease, 4, 6, 32, 71, 85, 121, 234
heart rate, 244
height, ix, 6, 12, 14, 15, 18, 19, 20, 22, 23, 24, 25, 27, 32, 36, 42, 46, 48, 49, 54, 56, 58, 74, 75, 77, 85, 89, 90, 91, 94, 102, 105, 112, 121, 125, 131, 170, 175, 186, 193, 204, 209, 210, 232, 245
heredity, 71
heterogeneity, 7, 57
high fat, 68, 95, 112, 133, 189
high school, 14, 79, 91, 97, 107, 114, 115, 119, 121, 124
hip, 10, 35, 53, 170, 171, 202
Hispanics, 184, 200, 248
HIV, 30
homeostasis, 18, 134
homework, 206, 225, 228
Hong Kong, 16, 41, 93
hormone, x, 19, 127, 128, 129, 132, 134, 149, 177, 178, 179, 183, 195
host, 140, 142, 193
House, 151, 176, 194
household income, 7, 112
housing, 56, 145, 180
human milk, 73, 133, 136
Hungary, 175
husband, 57
hygiene, 30
hyperinsulinemia, 71, 133, 198
hypertension, 6, 17, 27, 71, 83, 90, 100, 111, 126, 132
hyperventilation, 187
hypothalamus, 111, 128, 129, 132, 133, 177, 178
hypothesis, 27, 73, 157, 158, 215, 252

I

ideas, 144, 214, 215
identification, 9, 251
identity, 202, 203, 248, 249, 250, 252
immigrants, 176, 211
impaired immune function, 27
implementation, 79, 118, 122, 247
imprinting, x, 127, 131, 132, 133, 135
in transition, 2, 3, 10, 12, 125
incentives, 30, 208, 243
incidence, viii, 9, 19, 23, 69, 70, 100, 121, 183, 188, 198
inclusion, 57
income, 5, 12, 14, 19, 20, 26, 29, 31, 39, 45, 52, 53, 54, 56, 57, 58, 66, 75, 84, 86, 90, 94, 97, 102, 112, 114, 124, 135, 176, 184, 204, 249, 252
India, vii, 1, 67, 94
Indians, 27, 38, 173, 243
indication, viii, 18, 51, 95
indicators, 16, 17, 203
indices, 18, 35
indigenous, 109, 201, 211, 213
indirect measure, 10, 170
individual character, 202, 231, 243
individual characteristics, 202, 231, 243
individual differences, 110
Indonesia, vii, 1
induction, 129, 132
industrialized countries, viii, 13, 52, 69
industry, 57
infancy, xi, 8, 9, 22, 23, 25, 26, 35, 36, 84, 96, 135, 137, 155, 156, 157, 158, 167
infants, 23, 25, 26, 36, 46, 48, 84, 137, 156, 157, 158, 159, 165, 166, 168, 182, 193, 196
infarction, 194
infection, 19, 21, 31, 50, 84
infectious disease, 3, 5, 109
infertility, 17
inflammation, 71
influence, x, xii, 6, 8, 17, 27, 52, 54, 65, 73, 121, 131, 135, 139, 144, 146, 150, 151, 158, 160, 162, 167, 177, 200, 201, 202, 203, 204, 205, 207, 214, 216, 224, 230, 232, 238, 241, 243, 245, 248
information seeking, 253
informed consent, 90
infrastructure, 29
ingestion, 129, 133, 166
inhibition, 129, 132, 178
inhibitor, 192
initiation, 23
injury, 179, 180
INS, 84
insecurity, 32, 112
insight, 134, 135, 143, 200, 248
institutions, 141, 151
instruction, 245
insulin, 18, 19, 39, 47, 71, 72, 73, 84, 126, 133, 138, 179, 184
insulin resistance, 18, 47, 71, 72, 126, 184
insulin sensitivity, 133, 138
intelligence, 28
intensity, 22, 48, 117, 150, 181, 208, 243, 244, 250
intentions, 142
interaction, 11, 52, 65, 66, 73, 74, 131, 158, 202, 204, 213, 214
interaction effect, 65

interactions, x, xi, 2, 56, 127, 134, 169, 178, 203, 205
interest, 11, 54, 56, 143, 144, 173, 177, 178, 191, 216
international standards, 78, 174
internet, 228
interpretation, 48, 49, 215, 237
intervention, xi, 6, 29, 32, 41, 93, 95, 116, 117, 118, 122, 125, 139, 140, 141, 142, 143, 148, 149, 150, 151, 155, 157, 162, 169, 181, 182, 190, 191, 192, 198, 201, 210, 211, 216, 228, 232, 233, 237, 238, 239, 240, 241, 242, 243, 244, 245, 247, 248, 250, 251
intervention strategies, 29, 140, 141, 142, 148, 149, 151, 201, 216, 233, 241, 247
interview, vii, 51, 52, 54, 144, 153, 212, 213
intestinal tract, 177
intrauterine growth retardation, 22, 23
invitation to participate, 213
Iran, viii, ix, x, 40, 69, 70, 79, 80, 81, 87, 99, 100, 101, 103, 105, 106, 107, 108, 109, 111, 113, 114, 115, 116, 117, 118, 119, 120, 121, 122, 123, 124, 125, 126
Ireland, 124
iron, 5, 25, 123, 176
irradiation, 179, 180
isolation, 31, 71
Israel, 93
Italy, 101, 120, 123, 124, 175

J

Jamaica, 173
Japan, 16
jejunum, 138
jobs, 11, 145
judgment, 232, 245
junior high school, 14, 119

K

kidney, 71
kindergarten, 86, 144, 162
kindergarten children, 86
knees, 183
knowledge, x, 47, 50, 116, 118, 127, 128, 140, 142, 143, 149, 162, 168, 180, 201, 202, 210, 212, 234, 237, 244, 246, 247, 248
Kuwait, viii, 69, 75, 77, 102, 103

L

labeling, 90
labor, 27, 53, 57
land, 211
language, 187, 213, 225
later life, 27, 135
Latin America, 4, 41, 102, 123
LDL, 78
lead, vii, x, 1, 14, 19, 22, 26, 73, 90, 113, 114, 117, 118, 127, 134, 135, 141, 149, 150, 179
lean body mass, 24
learning, 157, 158, 166, 168, 178, 179, 220, 227, 228, 235, 236, 246
learning difficulties, 178, 179
Lebanon, 76, 86, 102, 103
legislation, 29
leisure, 6, 10, 47, 180, 200, 207
leisure time, 10, 47
lens, 215
leptin, 11, 73, 84, 111, 123, 128, 129, 132, 133, 134, 135, 137, 138, 177, 178, 195, 249
life course, 29
life cycle, 28
life expectancy, 100, 124, 193
lifestyle, viii, ix, 2, 28, 45, 69, 70, 71, 73, 74, 75, 79, 98, 109, 113, 115, 116, 141, 142, 149, 151, 176, 180, 185, 186, 187, 190, 191, 192, 193, 198, 235, 247
lifestyle changes, 45, 185, 186, 190, 192, 235, 247
lifetime, 38, 133
likelihood, 181, 193, 206
limitation, 114, 115, 205
linear programming, 112
links, 117
lipid oxidation, 131
lipids, 97, 122, 179
lipolysis, 177
lipoproteins, 39
liver, 96
living conditions, 57
location, 65, 66, 110
loneliness, 71
longevity, xi, 169
longitudinal study, 23, 42, 46, 96, 123, 204
loss of appetite, 134
love, 160, 222

M

macronutrients, 78
magazines, 235, 246

malabsorption, 134
Malaysia, 102, 123
males, 3, 8, 12, 14, 15, 16, 74, 77, 78, 93, 174, 203, 204, 206, 207
malignancy, 92
malnutrition, vii, ix, 1, 3, 4, 20, 21, 23, 24, 26, 32, 35, 38, 40, 41, 46, 47, 50, 67, 70, 74, 82, 105, 111, 113, 131
management, 28, 30, 95, 121, 179, 184, 191, 197, 230, 231
manners, 90
marginalization, 90
marital quality, 203
marital status, 204
market, 12
marketing, 29, 114, 115, 240
marketing strategy, 115
Mars, 167
mass, xi, 6, 14, 15, 17, 20, 24, 25, 36, 37, 38, 40, 83, 86, 98, 110, 118, 119, 125, 126, 133, 155, 170, 173, 177, 183, 191, 203, 209, 210
mass media, xi, 6, 155
maturation, 13, 14, 17, 26, 27, 39, 48, 49, 133
maturation process, 14, 26
meals, 5, 20, 77, 111, 114, 142, 147, 160, 185, 188, 189, 193
meanings, 144, 214
measurement, 15, 17, 52, 54, 170, 171, 209
measures, 7, 15, 16, 25, 31, 36, 54, 56, 185, 192, 193, 209, 210, 212, 214, 229, 232, 242, 245
meat, ix, 5, 12, 90, 93, 189
media, 30, 141, 151, 176, 178, 180, 203, 229, 234, 242, 246
median, 5, 6, 18, 118
medication, 192
Mediterranean, viii, ix, 69, 71, 73, 74, 75, 77, 79, 81, 83, 85, 87, 90, 93, 101, 175
melanin, 129
membership, 203
men, vii, 1, 11, 12, 17, 47, 53, 72, 76, 78, 112, 194, 204
menarche, 9, 17, 22, 25, 26, 27, 37, 47
menopause, 8
menstruation, 22, 27
mental health, 48, 126
meta analysis, 38
metabolic dysfunction, 195
metabolic syndrome, 19, 32, 45, 47, 71, 179, 196
metabolism, 20, 42, 73, 110, 125, 145, 150, 177, 195, 231, 243
metformin, 192, 198
methodology, 107, 114, 202, 212, 214
Mexico, vii, 1, 3, 7, 26, 46, 48, 125, 181, 196
mice, 133, 138, 195
micronutrients, 5, 25, 103
Middle East, vii, 1, 4, 74, 75, 86, 93, 103
migrants, 204
migration, 201
military, 126, 207
milk, 5, 157, 158, 166, 182
mining, 10
minorities, 7, 29, 101, 176
minority, 12, 72, 173, 174, 203
minority groups, 173, 174, 203
modeling, xi, 155, 159, 160, 162, 163, 166, 167, 233
models, 56, 57, 110, 112, 122, 131, 132, 135, 160, 165, 167
moderate activity, 190
modernisation, 7
modernization, 12, 77
money, 114, 117
Mongolia, vii, 1
monitoring, 7, 9, 30, 31, 82, 208, 229, 233, 234, 236, 241, 242, 244, 245
monozygotic twins, 131
mood, ix, 89
morbidity, 4, 8, 9, 17, 26, 27, 31, 38, 43, 48, 70, 72, 74, 82, 90, 93, 96, 97, 187, 191, 193
morning, 91, 219, 220, 225
Morocco, 55, 57, 78, 102
mortality, xi, 3, 4, 8, 13, 27, 31, 38, 43, 48, 70, 72, 74, 79, 81, 82, 83, 84, 90, 109, 115, 124, 169, 171, 182, 191, 192, 194, 242
mortality rate, 13
mothers, viii, 2, 5, 19, 48, 51, 52, 53, 54, 55, 64, 65, 66, 73, 81, 84, 112, 114, 115, 118, 132, 137, 158, 160, 163, 168, 175, 176, 185, 203, 204, 205, 213, 216, 222, 233, 234, 235, 239, 245, 246, 249
motivation, 148
motives, 148
movement, 122, 209, 217, 221, 236, 238
multidimensional, 202, 207
multi-ethnic, 197, 201, 202
muscle mass, 10, 16, 23
muscles, 244
mutation, 110, 132
myocardial infarction, 171, 192

N

NaCl, 156
National Health Service, 176
national income, 54, 58, 78
national product, 26
Native Americans, 173, 248

needs, 21, 28, 30, 33, 75, 115, 140, 149, 151, 176, 185, 190, 191, 193, 201, 221, 227, 246, 248
negative consequences, 12, 90
negative relation, 53
neglect, 180
neonates, 111
Nepal, vii, 1
nervousness, 71
Netherlands, 93, 162, 175
network, 128, 133, 232, 245, 253
neuroendocrine system, 42, 128
neurons, 129
neuropeptides, 179
neurotransmitters, 110, 131, 134, 177
New South Wales, 36
New Zealand, 252
newspapers, 115, 124, 235, 246
niacin, 5
Nicaragua, 55
nicotine, 138
Nigeria, 55, 173
nonsmokers, 76
norepinephrine, 129
normal children, 9
North Africa, 56, 59, 64, 66
North America, 42, 135, 248
Norway, 175
nucleus, 178
nurses, 147, 235
nutrients, 23, 73, 111, 128, 132, 167, 177, 181, 234, 246
nutritional deficiencies, vii, 1, 109

O

obesity, vii, viii, ix, x, xi, xii, 1, 2, 3, 4, 5, 6, 7, 8, 9, 10, 11, 12, 13, 14, 15, 16, 17, 18, 19, 20, 21, 23, 26, 27, 28, 29, 30, 31, 32, 33, 35, 36, 37, 38, 39, 40, 41, 42, 43, 44, 45, 46, 49, 51, 52, 53, 54, 66, 67, 68, 69, 70, 71, 72, 73, 74, 75, 76, 77, 78, 79, 80, 81, 82, 83, 84, 85, 86, 87, 89, 90, 91, 92, 93, 94, 95, 96, 97, 98, 99, 100, 101, 102, 103, 104, 106, 107, 108, 109, 110, 111, 112, 113, 114, 115, 116, 117, 118, 119, 120, 121, 122, 123, 124, 125, 126, 127, 128, 129, 130, 131, 132, 133, 134, 135, 136, 137, 138, 139, 140, 141, 142, 143, 144, 145, 146, 147, 148, 149, 150, 151, 152, 162, 169, 170, 171, 173, 174, 175, 176, 177, 178, 179, 180, 181, 182, 183, 184, 185, 186, 187, 188, 189, 190, 191, 192, 193, 194, 195, 196, 197, 198, 199, 200, 201, 202, 203, 204, 205, 206, 207, 208, 209, 210, 211, 212, 214, 216, 229, 230, 232, 233, 234, 236, 237, 238, 239, 240, 242, 243, 244, 245, 246, 247, 248, 249, 250, 251, 252, 253, 254
obesity prevention, 30, 117, 118, 126, 191, 208, 211, 243
observations, 20, 101, 177, 215
oil, 237
older adults, 76, 251
omega-3, 182, 191, 196
online information, 142
organ, 128
organization, 70
organizations, vii, 1, 29, 30, 208
output, 65
overnutrition, vii, 1, 3, 22, 26, 29, 41
overweight, vii, viii, ix, x, xi, 1, 2, 3, 4, 5, 6, 7, 8, 9, 11, 12, 13, 14, 15, 16, 17, 18, 19, 20, 21, 22, 23, 25, 26, 27, 28, 29, 30, 31, 32, 33, 35, 37, 38, 39, 40, 41, 42, 43, 44, 45, 49, 51, 52, 53, 54, 56, 57, 58, 59, 64, 65, 66, 67, 68, 69, 70, 71, 72, 74, 75, 76, 77, 78, 79, 80, 81, 82, 83, 84, 85, 86, 87, 89, 90, 91, 92, 93, 94, 95, 96, 97, 98, 99, 100, 101, 102, 103, 105, 106, 107, 108, 109, 110, 111, 112, 113, 114, 115, 116, 117, 118, 119, 120, 121, 122, 123, 124, 125, 126, 132, 137, 139, 140, 141, 161, 162, 169, 170, 173, 174, 175, 176, 180, 181, 182, 184, 185, 187, 190, 192, 193, 194, 195, 197, 198, 200, 201, 203, 204, 205, 207, 216, 218, 229, 230, 231, 233, 234, 236, 237, 238, 241, 242, 243, 244, 245, 247, 248, 249, 250, 251, 252, 253
ownership, 56
oxidation, 20, 24, 27, 40, 136, 177
oxygen, 177, 244
oxygen consumption, 177

P

Pacific, xi, 46, 47, 122, 199, 204, 205, 211, 238, 248, 252
pain, 129
Pakistan, viii, 69, 75, 86
paradigm shift, x, 31, 127, 134
parasitic infection, 36
parental control, 207
parental influence, 207
parental involvement, 216, 222, 230, 233, 234, 240, 242, 243, 245
parenting, xi, 155, 159, 160, 167, 180, 186, 202, 203, 204, 205
parenting behaviours, 186
parenting styles, xi, 155, 159, 160, 202, 203, 204
parents, x, 6, 11, 19, 30, 39, 59, 65, 73, 74, 77, 90, 109, 110, 112, 115, 116, 117, 118, 119, 121, 123, 130, 135, 139, 140, 143, 144, 145, 146, 147, 150,

158, 159, 162, 163, 167, 173, 180, 184, 186, 187, 191, 192, 193, 197, 202, 203, 204, 205, 207, 208, 209, 213, 215, 216, 217, 220, 222, 224, 226, 227, 228, 229, 230, 231, 233, 234, 235, 239, 240, 242, 243, 245, 246, 251
passive, 94
pasta, 113, 189
pathways, 111, 129, 133
pediatrician, 235
peer group, 190
peer influence, 160
peers, 73, 159, 160, 180, 184
penalties, 184
peptides, 129, 178, 179
per capita income, 12
percentage of fat, 118
percentile, 18, 74, 76, 77, 78, 97, 102, 103, 114, 116, 174
perceptions, x, xi, 139, 140, 141, 143, 145, 148, 149, 151, 199, 200, 201, 216, 217, 220, 238, 249, 251
perinatal, 72, 73, 133
personal responsibility, 146
personality, 251
perspective, 4, 7, 46, 49, 74, 83, 110, 121, 134, 148, 149, 197, 201, 211, 231, 248, 252
Peru, 55, 102, 173
PGN, 134
pharmacotherapy, 134
phenotype, 128, 131, 180
Philippines, 3, 16
photographs, 165
physical activity, vii, xi, xii, 2, 4, 5, 6, 10, 11, 12, 13, 19, 22, 24, 29, 30, 31, 32, 47, 48, 71, 72, 73, 75, 76, 77, 94, 95, 96, 97, 106, 109, 111, 112, 113, 115, 116, 117, 118, 123, 128, 130, 140, 141, 142, 143, 144, 147, 148, 149, 150, 151, 173, 176, 180, 181, 186, 188, 190, 196, 197, 199, 200, 201, 202, 203, 205, 206, 207, 208, 209, 210, 211, 212, 214, 215, 216, 217, 218, 219, 220, 221, 222, 229, 230, 232, 233, 234, 236, 237, 238, 239, 240, 241, 242, 243, 244, 245, 246, 248, 249, 250, 251, 252, 253
physical education, 11, 118, 214, 217, 220, 239
physical environment, 206
physical exercise, 142, 147
physical fitness, 207, 238, 239, 248
physical health, 17
physiology, 39, 179, 231, 243
physiopathology, 129
placebo, 25, 36
placenta, 73, 129, 177
planning, 29, 31, 122, 247
plants, 163, 219
plasma, 97, 122, 128, 131, 133, 134
plasma levels, 128
PM, 42, 44, 119, 126, 138
Poland, 175
policy makers, ix, 4, 70, 82
pollution, 106, 115
polydactyly, 179
poor, viii, 3, 17, 18, 19, 20, 21, 23, 26, 37, 51, 53, 54, 65, 66, 90, 107, 109, 112, 148, 170, 173, 176, 177, 183, 184
population, viii, ix, x, 2, 4, 5, 12, 14, 15, 16, 18, 23, 25, 36, 39, 42, 44, 47, 53, 57, 68, 69, 72, 75, 76, 77, 78, 79, 81, 86, 89, 90, 91, 92, 95, 96, 97, 99, 100, 101, 102, 107, 109, 110, 113, 117, 119, 121, 124, 125, 126, 141, 173, 176, 184, 193, 194, 201, 203, 207, 210, 211, 237, 241, 244, 248, 250, 252
population density, 25
positive correlation, 12, 158, 204
positive relation, 148, 159, 204, 206, 210
positive relationship, 159, 204, 206, 210
potassium, 15
potatoes, 189, 253
Potchefstroom, 1
poverty, viii, 13, 21, 26, 29, 31, 51, 52, 57, 66, 120, 184
power, 187, 216
Prader-Willi syndrome, 178
prediction, 39, 178
predictor variables, 209
predictors, 56, 59, 64, 65, 83, 84, 121, 160, 207
preference, 14, 115, 156, 157, 158, 159, 160, 163, 165, 166, 181, 206, 208, 224, 230, 238, 241, 243
pregnancy, 8, 132, 133, 185, 205
preparation, 114
pre-school, 119
preschool children, viii, 6, 14, 31, 67, 68, 69, 82, 85, 96, 102, 121, 136, 137, 159, 160, 167, 181, 204, 249, 251, 253
preschoolers, 249
pressure, 42, 49, 72, 73, 110, 117, 157, 163, 179, 183, 190, 208, 242
prevention, vii, x, xii, 2, 28, 29, 31, 32, 35, 37, 41, 49, 50, 73, 74, 82, 85, 93, 99, 116, 117, 118, 119, 120, 123, 125, 126, 141, 184, 185, 192, 197, 198, 200, 201, 208, 214, 216, 230, 233, 237, 238, 243, 244, 245, 247, 248, 252
primary data, 27
primary school, 21, 25, 27, 30, 31, 41, 42, 57, 125, 126, 175, 187, 250
primary school age children, 187
principle, 149
private sector, 180
probability, 56, 65
problem solving, 247

production, 19, 114, 132, 177, 192
productivity, 27, 28, 46, 100
program, 76, 131, 142, 143, 150, 207, 214, 218, 221, 223, 239, 244, 247, 250
programming, 23, 123, 132, 133, 138, 161, 167
proliferation, 132, 133
protective role, 133
protein synthesis, 14, 25
proteins, 25
protocol, 212, 213, 214
psychological distress, 184
psychological health, 71, 96
psychological problems, 150
psychologist, 142
psychology, 121, 123, 215
pubertal development, 17, 207
puberty, 9, 14, 15, 23, 27, 43, 94, 170, 219, 238, 239
public health, vii, viii, ix, 4, 5, 6, 28, 29, 30, 31, 32, 49, 69, 70, 72, 81, 82, 83, 93, 103, 111, 118, 135, 201, 235, 247, 248, 253
public schools, 74, 76, 212

Q

qualitative research, 140, 205, 214
quality of life, 90, 100
questioning, 220, 239

R

race, 13, 83, 126
radio, 235, 246
Rainbow Nation, 2
range, 8, 13, 19, 30, 32, 52, 58, 101, 102, 107, 110, 117, 128, 144, 183, 203
reading, 142, 206, 224, 229, 241, 242
reality, 250
reasoning, 149
receptors, 129, 130, 131, 132, 134, 136, 177
recognition, 239
recovery, 112
reduction, 21, 23, 72, 112, 116, 117, 140, 149, 177, 181, 182, 185, 190, 191, 192, 193, 208, 210
reflection, 21, 23, 176
regression, 56, 57, 59, 64, 65, 77
regression analysis, 77
regulation, x, 6, 20, 35, 110, 111, 123, 127, 128, 129, 131, 134, 135, 137, 177, 179, 182, 195, 196
rehabilitation, 121
reinforcement, 166
reinforcers, 208, 243
rejection, 156, 157, 165
relationship, vii, 1, 3, 10, 12, 13, 16, 17, 18, 19, 21, 28, 30, 31, 52, 53, 65, 68, 73, 85, 110, 111, 113, 119, 120, 125, 135, 159, 167, 181, 182, 184, 204, 205, 207, 209, 210, 229, 243, 248, 249
relationships, viii, 8, 51, 52, 54, 56
relatives, 221, 239
relativity, 54
relaxation, 164, 165
relevance, 27, 30, 143, 149, 192, 229
reliability, 215, 241
remission, 117
renal failure, 92
reserves, 128, 177
resistance, 71, 132, 135, 177, 179, 183, 190
resources, 29, 31, 32, 95, 143, 146, 150, 201, 202
respiratory, 4, 17, 20, 71, 72, 83, 84, 90
respiratory disorders, 17, 71
responsibility, 148, 187, 193, 216, 233, 245
responsiveness, 6, 156, 157
retardation, 5, 18, 19, 21, 23, 25, 26, 27, 34, 44, 49, 111
retinopathy, 179
returns, 22
reward conditions, 160
rewards, 229, 242
rhythm, 129
riboflavin, 5
ricc, 113, 189
rickets, 176
risk, vii, viii, ix, 2, 6, 7, 8, 9, 10, 11, 17, 18, 20, 21, 22, 23, 25, 26, 27, 28, 29, 31, 32, 36, 40, 42, 43, 44, 46, 51, 52, 53, 54, 57, 58, 59, 64, 65, 66, 67, 69, 71, 72, 73, 74, 75, 78, 79, 82, 83, 84, 85, 86, 87, 89, 90, 93, 100, 109, 111, 112, 113, 114, 115, 116, 118, 122, 123, 124, 125, 130, 133, 135, 136, 137, 170, 171, 173, 174, 175, 181, 182, 183, 184, 187, 192, 194, 196, 200, 201, 203, 204, 205, 206, 207, 210, 213, 249, 250, 254
risk factors, viii, 2, 6, 7, 9, 28, 32, 36, 42, 44, 57, 69, 71, 73, 74, 75, 79, 82, 83, 85, 86, 87, 115, 116, 118, 123, 125, 182, 187, 249
rodents, 133
rotavirus, 50
routines, 225
rugby, 180
rural areas, 13, 21, 25, 26, 79, 90, 91
rural women, 11
Russia, 3, 5, 7, 16, 21, 38, 49

S

sadness, 71
safety, 163, 168, 191, 197, 226, 236, 237, 238, 240

sales, 57
sample, ix, 52, 53, 54, 55, 56, 57, 58, 64, 65, 66, 74, 76, 77, 78, 79, 80, 89, 90, 91, 92, 105, 107, 173, 207, 214, 239, 241
sampling, 52, 54, 56, 58, 77
saturated fat, 177, 193
Saudi Arabia, viii, 69, 76, 86, 93, 94, 95, 103, 119
school, 2, 4, 6, 10, 11, 28, 30, 31, 34, 43, 49, 57, 67, 74, 75, 76, 77, 79, 81, 86, 87, 91, 93, 98, 115, 116, 117, 118, 119, 120, 122, 125, 141, 142, 144, 145, 147, 151, 173, 176, 180, 181, 184, 185, 188, 189, 190, 193, 194, 201, 207, 208, 210, 212, 213, 214, 219, 220, 221, 222, 225, 227, 228, 229, 235, 236, 237, 239, 241, 242, 246, 247, 250, 253
school achievement, 67
school community, 237, 247
school work, 222
schooling, 12, 15, 180
scientific understanding, 140
scores, 18, 23
sea level, 32
search, 70, 121
searches, 179
second language, 225
secretion, 123, 128, 129, 133
security, 29, 118, 122, 236, 237
sedentary behavior, 6, 249, 253
sedentary lifestyle, 13, 77, 145, 240
self, 57, 65, 71, 83, 90, 142, 160, 163, 182, 184, 186, 188, 192, 203, 205, 213, 227, 249, 252, 253
self esteem, 186, 205
self-concept, 83
self-definition, 203
self-employed, 57, 65
self-esteem, 71, 90, 184
self-image, 71
self-monitoring, 188
sensitivity, 47, 248
series, 8, 11, 19, 121, 122, 160, 162, 192, 194, 247
serotonin, 129
serum, 17, 39, 72, 83, 137
services, 12, 29, 40, 57, 90, 96, 125, 170
SES, 12, 13, 32, 33, 53, 54, 77
severity, 40, 48
shame, 100, 125
shape, 111, 148, 159
shaping, 159, 160
shortage, 10, 19
sibling, 65, 72, 159, 203
siblings, 58, 65, 66, 72, 84, 159, 216, 219, 229, 233, 239, 242, 245
sign, ix, 70, 74, 79, 213
signals, 128, 129
similarity, 110
Singapore, 16, 38
sites, 20, 23, 179
skills, 202
skin, 98, 132, 170, 190
skinfolds, 9, 14, 15, 16, 37, 42, 77
sleep apnea, 71, 90
Slovakia, 175
smoking, 30, 47, 91, 140, 185, 194
social change, 21
social class, 43, 74, 85, 112, 204
social control, 233, 245
social group, 173
social learning, 203
social status, viii, 51, 52, 57, 59, 61, 64, 65, 66
social support, 112, 122
socioeconomic background, 8
socioeconomic standard, 26
socioeconomic status, 12, 13, 52, 111, 112, 121, 203, 207, 222
sodium, 156, 179
software, 223
South Africa, vii, 1, 2, 3, 4, 5, 7, 11, 12, 13, 14, 15, 17, 19, 21, 22, 23, 24, 26, 27, 28, 29, 31, 32, 33, 34, 36, 41, 173
South Asia, 54, 86, 184
South Korea, 41
Spain, 175
specialisation, 142
spectrum, 28
speculation, 178
sports, 122, 142, 147, 180, 207, 217, 218, 221, 233, 238, 239, 244
stability, 252
stages, vii, 1, 21, 27, 45, 73, 118, 197, 239
stakeholders, 29, 117, 237
standard deviation, 56, 58
standard of living, 12
standards, 16, 95, 173
starvation, 45
state schools, 180
statistics, x, 55, 56, 91, 99
sterile, 156
steroids, 133
stigmatized, 204
stimulant, 192
stimulus, 135, 158
stomach, 128, 129, 134, 177, 178
storage, 14, 72, 94, 129
strategies, ix, x, xi, xii, 28, 29, 30, 32, 37, 70, 72, 95, 99, 115, 116, 117, 118, 123, 139, 141, 142, 143, 150, 151, 160, 162, 169, 184, 188, 200, 202, 208,

216, 222, 229, 230, 233, 234, 236, 237, 238, 242, 243, 244, 246, 248
strategy use, 142
stratification, 145
strength, 217, 234, 246
stress, 19, 129
structuring, 149
students, 47, 76, 77, 79, 81, 87, 91, 97, 107, 114, 115, 116, 117, 119, 120, 122, 123, 124, 126, 148, 208, 212, 239
sub-Saharan Africa, viii, 4, 51, 56, 64, 65
subsistence, 53, 109
subsistence farming, 109
substitutes, 91
substitution, 234, 246
sucrose, 156, 157, 162, 165, 166
sugar, 4, 12, 109, 111, 112, 114, 140, 147, 156, 158, 162, 163, 166, 167, 177, 181
summer, 227
supervision, 114, 188, 201, 226, 240
supply, 31, 201
suppression, 177
surgical intervention, xi, 169
surplus, viii, 69, 75
surveillance, 37, 79, 82
survival, 81, 170, 193
survival rate, 193
susceptibility, 11, 15, 19, 25, 30, 44, 47, 68, 111, 131, 132
sweat, 217
Sweden, 84, 97, 175, 192
Switzerland, 49, 126, 166, 175
sympathetic nervous system, 129
syndrome, ix, 70, 71, 72, 73, 89, 90, 94, 111, 132, 179, 180, 183, 187, 195
synthesis, 24, 25, 123, 129, 177
systems, 53, 109, 114, 212
systolic blood pressure, 78

T

T cell, 195
tactics, 188
Taiwan, 93, 94, 96
Tanzania, 251
targets, 142, 196
teachers, 30, 147, 159, 160
technology, 113, 120, 142
teenagers, xi, 143, 169, 180
television, 37, 54, 55, 56, 85, 94, 111, 116, 119, 143, 161, 167, 180, 181, 185, 188, 189, 190, 193, 196, 200, 206, 207, 209, 210, 214, 215, 219, 223, 224, 225, 226, 227, 228, 229, 237, 238, 239, 240, 241, 242, 248, 249, 251
television advertisements, 161, 167
television viewing, 37, 143, 181, 190, 196, 200, 206, 207, 209, 210, 214, 215, 219, 223, 224, 225, 226, 228, 229, 238, 240, 241, 242, 248, 251
temperature, 110, 115, 177
tertiary education, 57
Thailand, 12, 41, 43, 102, 175, 194
theory, 39, 44, 110, 123, 124, 203, 208, 244, 251
therapeutic targets, 134
therapists, 151
therapy, xi, 30, 92, 138, 169, 198
thermodynamics, 244
thinking, 146, 226
threat, 9, 115
threats, 140
thyroid, 179
tibia, 84
time, 10, 12, 14, 22, 33, 53, 57, 73, 82, 108, 111, 114, 116, 118, 119, 121, 138, 140, 142, 145, 147, 151, 156, 157, 159, 160, 165, 170, 179, 180, 181, 184, 186, 188, 189, 190, 200, 206, 207, 209, 214, 215, 217, 218, 220, 222, 225, 227, 228, 229, 234, 235, 236, 238, 239, 240, 241, 242, 243, 248, 249, 250
timing, 7, 8, 17, 43, 170
tissue, 9, 138
tobacco, 140
total energy, 20, 72, 113, 129, 180, 210
toys, 219
tracking, 70, 72, 236, 241
trade, 12, 32
traffic, 114, 115, 124
training, 112, 221, 233, 237, 244, 245, 247, 252
training programs, 244
traits, 202
trajectory, 10, 32, 66
transformation, 2
transition, vii, viii, 1, 2, 3, 4, 5, 7, 9, 12, 13, 17, 19, 20, 21, 25, 26, 28, 29, 31, 32, 36, 38, 40, 41, 43, 44, 45, 46, 67, 68, 69, 73, 75, 84, 87, 99, 103, 109, 113, 118, 120, 122, 124, 125
transition to adulthood, 9
transitional countries, 21
transitions, 2, 79, 108, 109, 125
translation, 41, 144
transmission, 84, 202, 203, 211
transmits, 178
transplantation, 133, 138
transport, 117
transportation, 6, 10, 35, 109, 115

trend, x, 10, 22, 30, 76, 79, 94, 99, 102, 109, 112, 173, 209, 252
trial, 25, 36, 123, 125, 167, 192, 196, 198
triangulation, 212, 214
triceps, 13, 14, 37, 43, 49, 98, 118, 121, 170, 190, 193
triggers, 188
Turkey, ix, 74, 89, 90, 93, 95, 96, 103, 203
twins, 110, 131
type 2 diabetes, 27, 32, 41, 71, 100, 111, 122, 198

U

UK, 37, 83, 98, 101, 170, 171, 172, 175, 176, 180, 181, 184, 186, 192, 197
umbilical cord, 128, 129, 134
UN, 125
undernutrition, 3, 4, 5, 7, 12, 19, 20, 21, 22, 23, 25, 26, 27, 30, 32, 35, 39, 43, 51, 85, 103, 133
unemployment, 12, 13
uniform, 82
United Kingdom, 101, 140, 176
United Nations, 20, 33
United States, 7, 10, 39, 49, 68, 76, 84, 97, 100, 101, 124, 126, 136, 141, 174, 182, 196, 254
urban areas, 2, 4, 8, 13, 18, 25, 53, 78, 90, 91, 109, 113
urban population, 2, 87
urbanisation, 109, 120
urbanization, 48, 66, 67, 74, 75, 79, 200
urea, 157, 165
US Department of Health and Human Services, 18
Uzbekistan, 102, 173

V

vacuum, 150
values, 5, 9, 12, 14, 56, 74, 75, 76, 77, 83, 91, 94, 97, 101, 103, 200, 201, 202, 203, 209, 248
variable, 56, 57, 58, 66, 72, 73, 179, 206, 209
variables, viii, x, 45, 51, 52, 54, 56, 58, 59, 99, 113, 204, 205, 206, 209
variation, 2, 13, 18, 54, 56, 57, 65, 76, 83, 94, 131
vegetables, ix, 5, 90, 93, 109, 114, 118, 158, 160, 163, 167, 181, 182, 187, 189, 210, 235, 246
velocity, 15, 18, 22, 23, 25, 27, 44
verbal praise, 160
video games, 180, 185, 207, 224
village, 31, 234, 246
violence, 225, 226, 240
vitamin A, 5, 123
vitamin B12, 5
vitamin B6, 5
vitamin C, 5
vitamin D, 123
vitamins, 167
voice, 219, 229, 242
voting, 114

W

walking, 142, 181, 217, 222, 242
war, 226
warrants, 82
water, 54, 56, 156, 187, 189
wealth, viii, 51, 52, 54, 56, 57, 58, 59, 60, 64, 65, 66, 67, 232, 245
wealth effects, 67
websites, 114
weight control, 179, 212, 214, 218, 229, 232, 242, 245
weight gain, xi, 9, 10, 11, 19, 22, 24, 27, 30, 37, 66, 71, 113, 117, 118, 129, 131, 133, 142, 169, 179, 182, 251
weight loss, x, xi, 10, 32, 110, 116, 120, 122, 129, 138, 139, 142, 143, 144, 150, 151, 177, 186, 191, 192
weight management, 122, 186
weight reduction, 146, 147, 149, 150, 151, 192, 195
weight status, xii, 25, 47, 53, 57, 66, 94, 200, 201, 204, 205, 207, 214, 216, 230, 231, 232, 235, 238, 239, 243, 245, 246
welfare, 32
Western countries, 70
Western Europe, 175
wives, 245
women, vii, 1, 11, 12, 13, 14, 16, 17, 28, 46, 52, 53, 54, 56, 57, 66, 76, 78, 112, 114, 123, 166, 174, 175, 176, 184, 194, 196, 203, 204
words, 90, 143, 147, 149, 170, 214, 223, 226, 240
work, 6, 11, 19, 28, 30, 35, 100, 151, 185, 193, 197, 217, 224, 226, 233, 241, 244, 245, 247, 250
work absenteeism, 100
workers, 5, 8, 11, 16, 18, 23, 24, 25, 32, 65
workload, 93
World Bank, 58, 68, 254
World Health Organisation, 121
World Health Organization, vii, 6, 33, 46, 49, 50, 56, 68, 75, 82, 152, 209, 250, 251
World War I, 94
worry, 249
writing, 212, 214, 215, 217, 223, 226, 240

Y

yield, 19
young adults, 71
young men, 84, 135
Yugoslavia, 175

Z

zinc, 25, 44, 123